MCBU
Molecular and Cell Biology Updates

Series Editors:

Prof. Dr. Angelo Azzi
Institut für Biochemie
und Molekularbiologie
Bühlstr. 28
CH–3012 Bern
Switzerland

Prof. Dr. Lester Packer
Dept. of Molecular
and Cell Biology
251 Life Science Addition
Membrane Bioenergetics Group
Berkeley, CA 94720
USA

Molecular Aspects of Cancer and its Therapy

Edited by   A. Mackiewicz
P.B. Sehgal

Springer Basel AG

Volume editors' address:

Prof. Dr. A. Mackiewicz
Department of Cancer Immunology
University School of Medical Sciences
15 Garbary St.
PL-61-866 Poznan
Poland

Dr. P.B. Sehgal
Dept. of Cell Biology and Anatomy,
and Medicine
New York Medical College
Basic Science Building
Valhalla, NY 10595
USA

Library of Congress Cataloging-in-Publication Data

Molecular aspects of cancer and its therapy / edited by A. Mackiewicz,
    P.B. Sehgal.
        p.   cm. – (Molecular and cell biology updates)
    Includes bibliographical references and index.
    ISBN 978-3-0348-9839-3   ISBN 978-3-0348-8946-9 (eBook)
    DOI 10.1007/978-3-0348-8946-9
    1. Cancer – Genetic aspects. 2. Cancer – Gene therapy. 3. Cancer –
    Molecular aspects. I. Mackiewicz, Andrzej. II. Sehgal,
    Pravinkumar B. III. Series.
    RC268.4.M633 1998
    616.99'4042 – dc21

Deutsche Bibliothek Cataloging-in-Publication Data

Molecular aspects of cancer and its therapy / ed. by A.
    Mackiewicz ; P.B. Sehgal. - Basel ; Boston ; Berlin : Birkhäuser,
    1998
    (Molecular and cell biology updates)
    ISBN 978-3-0348-9839-3

Table of contents

List of contributors

Joseph M. Backer, Department of Microbiology and Immunology, New York Medical College, Valhalla, NY 10595, USA

Bruno Calabretta, Thomas Jefferson University, Microbiology and Immunology, Kimmel Cancer Institute, Bluemle Life Sciences Bldg., Rm. 630, 233 South 10th Street, Philadelphia, PA 19107, USA

Irma Cardinale, The Rockefeller University, 1230 York Avenue, New York, NY 10021, USA

Angus G. Dalgleish, Division of Oncology, Department of Cellular and Molecular Sciences, St. George's Hospital Medical School, Jenner Wing, Cranmer Terrace, London SW17 ORE, UK

Alan M. Gewirtz, Department of Internal Medicine, University of Pennsylvania School of Medicine, Philadelphia, PA 19104, USA

Carl V. Hamby, Department of Microbiology and Immunology, New York Medical College, Valhalla, NY 10595, USA

George P. Hemstreet, III, Department of Urology, University of Oklahoma Health Sciences Center, P.O. Box 26901, Oklahoma City, OK 73190, USA

David Hrouda, Division of Oncology, Department of Cellular and Molecular Sciences, St. George's Hospital Medical School, Jenner Wing, Cranmer Terrace, London SW17 0RE, UK

Anna Jasinska, Laboratory of Cancer Genetics, Institute of Bioorganic Chemistry, Polish Academy of Sciences, Noskowskiego St. 12/14, PL-71-604 Poznan, Poland

Ewa Jassem, Department of Pneumonology, Medical University of Gdansk, Debinki 7, PL-80-211 Gdansk, Poland

Jacek Jassem, Department of Oncology and Radiotherapy, Medical University of Gdansk, Debinki 7, PL-80-211 Gdansk, Poland

Toyoko Kikuchi, The Rockefeller University, 1230 York Avenue, New York, NY 10021, USA

Piotr Kozlowski, Laboratory of Cancer Genetics, Institute of Bioorganic Chemistry, Polish Academy of Sciences, Noskowskiego St. 12/14, PL-71-604 Poznan, Poland

James G. Krueger, The Rockefeller University, 1230 York Avenue, New York, NY 10021, USA

Wlodzimierz J. Krzyzosiak, Laboratory of Cancer Genetics, Institute of Bioorganic Chemistry, Polish Academy of Sciences, Noskowskiego St. 12/14, PL-71-604 Poznan, Poland

Andrzej Mackiewicz, Department of Cancer Immunology, University School of Medical Sciences at Great Poland Cancer Center, 15 Garbary St., PL-61-866 Poznan, Poland

Anthony Maraveyas, Division of Oncology, Department of Cellular and Molecular Sciences, St. George's Hospital Medical School, Jenner Wing, Cranmer Terrace, London SW17 0RE, UK

James S. Murphy, The Rockefeller University, 1230 York Avenue, New York, NY 10021, USA

Marek Napierala, Laboratory of Cancer Genetics, Institute of Bioorganic Chemistry, Polish Academy of Sciences, Noskowskiego St. 12/14, PL-71-604 Poznan, Poland

Mariusz Z. Ratajczak, Department of Pathology and Laboratory Medicine, University of Pennsylvania School of Medicine, Room 515 Stellar Chance Building, 422 Curie Boulevard, Philadelphia, PA 19104, USA

Stefan Rose-John, Abteilung Pathophysiologie, I Med. Klinik, Johannes-Gutenberg-Universität, Obere Zahlbacher Str., D-55101 Mainz, Germany

Pravin B. Sehgal, Departments of Cell Biology and Anatomy and of Medicine, New York Medical College, Valhalla, NY 10595, USA

Tomasz Skorski, Thomas Jefferson University, Microbiology and Immunology, Kimmel Cancer Institute, Jefferson Alumni Hall, Rm. 372, 1020 Locust Street, Philadelphia, PA 19107, USA

Krzysztof Sobczak, Laboratory of Cancer Genetics, Institute of Bioorganic Chemistry, Polish Academy of Sciences, Noskowskiego Str. 12/14, PL-71-604 Poznan, Poland

Cezary Szczylik, Department of Oncology, CSK WAM, Warsaw, Poland

Igor Tamm, The Rockefeller University, 1230 York Avenue, New York, NY 10021, USA

Maciej Wiznerowicz, Department of Cancer Immunology, University School of Medical Sciences at Great Poland Cancer Center, 15 Garbary St., PL-61-866 Poznan, Poland

Preface

On the basis of the agreement signed between UNESCO and the Government of the Republic of Poland the International Institute for Cell and Molecular Biology of UNESCO was officially inaugurated in October 1995 in Warsaw, Poland, as part of the activity of the Global Network for Molecular and Cell Biology (MCBN) of UNESCO. The occasion was marked by the bringing together in Warsaw of a broad spectrum of cell and molecular biologists from around the world under the auspices of the Global MCBN UNESCO. At the conclusion of that week-long celebration it became clear that Polish cell and molecular biology had come of age in terms of its depth, vigor and impact on the global scene. At the suggestion of Professor Angelo Azzi, chairman of Global MCBN UNESCO, we considered the challenge of compiling a volume in the Molecular and Cell Biology Updates (MCBU) Series that would address the molecular basis of cancer and its therapy, but one that would additionally serve to highlight Polish contributions to this field of research. We accepted the challenge presented to us by Professor Azzi and are grateful to all contributors of the present volume for making this a pleasant and stimulating project.

We requested each contributor to present his personal perspective of respective topics. As a consequence, we hope that each contribution has a distinctive individual flavor which reflects the role played by individual research groups in advancing science. We believe that this approach to the preparation of the contributions serves to distinguish this volume from many of the more archival review volumes. This approach also serves to foster the objective of highlighting the various Polish contributions from their respective individual perspectives.

The scope of a topic such as the molecular aspects of cancer and its therapy is clearly very broad. While we have sought to make the scope of this volume as broad as possible by inviting contributions from diverse scientists engaged in cancer research today, we realize that no one compendium of this kind can do full justice to the subject matter at hand. To the editors goes the blame for any omissions and oversights.

September 11, 1997   Andrzej Mackiewicz
                                                                        Pravin B. Sehgal

Molecular Aspects of Cancer and its Therapy
A. Mackiewicz and P.B. Sehgal (eds)
© 1998 Birkhäuser Verlag Basel/Switzerland

Genetic control of metastasis

J.M. Backer and C.V. Hamby

Department of Microbiology and Immunology, New York Medical College, Valhalla, NY 10595, USA

Introduction

The major cause of cancer mortality is metastatic dissemination of primary tumors. Our ability to develop effective antimetastatic therapeutics depends on knowledge of the underlying molecular processes. Even more pressing is the necessity to identify patients at risk of metastatic disease. It is estimated that by the time of diagnosis, approximately 30% of patients with breast or prostate cancer are already the victims of metastatic disease [1, 2]. Reliable identification of these patients would permit the administration of systemic therapies at the earliest possible time, and would avoid subjecting patients with localized disease to harmful and expensive procedures.

Metastatic dissemination of primary tumors is a complex, multistep process (see [3, 4] for recent reviews). Animal models, including the nude mouse model for metastatic dissemination of human tumor cells, have been developed to study this process (see [5] for review). In these models, tumor cells are injected into animals in order to form primary tumors, which subsequently metastasize to distant organs. Experimental evidence indicates that injection of tumor cells into the organ corresponding to their origin (orthopic injection) yields more relevant results than subcutaneous (ectopic) injection [6]. A supplementary approach is to determine the ability of tumor cells to colonize various organs after intravenous or intracardial injection of cells into animals. Unfortunately, it is not known to what extent colonization assay measures the metastatic potential of tumor cells which were selected in primary tumors. For example, it is possible that cells which colonize lungs in an intravenous injection assay do not have the traits necessary for leaving the primary tumor or for intravasation. Thus, the 'true' measure of the metastatic potential of tumor cells may be obtained only in experiments where metastases are the result of the dissemination of cells from the primary tumor.

Animal studies of metastatic dissemination have revealed several crucial steps in this process [3, 4]. Tumor cells must leave the primary tumor, enter the blood circulation (intravasate), travel to a distant organ, exit the circulation (extravasate), grow to form an avascular micrometastasis in a new environment, induce a host angiogenic response, and grow further to form a vascularized macrometastatic lesion. Some steps in this process are similar to those which occur in primary tumor growth, and many of the molecular mechanisms underlying tumor growth are most likely to be operational in metastatic lesions. For example, invasion of the surrounding tissue [7], remodeling of the extracellular matrix [8], and the induction of the host's angiogenic response [9] take place in both primary tumors and metastatic lesions. Thus, it was thought possible that the same set of genes may control both the tumorigenic and metastatic phenotype of cancer cells.

However, experiments in the early 1980s demonstrated that the fusion of metastatic and non-metastatic tumor cells yielded non-metastatic but tumorigenic hybrid cells. These experiments suggested that the metastatic phenotype is controlled by metastasis suppressor gene(s) which are inactivated in metastatic tumor cells. The existence of separate negative regulators of the metastatic phenotype was further substantiated in experiments with microcell-mediated transfer of individual chromosomes in metastatic tumor cells. The hybrids obtained in these experiments formed non-metastatic tumors. Further research led to the identification of at least three putative metastasis suppressor genes, whose transfection into metastatic cells yielded clones that in animal models formed non- or weakly metastatic tumors. Very recently, three different genes were implicated in the positive regulation of the metastatic phenotype, since inhibition of their expression *via* ribozymes significantly decreased the ability of cells to colonize various organs in animal experiments.

Taken together, experimental research on the genetic control of metastasis may be summarized in two very general statements:
(1) There are genes which control the metastatic phenotype independently of the tumorigenic phenotype.
(2) The genetic control of metastasis may involve both positive and negative regulatory genes.
The present review will summarize experimental evidence for genetic control of metastasis and discuss molecular characteristics of putative metastasis control molecules.

Suppression of metastatic potential in cell fusion experiments

Early evidence that the tumorigenic and metastatic capabilities of tumor cells derived from solid tumors may be controlled by different genes were provided by cell fusion experiments with murine cells. In these experiments metastatic and non-metastatic cells were tagged with different selectable markers, fused, and hybrid cells carrying both markers were selected and assayed. The hybrids obtained with five different systems were tumorigenic but non- or weakly metastatic. Selective suppression of metastatic potential observed in these experiments was explained by the existence of metastasis suppressor gene(s), which are active in non-metastatic cells. The operational definition of metastasis suppressor genes implies that their loss, inactivation or underexpression led to acquisition of the metastatic phenotype.

In the first experiment of this kind, Ramshaw et al. [10] fused a tumorigenic and highly metastatic clone of 13762 MAT rat mammary adenocarcinoma with a tumorigenic but non-metastatic clone of DMBA-8 rat mammary adenocarcinoma. Three hybrid clones were tested and found to be tumorigenic upon injection of $1-5 \times 10^6$ cells in the footpads of normal rats. However, no tumor cells were found in popliteal lymph nodes, as tested by the ability of collagenase-dissociated cells from lymph nodes to form colonies in soft agar.

Sedebottom and Clark [11] fused the metastatic derivative of a C57B1 mouse melanoma cell line with either a non-metastatic derivative of the same cell line or with diploid CBA T6T6 lymphocytes. The tumorigenicity and metastatic dissemination of hybrid cells were tested by injecting 5×10^4 cells subcutaneously into the backs of newborn sublethally-irradiated syngeneic mice. Testing of ten melanoma/melanoma clones revealed a 98.5 % tumor take incidence, but only

3.8% incidence of metastasis (calculated from Table III in [11]). Testing of seven melanoma/lymphocyte hybrids revealed a 100% tumor take, but only 3.2% incidence of metastasis (calculated from Table II in [11]).

Layton and Franks fused highly metastatic CMT 167 mouse lung cell carcinoma cells and non-metastatic L-M mouse cells of mesenchymal origin [12]. Of nine hybrid clones that were tumorigenic only one produced a few lung metastases upon subcutaneous injection of 5×10^5 cells into nude mice.

Turpeenniemi-Hujanen et al. [13] fused a highly metastatic subclone (B16-F10^{RR}) of mouse B16 melanoma either with C3H mouse embryo fibroblasts or with mouse peritoneal macrophages, and also fused a highly metastatic subclone (UV-2237^{RR}) of a mouse fibrosarcoma with mouse peritoneal macrophages. The hybrids were tumorigenic in both syngeneic and nude mice after subcutaneous injection of 10^5 cells. The same hybrids, unlike parental metastatic cells, did not form lung metastases upon tail vein injection of 10^5 cells [12].

Ichikawa et al. [14] fused highly metastatic and non-metastatic subclones of Dunning rat prostatic cancer cells derived from a prostatic adenocarcinoma of a Copenhagen rat. This group found two hybrids were tumorigenic but non-metastatic upon subcutaneous injection of 10^6 cells into the legs of Copenhagen rats. Passage of non-metastatic tumors *in vivo* led to the appearance of metastatic variants. Cytogenetic analysis of these new metastatic variants revealed a consistent loss of chromosome 2, which suggests that a metastasis suppressor gene for prostate cancer may be localized on this chromosome. It should be noted that this work was the first to demonstrate that suppression of metastatic potential in cell fusion experiments may be attributed to a specific chromosome. These experiments paved the way to a new approach to the search for metastasis suppressor genes: chromosome transfer-mediated suppression of metastatic potential of tumor cells.

Suppression of metastatic potential in chromosome transfer experiments

In order to determine the chromosomal location of putative metastasis suppressor genes, two groups employed microcell-mediated chromosome transfer. In these experiments, mouse A9 cells containing a single human chromosome tagged with the selectable neomycin resistance gene were used as a source of microcells. Microcells are subnuclear particles containing a limited amount of genetic material packaged in a micronucleus surrounded by a rim of cytoplasm and intact plasma membrane. The micronucleation of cells is induced by colcemid treatment, and enucleation of micronucleate cells is induced by cytochalasin B [15]. Fusion of microcells with target cells and selection of hybrids for neomycin resistance allows the introduction of a specific human chromosome carrying a selectable marker into appropriate host cells. The chromosomes for a transfer are selected on the basis of frequency of chromosomal abnormalities in a particular type of cancer.

In experiments with rat prostate tumor cells, Ichikawa et al. [16] found that introduction of human chromosome 11 into a highly metastatic subclone of Dunning rat prostate tumor cells yielded hybrids which were tumorigenic but non-metastatic upon injection (5×10^5 cells/mouse) into nude mice. Detailed analysis of human chromosome 11 fragments retained in hybrids revealed that putative metastasis suppressor gene(s) may be localized to the region 11p11.2–13 [16]. Similarly, tumorigenic but non-metastatic clones were obtained after introduction of human chromosomes 8, 17 or 10 into highly metastatic subclones of Dunning rat prostate tumor cells [17–19]. Introduction of the pter-q14 region of human chromosome 11 into rat mammary carcinoma cells did not affect either tumorigenicity or the metastatic potential of these cells [18]. The latter result suggested that at least some metastasis suppressor genes may be either tumor specific or species specific.

Welch et al. [20] found that introduction of human chromosome 6 into metastatic c8161 human melanoma cells suppresses their metastatic potential, but not tumorigenicity, in a nude mouse assay. The same group reported that that introduction of human chromosome 11 into highly metastatic MDA-MB-435 human breast carcinoma cells yielded tumorigenic, but weakly metastatic clones [21]. Human chromosome 11 did not suppress the metastatic potential of rat mammary carcinoma cells [16]. Taken together, the suppressive potential of human chromosome 11 in rat prostate tumor cells and human breast carcinoma cells strongly suggests the presence of a common metastasis suppressor gene. Indeed, further studies revealed that a gene named *KAI1* located on 11p11.2 may be responsible for the suppression of metastatic dissemination of different tumor cells.

Suppression of metastatic potential in transfection experiments

Transfection experiments provide direct proof that a certain gene can act as a metastasis suppressor gene. In these experiments the cDNA of a putative metastasis suppressor gene is transfected into highly metastatic tumor cells, and the tumorigenicity and metastatic dissemination of transfected cells is assayed in animal models. The underlying assumption for these experiments is that the levels of expression of the active metastasis suppressor genes are low in highly metastatic cells, and that this defect may be compensated by introduction of an intact transgene. However, three points must be kept in mind. First, phenotypic effects observed with a particular clone, or even few clones of transfected cells, may still be attributed to a fortuitous integration of a transgene. Second, the effect of the transgene may be specific for a given type of tumor cell. Third, it appears that in transfected cells the suppression of metastatic potential is not always associated with enhanced production of the protein encoded by the transgene (see discussion below).

Hypothetically, candidates for testing as metastasis suppressor genes may be obtained by subtractive hybridization [22] or mRNA differential display screening of cDNA prepared from highly metastatic and weakly metastatic subclones of the same cell line [23]. It is possible to narrow the search to chromosomes that suppress metastatic potential in chromosome transfer experiments [24]. Finally, it is possible to hypothesize that a known gene may act as a metastasis suppressor, based on the activity of its product, and to test this hypothesis in direct transfection experiments.

With all these technical capabilities by the end of 1996 only three genes, namely *nm23*, *KAI*1, and *SOD2* passed the transfection test. The history of discovery, the accumulated knowledge and hypotheses related to the mechanisms of action are quite different for these three putative metastasis suppressor genes and we will discuss them separately.

Nm23 *genes and metastasis control*

The mouse *nm23* gene was originally cloned using a subtractive hybridization strategy applied to highly metastatic and weakly metastatic subclones of murine K-1735 melanoma cells [22]. The original discovery of the *nm23* gene was quite a serendipitous event, since a subsequent study of a broader panel of K-1735 subclones did not confirm an inverse correlation between metastatic potential and the level of the *nm23* gene expression [25]. However, results from many laboratories from 1988 to 1996 support the involvement of *nm23* in metastasis control. The research on *nm23* can be summarized as follows:

Nm23 *genes and proteins*
There are two highly homologous human genes, *nm23-H1* and *nm23-H2* (formally assigned as *NME1* and *NME2*), that are mapped, 4 kb apart, to the region 17q21.3 [26, 27]. *Nm23* genes encoding evolutionary conserved proteins were also found in other species. The genomic structure of the *nm23-H1* gene has been reported [28]. Two new human *nm23*-related genes (*DR-nm23* and *nm23-H4*), which encode proteins that are 70% and 55% identical to *nm23-H1* and *nm23-H2* gene products, have been discovered recently and mapped to chromosome 16 [29, 30].

Nm23-H1 and *nm23-H2* genes encode two highly homologous enzymes which were discovered and characterized decades ago as nucleoside diphosphate kinase (NDPK) A and B, respectively. A review of published data and our own experiments with approximately 20 human tumor cell lines indicate that the amount of cellular NDPK B as a rule is several times higher than the amount of NDPK A. The regulation of *nm23* gene expression is not well understood. In human cells the expression of these genes is controlled by independent promoters [27]. In rat cells transcription of the rat homologue of *nm23-H2* is initiated from a wide range of sites and different transcripts are translated with different efficiency [31]. So far, a correlation between the levels of *nm23* mRNA and proteins has been reported only by one group [32]. However, in several systems there was no correlation between *nm23* mRNA and protein levels [32–36] suggesting that NDPK protein levels may be regulated post-transcriptionally [36–38].

NDPK A and NDPK B are 153 amino acids long, 17 kDa proteins with 88% identity and two distinct regions of sequence divergency at aa37–53 and aa124–150. NDPKs from several organisms, including human NDPK B, have been crystallized as hexamers with regions of sequence divergency exposed on the outer surface of the hexamer [39]. In solution, in the presence of DTT, recombinant NDPK A and B form hexamers [40]. The proteins readily form heteromers in solution.

Subcellular localization of NDPK
NDPK appears to be present in different cellular compartments. Part of cytosolic NDPK is associated with microtubules [34, 41]. Part of cellular NDPK is associated with various membranes [42]. Urano et al. [43] reported expression of NDPK A, or of both NDPK A and B, but not of NDPK B alone, on the cell surface in several cell lines. Recently, a substantial part of the cellular NDPK B was found to be associated with chromatin in the nuclei of cultured cells [44]. NDPK is also a marker enzyme for the intermembrane space between the inner and outer

mitochondrial membranes, and was found in contact points between inner and outer mitochondrial membranes (see [45] for review).

Biochemical activities of NDPK A and B

A well-established enzymatic function of NDPKs is to catalyse the transfer of terminal phosphoryl groups from ATP to nucleoside- and deoxynucleoside diphosphates *via* a phosphohistidine protein intermediate according to the following scheme:

$$ATP + NDPK(^{118}his) = ADP + NDPK(^{118}his\text{\textasciitilde}P)$$

$$GDP + NDPK(^{118}his\text{\textasciitilde}P) = GTP + NDPK(^{118}his)$$

It has been suggested that NDPK may control different signal transduction pathways by modulating the supply of GTP to various GTP-binding proteins [42]. Two recent reports indicated that NDPK may act as a phosphotransferase, by transferring phosphate groups to other proteins. The reported targets were a histidine in ATP-citrate lyase [46] and serine/threonine residues of some proteins in cell extracts [47]. It remains to be established whether in eukaryotic cells, phosphotransferase activity of NDPK plays a role in signal transduction similar to that of bacterial histidine kinases [48].

Several additional activities were reported for NDPK B, indicating that it may be a multifunctional protein. A recently discovered activity of recombinant NDPK B is its ability to act as a transcription factor by making contact with the GGGTGGG sequence motif [49]. This motif is present in the c-*myc* promoter and it was reported that NDPK B binds to and activates the translocated c-*myc* allele in Burkitt's lymphoma [50]. Further studies suggested that, at least *in vitro*, this activity does not depend on the catalytic activity of NDPK B [51] and may reflect the ability of NDPK B to bind single-stranded polypyrimidine sequences [52]. Mutational analysis of NDPK B identified arg-34, asn-69 and lys-135 as critical for DNA binding and suggested a structural model for it [40].

Another recently discovered activity of NDPK is the ability to inhibit differentiation of mouse myeloid leukemia cells induced by dexamethasone [53, 54]. This activity was observed with mouse, rat and human NDPK A and B, with catalytic inactive human NDPK B (118cys), and, paradoxically, with both N-terminal [1−60 and 1−108] and C-terminal [61−152] peptides. Finally, a yeast two-hybrid system screen revealed that NDPK B, but not NDPK A specifically interacts with members of the ROR/RZR nuclear orphan receptor subfamily [55]. This activity appears to be retained by the N-terminal 60 amino acid portion of NDPK B.

Clinical and experimental correlations between nm23 *gene expression and metastatic potential of tumor cells*

Both the enzymatic activity of NDPK and the level of mRNAs are frequently increased in rapidly proliferating cells and in many human tumors in comparison with surrounding normal tissues [56]. However, the interest in *nm23* genes is driven by the finding that in some tumors and tumor cell lines, particularly in human breast tumors, progression towards a more metastatic phenotype has been associated with a decrease in nm23 mRNA level and NDPK immunostaining [56]. It should be noted, however, that the statistical significance of this association for breast cancer is currently a matter of controversy [57, 58]. It was also found that loss or low levels of expression of NDPK proteins are associated with abnormal differentiation in some tumors and cancer cells [59–62] and with abnormal postembryonic development in *Drosophila* [34, 63].

Transfection experiments with nm23
There are three reports on the transfection of nm23 cDNAs in mouse and human tumor cells. Leone et al. [64] transfected a mouse nm23-1 cDNA into a highly metastatic subclone of mouse K-1735 melanoma cell line, and assayed the metastatic dissemination of transfected cells after either tail vein (2×10^4 cells/mouse) or subcutaneous injection (1×10^4 cells/mouse). Five randomly selected transfected clones and two clones selected for high level of expression of the *nm23-1* gene were compared with a corresponding number of vector-transfected clones. The growth rate and the ability of cells to grow in soft agar were not affected by *nm23-1* transfection. However, tumor take and tumor growth were lower for *nm23-1*-transfected cells as compared with vector-transfected cells [64]. In addition, a significant reduction in metastatic dissemination of *nm23-1*-transfected cells as compared with vector-transfected cells was found in both tail vein and subcutaneous injection experiments. Thus, in this system, transfection of *nm23-1* affected both tumorigenic and metastatic potential of mouse melanoma cells.

In the first experiment with a human tumor cell line, Leone et al. [65] transfected nm23-H1 cDNA and nm23-H2 cDNA into human breast carcinoma MDA-MB–435 cells. Pooled transfected clones (bulk transfectants) were as tumorigenic as control (vector-transfected) cells, and displayed unaltered tumor growth rates upon injection of 1×10^5 cells/mouse either into mammary fat pad or subcutaneously. However, tumors formed by bulk *nm23-H1*-transfected cells produced significantly fewer metastatic lesions than control tumors. Thus, the *nm23-H1* gene appeared to fit the operational definition of a metastasis suppressor gene, capable of inhibiting metastatic potential of cells without affecting their tumorigenicity.

The metastatic potential of bulk *nm23-H2*-transfected cells was similar to that of control cells, suggesting distinctively different functions for *nm23-H1* and *nm23-H2* genes in human breast carcinoma cells. The diminished metastatic potential of the *nm23-H1*-transfected cells was confirmed in experiments with two individual clones selected for their high level of expression of a transgene. The same clones also displayed diminished tissue culture characteristics usually associated with the metastatic phenotype such as growth in agar, responsiveness to chemotactic stimuli, and inhibition of differentiation [65–67]. According to Leone et al. [65] no individual clone with high levels of expression of the *nm23-H2* transgene were found among over 50 individual transfected cell lines' clones. Direct measurements of NDPK activity in bulk and individual transfected cell lines did not correlate with the amount of protein as assessed by Western blot analysis.

The results of the transfection of mouse nm23-1 cDNA into mouse cells [64] and human nm23-1 cDNA into human cells were different in two respects. First, the ability to grow in soft agar was inhibited only in transfected human cells. Second, tumorigenicity was inhibited only in transfected mouse cells. However, the latter effect may be specific for mouse K-1735 melanoma cells. In recent experiments with another murine melanoma cell line, Baba et al. [68] transfected either mouse nm23-1 cDNA, or mouse nm23-2 cDNA, or both nm23-1 and nm23-2 cDNAs, into highly metastatic subclones of the mouse B16 melanoma cell line. Two clones were selected from each transfection for further studies. The growth rate and the ability of cells to grow in soft agar were not affected by transgenes, individually or together. Furthermore, unlike transfected murine K-1735 melanoma cells [64], the presence of a transgene in B16 cells did not affect tumor growth after subcutaneous injection of 5×10^5 cells/mouse. However, in a lung colonization assay, the number of pulmonary metastases formed by transfectants after tail vein injection of 2×10^5 cells/ mouse was significantly lower than that formed by vector-transfected cells. With the usual reservations about the relevance of lung colonization assays, these results suggest that in mouse melanoma cells both *nm23-1* and *nm23-2* genes may act as negative regulators of certain functions related to metastatic dissemination.

Transfection of human nm23-H1, or nm23-H2, or both nm23-H1 and nm23-H2 cDNA into the same subclone of mouse B16 melanoma cells failed to affect primary tumor growth and metastatic dissemination of cells in the lung colonization assay. Baba et al. [68] noted that mouse NDPK B protein encoded by nm23-2 and human NDPK B protein encoded by nm23-H2 proteins differ only in amino acid residues 124, 131, and 140 clustered at the C-terminus of the molecule. These residues are not crucial for catalytic activity of NDPK B [39], or DNA-binding activity of NDPK B [40]. One possible explanation for these results is that the difference in three amino acid residues between mouse and human NDPK Bs is recognized by as yet unknown protein(s) that interact with NDPK B and mediate its phenotypic effects.

Further evidence that functions of *nm23-H1* and *nm23-H2* are different was obtained in experiments with *Drosophila* [69]. Null mutations in the *Drosophila awd* gene encoding NDPK cause lethality after puparium formation. Although *Drosophila*'s NDPK is 78% identical to either human NDPK, only NDPK B (*nm23-H2*) can rescue phenotypes caused by *awd* null mutations (although at different doses of transgene for rescuing different phenotypic characteristics of the *awd* null mutants). Neither NDPK A nor catalytically inactive NDPK B were effective, suggesting that catalytic activity of NDPK is necessary but not sufficient for biological functions in this system.

Opposite effects of NDPK A and NDPK B?

Transfection of human nm23-H1 cDNA in human breast carcinoma cells suppresses their metastatic potential without affecting tumorigenicity in a nude mouse model [65]. Thus, human *nm23-H1* appears to act as a true metastasis suppressor gene in breast carcinoma cells. Correlation data support this role of the *nm23-H1* gene in at least some tumors (see [56] for review). It is possible that the product of *nm23-H1* gene, NDPK A, acts as a negative regulator of the metastatic phenotype by affecting as yet unknown regulatory circuits in tumor cells. However, NDPK A readily binds NDPK B, the product of the *nm23-H2* gene, for which a host of activities has been reported [51, 55, 69]. Thus, it is possible that the biological activity of NDPK A is based on its ability to sequester NDPK B in heteromers, while NDPK B acts as a positive regulator of the metastatic phenotype. Finally, it is possible that both NDPK A and NDPK B may act either independently, or titrate each other out depending on the cell type.

In order to analyse these alternatives experimentally, we have created a panel of human breast carcinoma MDA-MB-435 cells transfected with cDNAs for catalytically active NDPK A and NDPK B, and with cDNAs for catalytically inactive NDPK A/T and NDPK B/T created by substituting his[118] with tyrosine. The MDA-MB-435 cell line has been used by Leone et al. [65] for transfection of cDNA for catalytically active NDPK A and NDPK B. We also created a similar panel of human melanoma line IV Cl1 cells [36] transfected with the cDNAs for catalytically active NDPK A and NDPK B, and with cDNAs for catalytically inactive NDPK A/T and NDPK B/T. We reasoned that catalytically inactive NDPK A/T and NDPK B/T may act as dominant negative mutants for those functions of NDPK which are mediated by interactions with some protein(s) and which require catalytic activity of NDPK. In experiments described further, we have used bulk transfected cells (pooled transfected clones) in order to avoid possible bias in the selection of clones with fortuitous transgene integration sites.

Experiments are now in progress to evaluate the tumorigenic and metastatic potential of MDA-MB-345 cells and human melanoma line IV Cl1 cells transfected with catalytically active and catalytically inactive NDPK A and NDPK B. Preliminary results indicate that human breast carcinoma and human melanoma cells transfected with catalytically inactive NDPK B/T are tumorigenic, but have a significantly lower metastatic potential than control (vector-transfected) cells. Assuming that NDPK B/T acts as a dominant negative mutant we hypothesize that wildtype NDPK B may act as a positive regulator of metastatic potential.

Tetra span transmembrane protein superfamily (TM4SP) and metastasis control

Several recent publications indicate that members of the tetra span transmembrane protein superfamily (TM4SP) may act as metastasis suppressor genes. TM4SP proteins [70, 71] are integral membrane proteins with presumably four transmembrane domains, a major extracellular N-glycosylated loop and intracellular N- and C-termini. Most members of the family were identified as cell surface antigens in leukocytes and assigned names according to the CD nomenclature, although subsequent studies established their expression in various mammalian tissues and in some intracellular membranes. The functions of TM4SP proteins are not known, but indications are that they may be involved in cell-cell and cell-matrix interactions. Several members of this family are coupled to signal transduction pathways [71]. Members of this family form complexes with other cell surface molecules such as MHC class II antigens, CD4 and CD8, which are known to be involved in signal transduction. One of the TM4SP proteins (CD82) has recently been independently cloned by Dong et al. [24], as a metastasis suppressor gene for prostate cancer on human chromosome 11p11.2, and named KAI1 (for *kang ai*, anti-cancer in Chinese).

KAI1, a new metastasis suppressor gene
A putative metastasis suppressor gene for prostate cancer was mapped to the region p11.2–13 of human chromosome 11 by microcell-mediated chromosome transfer [16]. Dong et al., cloned the *KAI1* gene using Alu-PCR fragments [72] of p11.2–13 to screen a cDNA library prepared from a microcell hybrid of Dunning rat prostate cancer cells, AT6.1-11-1, containing a fragment of human chromosome 11 from centromere to region 11p13. The metastatic potential of AT6.1-11-1 cells is significantly lower compared to other microcell hybrids, AT6.1-11-2 and AT6.1-11-3, containing smaller fragments of human chromosome 11 from centromere to region p11.2. The 2.4 kb KAI1 cDNA obtained through this screening contained a sequence encoding a predicted

29.6 kDa member of TM4SP protein which was identical to three cDNA clones isolated independently in different laboratories. Transfection of KAI1 cDNA in highly metastatic ATF6.1 prostate
tumor cells yielded clones whose tumorigenicity in nude mice was similar to that of parental cells.
However, the ability of transfected cells to form lung metastasis in nude mice was significantly
lower than that of the vector-transfected cells ($p < 0.001$ for two clones and $p < 0.02$ for one
clone). Similar results were obtained in experiments with mice with severe immunodeficiency
disease (SCID). Thus, *KAI1* appeared to act as a true metastasis suppressor gene capable of
inhibiting the metastatic potential of cells without affecting their tumorigenicity.

The same group used immunohistochemical analysis to screen expression of the *KAI1* gene in
98 primary prostatic tumors and 32 metastases [73]. The expression of the *KAI1* gene was significantly decreased ($p < 0.05$) in the progression from normal prostatic tissue to localized prostate
cancer to metastatic prostatic cancer. It is interesting that expression of the *KAI1* gene was decreased in normal prostatic tissue of 20% patients with prostate cancer. The latter result suggests
that downregulation of *KAI1* gene may be driven by epigenetic factors rather than by genetic
alterations in the structure of this gene. Indeed, microsatellite analysis of 34 primary tumors and
12 metastases did not reveal a single instance of allelic loss of the *KAI1* gene. Likewise, SSCP
analysis of *KAI1* gene exons from ten prostatic metastasis did not reveal any mutations [73].

Two recent papers evaluated the role of *KAI1* gene expression in the progression of non-small
cell lung cancer [74] and pancreatic cancer (NSCLC) [75]. Adachi et al. [74] reported that the
overall survival rate of NSCLC patients with KAI1-positive tumors was higher than that for
patients with KAI1-reduced/negative tumors (77.4% vs 38.5%, $p = 0.002$). The level of *KAI1*
gene expression was determined by RT-PCR analysis of RNA purified from fresh and frozen
tumor samples. In fact, multivariate analysis with the Cox regression model revealed an
association of high *KAI1* gene expression with the overall survival rate ($p = 0.046$).

Guo et al. [75] reported that expression of the *KAI1* gene, as measured by Northern blot analysis, is upregulated in pancreatic cancer tissue in comparison with normal pancreatic tissue. *In
situ* hybridization experiments revealed that the *KAI1* gene was overexpressed in pancreatic cancer cells and not in normal cells within the cancer tissue. However, comparison of KAI1 mRNA
levels in stage I to IV pancreatic tumors revealed a significant ($p < 0.05$) negative correlation
between tumor progression and expression of the *KAI1* gene. It is noteworthy that there was no
correlation between *KAI1* gene expression and postoperative survival time, which was limited to a
median time of 5–6 months.

It should be noted that microcell-mediated transfer of the fragment of human chromosome 11
containing the *KAI1* gene into metastatic mammary rat carcinoma cells did not change their
metastatic potential [18]. This result suggests that the metastasis-suppressing function(s) of *KAI1*
gene may be tumor specific. In this respect, effects of *KAI1* are reminiscent of observations that
downregulation of *nm23* correlates with metastatic progression in some, but not all tumors [56].

The functions of *KAI1* in tumor cells are unknown. The cDNA for this gene has been cloned
by three independent groups [76–78]. Gaugitsch et al. [76] cloned KAI1 cDNA under the name
R2 by subtractive hybridization of a cDNA library of stimulated Jurkat cells. The homology
search revealed that R2 belongs to TM4SP proteins and that the level of R2 mRNA is elevated in
activated lymphoid cells. Gil et al. [77] cloned KAI1 cDNA under the name IA4 using transient
expression of a monocytic U937 cell cDNA library in COS cells and a panning strategy with

anti-IA4 monoclonal antibody. This group established that expression of IA4 is a marker of lymphocyte activation with IL-2, PHA, and *Staphylococcus aureus* Cowan I. In human monocytic U937 cells, tumor necrosis factor α (TNF-α) and IL-6 upregulated expression of IA4. Exposure of U937 cells to saturating doses of IA4 antibody led to a rapid (seconds) increase in cytosolic free Ca^{2+}, suggesting that IA4 may be involved in Ca^{2+} regulation. Finally, Imai et al. [78] cloned KAI1 cDNA under the name C33 by screening an expression library with antibody against C33 antigen. C33 antigen was originally identified as a target for antibody which inhibited syncytium formation, induced by the human T cell leukemia virus type 1 (HTLV-1) in human T cell line MOLT-4. This group established that C33 is heavily N-glycosylated and that the pattern of glycosylation is different in HTLV-1$^+$ and HTLV-1$^-$ cells.

Although the biological functions of TM4SP proteins are unknown, two other members of this family were recently implicated in the development of malignant and metastatic phenotypes.

CD63 glycoprotein

Two groups reported that another member of TM4SP family, a melanoma-specific antigen CD63 (ME491), may function as a tumor suppressor gene. CD63 is a lysosomal membrane glycoprotein which is also expressed on the surface of melanoma cells and platelets [79, 80]. It was found that transfection of CD63 cDNA in H-*ras*-transformed NIH 3T3 cells yielded clones with decreased ability to grow in nude mice after subcutaneous injection [81]. Similar results were obtained when a genomic CD63 clone (in an episomal vector) was transfected into KM3, a human melanoma cell line negative for CD63 [82]. One of the transfected clones was assayed for its ability to grow in a nude mice after intradermal injection and was found to grow significantly less vigorously than a control (vector-transfected) clone. In addition, after tail vein injection of 3×10^6 cells the CD63 transfectant formed significantly fewer subcutaneous and peritoneal metastatic nodules than control cells.

MRP-1/CD9 glycoprotein

Ikeyama et al. [83] reported that another member of the TM4SP superfamily, the MRP-1/CD9 protein, may be involved in control of metastatic phenotype. MRP-1/CD9 is a 24–27 kDa glycoprotein which is expressed in hemopoietic tissues, in many nonhemopoietic tissues and in human tumor cell lines [84]. Monoclonal antibodies to CD9 induce platelet activation and aggregation [85]. The M31-15 monoclonal antibody against MRP-1/CD9 inhibits motility of MAC10 cells derived from a human lung adenocarcinoma [84] and overexpression of MRP-1/CD9 protein in several type of cells suppressed their motility [83]. Somewhat contra-intuitively, overexpression of MRP-1/CD9 in highly metastatic mouse melanoma BL6 cells also resulted in the suppression of their ability to form lung metastasis upon intravenous injection of 10^5 cells into BALB/c *nu/nu* mice [83]. The potential ability of MRP-1/CD9 to suppress metastatic dissemination was further supported by the finding of a lower expression of this protein in breast cancer metastatic lymph nodes as compared with primary tumors [86].

Manganese superoxide dismutase and control of metastatic potential

Manganese superoxide dismutase (MnSOD) is a nuclear DNA-encoded mitochondrial enzyme that converts superoxide radicals formed in mitochondria into H_2O_2. Superoxide radicals are potent genotoxic agents and also apparently serve as second messengers in some signal transduction pathways [87]. MnSOD is encoded by the *SOD2* gene and there are indications that it may function as a tumor suppressor gene [88]. Safford et al. [89] reported that overexpression of human MnSOD in highly metastatic mouse fibrosarcoma cells (FSa-II) yielded clones which were tumorigenic, but weakly metastatic, upon injection of $1-2 \times 10^5$ cells into the feet of syngeneic mice. Thus, it appears that in this heterologous system MnSOD may function as a true metastasis suppressor capable of inhibiting metastatic potential of cells without affecting their tumorigenicity. Chromosome transfer experiments in human cells supported this possibility, since introduction of human chromosome 6 carrying *SOD2* [90] into highly metastatic human melanoma cell line c8161 yielded tumorigenic but weakly metastatic clones [20]. However, direct transfection of human SOD2 cDNA into c8161 cells did not change their metastatic potential [91]. The total amount of MnSOD protein and total antioxidant activity of MnSOD has not been altered in transfected cells as compared with control (vector-transfected) cells. The latter result suggests a highly regulated level of expression of the *SOD2* gene in human melanoma cells, which in turn may explain the difference between the results of transfection experiments with mouse [89] and human [91] cells.

E-cadherin and control of tumorigenicity and metastatic potential

Several reports suggest that E-cadherin molecules may be involved in control of the metastatic phenotype. Although these reports do not contain direct experimental evidence separating the effects of E-cadherin on tumorigenicity and metastatic dissemination of primary tumor, they nevertheless merit discussion in this review. The first step in tumor cell metastatic dissemination is separation from other tumor cells, for example the disruption of homophilic interactions between tumor cells. These interactions are mediated by cadherins, a family of transmembrane glycoproteins that provide for Ca^{2+}-dependent cell-cell adhesion [92]. The extracellular N-terminal 113 amino acid region apparently defines the specificity of the cell-cell binding, while the intracellular C-terminal domain interacts with cytoskeletal proteins and is necessary for mobilizing the ability of cells to bind to each other. Several lines of evidence indicate that the level of expression of E-cadherin (uvomorulin) may play a crucial role in the metastatic dissemination of certain types of tumor cells. First, low levels of expression of the E-cadherin gene correlate with the progression of human prostate cancer [93, 94]. Second, reduced expression of E-cadherin is associated with increased invasiveness of human colorectal carcinoma cell lines in tissue culture assays [95]. Third, transfection of mouse E-cadherin cDNA into human colon carcinoma cell line COKFu resulted in transfectants with decreased growth rates *in vitro* and in the subcutis of nude mice, and with decreased ability to form lymph node metastasis after intravenous injection [96]. However, ectopic expression of E-cadherin in mouse HaCa4 cells derived from a mouse skin carcinoma produced a clone (E62) which remains metastatic [97].

The regulation of expression of the E-cadherin gene occurs on several levels. Graff et el., [98] demonstrated that downregulation of E-cadherin in some prostate and breast tumors may be caused by hypermethylation of the promoter region. Yoshimura et al. [99, 100] demonstrated that increased expression of E-cadherin on the cell surface may be achieved by altering the pattern of glycosylation of this protein. The experiments were based on the notion that the beta-1-6 structure of N-linked oligosaccharides, formed by beta-1,6-N-acetylglucosaminyltransferase (GnT-V), is associated with metastatic potential. In order to decrease the level of beta-1-6 structures, Yoshimura et al. [99] overexpressed a competing enzyme, beta-1,4-N-acetylglucosaminyltransferase (GnT-III), in B16-hm, a highly metastatic subclone of mouse B16 melanoma cells. This experiment resulted in transfectants with decreased ability to form lung metastasis after intravenous injection into syngeneic and nude mice. Further study established that E-cadherin was glycosylated by GnT-III in transfectants, and that the turnover of E-cadherin in the GnT-III transfectants was slower, resulting in the increased presence on the cell surface.

Unfortunately, the metastatic dissemination of cells transfected with E-cadherin or GnT-III was assayed in intravenous injection experiments which do not allow for the separation of effects of E-cadherin on the growth of primary tumor and the ability of the primary tumor to metastasize.

Potential positive regulators of metastatic dissemination

To discover positive regulators of metastatic potential, which selectively enhance metastatic dissemination of tumor cells without affecting their tumorigenicity, appears to be even more difficult than the search for metastasis suppressor genes. It should be noted however, that positive regulators of metastatic dissemination would be more conventional targets for the development of antimetastasis therapeutics than negative regulators. Although several strategies for selective inhibition of target proteins are available (dominant negative mutants, ribozymes, antisense constructs, knockout constructs), all of them require prior knowledge of putative positive regulators of metastasis.

A ribozyme-based approach to inhibiting expression of proteins suspected to have a role in the control of metastatic dissemination has been tested recently by three groups. The approach is based on constructing ribozymes with the catalytic hammerhead RNA sequence flanked with RNA sequences complementary to a targeted mRNA. Expression of targeted ribozymes in mammalian cells leads to decreased expression of a targeted protein [101, 102]. Unfortunately, all three groups have chosen to test metastatic potential of constructed tumor cells in the colonization assay based on intravenous or intracardial injection of tumor cells, and therefore (as discussed above) it is impossible to establish whether their findings will be true for cells disseminating from primary tumors.

Hua and Muschel [103] expressed a ribozyme-targeting metalloproteinase 9 (MMP-9) in a metastatic rat embryo fibroblast line 2.10.10 that was transformed by ras^H and v-myc and constitutively expresses MMP-9. MMP-9, as well as other metalloproteinases, is implicated in invasion and metastasis [8]. Expression of MMP-9 ribozymes in 2.10.10 cells yielded clones which, upon subcutaneous injection into nude mice (5×10^5 cells/mouse), were as tumorigenic as parental cells, or cells overexpressing untargeted hammerhead ribozymes. However, the ability of these cells to colonize nude mouse lungs after tail vein injection of 5×10^4 cells was significantly lower in two tested clones than in control cells.

Melandsmo et al. [104] expressed a ribozyme targeting the mRNA of *CAPL* (*mts1*) gene in OHS, a human osteosarcoma cell line established from a patient with multiple skeletal metastases. When these cells were injected intracardially into immunodeficient nude rats the tumors were formed in spinal vertebrae and long bones. The *CAPL* gene encodes a protein which belongs to the S-100 family of Ca^{2+} binding proteins implicated in control of signal transduction pathway, and in control of cytoskeletal and motor functions *via* activation of giant protein kinases [105, 106]. Expression of CAPL ribozymes in OHS cells did not affect their tumorigenicity as measured by subcutaneous injection of 1×10^6 cells into nude mice. However, the expression of CAPL ribozymes significantly inhibited the ability of transfected cells (three clones tested) to form spinal tumors upon intracardial injection of 1×10^6 cells into nude rats.

Finally, Yamamoto et al. [107] designed a ribozyme targeting mRNA of the alpha 6 subunit of the VLA-6 ($\alpha 6\beta 1$) integrin receptor which recognizes laminin. Expression of this ribozyme in the human fibrosarcoma cell line HT1080 yielded clones with significantly reduced expression of VLA-6 and dramatically reduced ability to colonize lungs of nude mice upon tail vein injection. Unfortunately, the authors did not present evidence on the tumorigenicity of the selected clones and therefore it is impossible to establish whether inhibition of VLA-6 expression is related specifically to a metastatic phenotype. Hopefully, either a ribozyme-based strategy, or a recently reported dominant negative receptor strategy of downregulating VLA-6 expression [108], will discriminate the contribution of this receptor to tumorigenic and metastatic phenotypes.

Summary

Three types of experiments clearly demonstrated that different genes control the ability of cells to form a primary tumor and to metastasize from the primary tumor. First, there are three reports that fusion of metastatic and non-metastatic cells produced non-metastatic, but tumorigenic cells [10–12]. Second, there are six reports that introduction of specific normal human chromosomes into metastatic cells suppresses their metastatic potential, but does not affect tumorigenicity [16–21]. Third, there are three reports that transfection of cDNA for *nm23-H1*, *KAI1* and *SOD2* genes into metastatic cells suppresses their metastatic potential, but does not affect tumorigenicity [65, 24, 89]. In addition, there are several reports that transfection of cDNA for MRP-1/CD9, beta-1,4-N-acetylglucosaminyltransferase, and ribozymes for MMP-9, CAPL, and alpha 6 subunit of VLA-6 suppresses the metastatic potential of tumor cells in intravenous (or intracardial) injection assays.

Currently, the crop of identified metastasis control genes is much smaller than that of oncogenes or tumor suppressor genes. Perhaps activation of oncogenes and/or inactivation of tumor suppressor genes equipped cells with means nearly sufficient for formation of primary tumor and for metastatic dissemination. If this is the case, then alterations in only a few genes may be necessary for successful metastatic dissemination of tumor cells. However, it is possible that there are numerous metastasis control genes whose discovery has been hindered by at least three experimental problems. First, there are no tissue culture experiments that can separate effects of transgenes on tumorigenic and metastatic potential of tumor cells. Therefore, validation of putative metastasis control genes requires costly and lengthy *in vivo* experiments. Second, *in vivo* experiments are designed to detect inhibition of metastatic potential. Thus, positive regulators of metastatic potential can be detected only through strategies that lead to the 'loss-of-function' (dominant negative mutants, ribozymes, knockouts). These strategies in turn require pre-existing knowledge, or at least suppositions, about functions of the targeted gene. Third, strategies based on differential screening of highly metastatic and non-metastatic subclones of the same tumor cell line require validation of any findings on a large number of subclones in order to be considered statistically significant.

However, the results of transfection experiments suggest that manipulation of single genes (*nm23, KAI1, SOD2*) may be sufficient for dramatic decreases in metastatic capabilities of tumor cells. Given the reservations about translation of 'nude mouse' results to 'real' tumors, the results of transfection experiments suggest that identification of genetic control elements of metastatic dissemination may lead to new targeted anti-metastatic therapeutics.

Acknowledgements
This work was supported by the grant DAMD17-96-1-6078 from the Department of the Army, USA.

References

1. Steeg PS, De La Rosa A, Flatow U, MacDonald NJ, Benedict M, Leone A (1993) Nm23 and breast cancer metastasis. *Breast Cancer Res Treat* 25: 175–187.
2. Scardino PT, Weaver R, Hudson MA (1992) Early detection of prostate cancer. *Hum Pathol* 23: 211–222.
3. Aznavoorian S, Murphy AN, Stetler-Stevenson WG, Liotta LA (1993) Molecular aspects of tumor cell invasion and metastasis. *Cancer* 71: 1368–1383.
4. MacDonald NJ, Steeg PS (1993) Molecular basis of tumour metastasis. *Cancer Surv* 16: 175–199.
5. Fidler IJ (1986) Rationale and methods for the use of nude mice to study the biology and therapy of human cancer metastatis. *Cancer Metastasis Rev* 5: 29–49.
6. Kerbel RS, Cornil I, Theodorescu D (1991) Importance of orthotopic transplantation procedures in assessing the effects of transfected genes on human tumor growth and metastasis. *Cancer Metastasis Rev* 10: 201–215.
7. Mignatti P, Rifkin DB (1993) Biology and bichemistry of proteinases in tumor invasion. *Physiol Rev* 73: 161–195.
8. Powell WC, Matrisian LM (1996) Complex role of matrix metalloproteinase in tumor progression. *Curr Topics Microbiol Immunol* 213: 1–21.
9. Hanahan D, Folkman J (1996) Patterns and emerging mechanisms of the angiogenic switch during tumorigenesis. *Cell* 86: 353–364.
10. Ramshaw IA, Carlsen S, Wang HC, Badenoch-Jones P (1983) The use of cell fusion to analyze factors involved in tumour cell metastasis. *Int J Cancer* 32: 471–478.
11. Sidebottom E, Clark SR (1983) Cell fusion segregates progressive growth from metastasis. *Brit J Cancer* 47: 399–406.
12. Layton MG, Franks LM (1986) Selective suppression of metastasis but not tumorigenicity of a mouse lung carcinoma by cell hybridization. *Int J Cancer* 37: 723–730.
13. Turpeeniemi-Hujanen T, Thorgeirsson UP, Hart IR, Grant SS, Liotta LA (1985) Expression of collagenase IV (basement membrane collagenase) activity in murine tumor hybrids that differ in metastatic potential. *J Nat Cancer Inst* 75: 99–103.
14. Ichikawa T, Ichikawa Y, Isaacs JT (1991) Genetic factors and suppression of metastatic ability of prostate cancer. *Cancer Res* 51: 3788–3792.
15. Fournier REK, Ruddle FH (1977) Microcell-mediated transfer of murine chromosomes into mouse, Chinese hamster, and human somatic cells. *Proc Natl Acad Sci USA* 74: 319–323.
16. Ichikawa T, Ichikawa Y, Dong J, Hawkins AL, Griffin CA, Isaacs WB, Oshimura M, Barrett JC, Isaacs JT (1992) Localization of metastasis suppressor gene(s) for prostatic cancer to the short arm of human chromosome 11. *Cancer Res* 52: 3486–3490.

17. Ichikawa T, Nihei N, Suzuki H, Oshimura M, Emi M, Nakamura Y, Hayata I, Isaacs JT, Shimazaki J (1994) Suppression of metastasis of rat prostatic cancer by introducing human chromosome 8. *Cancer Res* 2299–2302.
18. Rinker-Schaeffer CW, Hawkins AL, Ru N, Dong J, Stoica G, Griffin CA, Ichikawa T, Barrett JC, Isaacs JT (1994) Differential suppression of mammary and prostate cancer metastasis by human chromosomes 17 and 11. *Cancer Res* 54: 6249–6256.
19. Nihei N, Ichikawa T, Kawana Y, Kuramochi H, Kugo H, Oshimura M, Killary AM, Rinker-Schaeffer CW, Barrett JC, Isaacs JT et al. (1995) Localization of metastasis suppressor gene(s) for rat prostatic cancer to the long arm of human chromosome 10. *Gene Chromosome Cancer* 14: 112–119.
20. Welch DR, Chen PC, Miele ME, Bower JM, McGary CT, Stanbridge EJ, Weismann BE (1994) Microcell-mediated transfer of chromosome 6 into metastatic human c8161 melanoma cells suppresses metastasis but does not inhibit tumorigenicity. *Oncogene* 9: 255–262.
21. Phillips KK, Welch DR, Miele ME, Lee JH, Wei LL, Weissman BE (1996) Suppression of MDA MB 435 breast carcinoma cell metastasis following the introduction of human chromosome 11. *Cancer Res* 56: 1222–1227.
22. Steeg PS, Bevilacqua G, Kopper L, Thorgeirsson UP, Talmadge JE, Liotta L, Sobel ME (1988) Evidence for a novel gene associated with low tumor metastatic potential. *J Nat Cancer Inst* 80: 200–204.
23. Hashimoto Y, Shindo-Okada N, Tani M, Takeuchi K, Toma H, Yokota J (1996) Identification of gene differentially expressed in association with metastatic potential of K-1735 murine melanoma by messinger RNA differential display. *Cancer Res* 56: 5266–5271.
24. Dong JT, Lamb PW, Rinker-Schaeffer CW, Vukanovic J, Ichikawa T, Isaacs JT, Barrett JC (1995) KAI1, a metastasis suppressor gene for prostate cancer on human chromosome 11p11.2. *Science* 268: 884–886.
25. Radinsky R, Weisberg HZ, Staroselsky AN, Fidler IJ (1992) Expression level of the *nm23* gene in clonal population of metastatic murine and human neoplasms. *Cancer Res* 52: 5808–5814.
26. Backer JM, Mendola CE, Kovesdi I, Fairhurst JL, O'Hara B, Eddy Jr RL, Shows TB, Mathew S, Murty VVVS, Chaganti RSK (1993) Chromosomal localization and nucleoside diphosphate kinase activity of human metastasis suppressor genes *NM23-1* and *NM23-2*. *Oncogene* 8: 497–502.
27. Seifert M, Seib T, Engel M, Dooley S, Welter C (1995) Characterization of the human nm23-H2 promoter region and localization of the microsatellite D17S396. *Biochem Biophys Res Commun* 215: 910–914.
28. Dooley S Seib T, Engel M, Theisinger B, Janz H, Piontek K, Zang K-D, Welter C (1994) Isolation and characterization of the human genomic locus coding for the putative metastasis control gene nm23-H1. *Hum Genet* 93: 63–66.
29. Venturelli D, Martinez R, Melotti P, Casella I, Peschle C, Cucco C, Spampinato G, Darzynkiewicz Z, Calabretta B (1995) Overexpression of DR-nm23, a protein encoded by a member of the nm23 gene family, inhibits granulocyte differentiation and induces apoptosis in 32Dc13 myeloid cells. *Proc Natl Acad Sci USA* 92: 7435–7439.
30. Milon L, Rousseau-Merck M-F, Munier A, Erent M, Lascu I, Capeau J, Lacombe M-L (1997) nm23-H4, a new member of the human nm23/nucleoside diphosphate kinase gene family localized on chromosome 16p13. *Hum Genet* 99: 550–557.
31. Ishikawa N, Taniguchi-Seto H, Munankata Y, Takagi Y, Shimada N, Kimura N (1997) Multiple transcripts for rat nucleoside diphosphate kinase A are structurally categorized into two groups that exibit cell-specific expression and distinct translational potential. *J Biol Chem* 272: 3289–3295.
32. Iizuka N, Oka M, Noma T, Nakazawa A, Hirose K, Suzuki T (1995) NM23-H1 and NM-23-H2 messenger RNA abundance in human hepatocellular carcinoma. *Cancer Res* 55: 652–657.
33. Ayhan A, Yasui W, Yokozaki H, Kitadai Y, Tahara E (1993) Reduced expression of nm23 protein is associated with advanced tumor stage and distant metastases in human colorectal carcinomas. *Virchows Arch B Cell Pathol* 63: 213–218.
34. Biggs J, Hersperger E, Steeg PS, Liotta LAShearn A (1990) A *Drosophilia* gene that is homologous to a mammalian gene associated with tumor metastasis codes for a nucleoside diphosphate kinase. *Cell* 63: 933–940.
35. Backer J, Murty VVVS, Potla L, Mendola CE, Rodriguez E, Reuter VE, Bosl GG, Chaganti RSK (1994) Loss of heterozygosity and decreased expression of *NME* genes correlate with teratomatous differentiation in human male germ cell tumors. *Biochem Biophys Res Commun* 202: 1096–1103.
36. Hamby CV, Mendola CE, Potla L, Stafford D, Backer JM (1995) Differential expression and mutation of NME genes in autologous cultured human melanoma cells with different metastatic potentials. *Biochem Biophys Res Commun* 211: 578–585.
37. Lascu I, Chaffotte A, Limbourg-Bouchon B, Veron M (1992) A pro/ser substitution in nucleosude diphosphate kinase of *Drosophilia melanogaster* (mutation *killer of prune*) affects stability but not catalytic efficiency of the enzyme. *J Biol Chem* 267: 12775–12781.
38. MacDonald NJ, De La Rosa A, Benedict MA, Freije JM, Krutsch H, Steeg PS (1993) A serine phosphorylation of Nm23, and not its nucleoside diphosphate kinase activity, correlates with suppression of tumor metastatic potential. *J Biol Chem* 268: 25780–25789.
39. Webb PA, Perisic O, Mendola CE, Backer JM, Williams RL (1995) The crystal structure of a human nucleoside diphosphate kinase, NM23-H2. *J Molec Biol* 251: 574–587.

40. Postel EH, Weiss VH, Beneken J, Kirtane A (1996) Mutational analysis of NM23-H2/NDP kinase identifies the structural domains critical to recognition of a c-myc regulatory element. *Proc Natl Acad Sci USA* 93: 6892–6897.
41. Lombardi D, Sacchi A, D Agostino G, Tibursi G (1995) The association of the nm23-M1 and α-tubulin correlates with cell differentiation. *Exp Cell Res* 217: 267–271.
42. Otero AD (1990) Transphosphorylation and G-protein activation. *Biochem Pharmacol* 39: 1399–1404.
43. Urano T, Furukawa K, Shiku H (1993) Expression of nm23/NDP kinase proteins on the cell surface. *Oncogene* 8 1371–1376.
44. Kreft S-K, Traincart F, Mesnildrey S, Bourdais J, Veron M, Chen LB (1996) Nuclear localization of nucleoside diphosphate kinase type B (*nm23-H2*) in cultured cells. *Exp Cell Res* 227: 63–69.
45. Saks VA, Khuchua ZA, Vasilyeva EV, Belikova OY, Kuznetsov AV (1994) III-1 Metabolic compartmentalization and substrate channeling in muscle cells. *Mol Cell Biochem* 133/134: 155–192.
46. Wagner PD, Vu N-D (1995) Phosphorylation of ATP-citrate lyase by nucleoside diphosphate kinase. *J Biol Chem* 270: 21758–21764.
47. Engel M, Veron M, Theisinger B, Lacombe M-L, Seib T, Dooley S, Welter C (1995) A novel serine/threonine-specific protein phosphotransferase activity of Nm23/nucleoside-diphosphate kinase. *Eur J Biochem* 234: 200–207.
48. Alex LA, Simon MI (1994) Protein histidine kinases and signal transduction in procaryotes and eucaryotes. *Trends Genet* 10: 133–138.
49. Postel EH, Ferrone CA (1994) Nucleoside diphosphate kinase enzyme activity of NM23-H2/PuF is not required for its DNA binding and *in vitro* transcriptional functions. *J Biol Chem* 269: 8627–8630.
50. Ji L, Arcinas M, Boxer LM (1995) The transcriptional factor Nm23H2, binds to and activates the translocated c-myc allele in Burkitt's lymphoma. *J Biol Chem* 270: 13392–13398.
51. Postel EH, Berberich SJ, Flint SJ, Ferrone CA (1993) Human c-myc transcription factor PuF identified as nm23-H2 nucleoside diphosphate kinase, a candidate suppressor of tumor metastasis. *Science* 261: 478–480.
52. Hildebrandt M, Lacombe M-L, Mesnildrey S, Veron M (1995) A human NDP-kinase B specifically binds single-stranded poly-pyrimidine sequences. *Nucl Acid Res* 23: 3858–3864.
53. Okabe-Kado J, Kasukabe T, Honma Y, Hayashi M, Henzel WJ, Hozumi M (1992) Identity of a differentiation inhibiting factor for mouse myeloid leukemia cells with NM23/nucleoside diphosphate kinase. *Biochem Biophys Res Commun* 182: 987–994.
54. Okabe-Kado J, Kasukabe T, Baba H, Urano T, Shiku H, Honma Y (1995) Inhibitory action of nm23 proteins on induction of erythroid differentiation of human leukemia cells. *Biochim Biophys Acta* 1267: 101–106.
55. Paravicini G, Steinmayr M, Andre E, Becker-Andre M (1996) The metastasis suppressor candidate nucleoside diphosphate kinase nm23 specifically interacts with members of the ROR/RZR nuclear orphan receptor subfamily. *Biochem Biophys Res Commun* 227: 82–87.
56. De La Rosa A, Williams RL, Steeg PS (1995) Nm23/nucleoside diphosphate kinase: Toward a structural and biochemical understanding of its biological functions. *BioEssays* 17: 53–62.
57. Sawan A, Lascu I, Veron M, Anderson JJ, Wright C, Horne CHW, Angus B (1994) NDP-K/nm23 expression in human breast cancer in relation to relapse, survival, and other prognostic factors: an immunohistochemical study. *J Pathol* 172: 27–34.
58. Russell RL, Geisinger KR, Mehta R, White W, Shelton B, Kute TE (1997) Nm23: relationship to the metastatic potential of breast cancer cell lines, primary human xenografts and node negative breast cancer patients. *Cancer; in press*
59. Engel M, Theisinger B, Seib T, Seitz G, Huwer H, Zang KD, Welter C, Dooley S (1993) High level of NM23-H1 and NM23-H2 messenger RNA in human squamous-cell lung carcinoma are associated with poor differentiation and advanced tumor stages. *Int J Cancer* 55: 375–379.
60. Konishi N, Nakaoka S, Tsuzuki T, Matsumoto K, Kitahori Y, Hiasa Y, Urano T, Shiku H (1993) Expression of nm23-H1 and nm23-H2 proteins in prostate carcinoma. *Jpn J Cancer Res* 84: 1050–1054.
61. Hsu S, Huang F, Wang L, Banerji S, Winawer S, Friedman E (1994) The role of nm23 in transforming growth factor β1 – mediated adherence and growth arrest. *Cell Growth Diff* 5: 909–917.
62. Backer J, Murty VVVS, Potla L, Mendola CE, Rodriguez E, Reuter VE, Bosl GG, Chaganti RSK (1994) Loss of heterozygosity and decreased expression of *NME* genes correlate with teratomatous differentiation in human male germ cell tumors. *Biochem Biophys Res Commun* 202: 1096–1103.
63. Zinyk DL, McGonnigal BG, Dearolf CR (1993) *Drosophila* awd K-pn, a homologue of the metastasis suppressor gene nm23, suppresses the Tum-1 haematopoietic oncogene. *Nat Genet* 4: 195–201.
64. Leone A, Flatow U, King CR, Sandeen MA, Margulies IM, Liotta LA, Steeg PS (1991) Reduced tumor incidence, metastatic potential, and cytokine responsiveness of nm23-transfected melanoma cells. *Cell* 65: 25–35.
65. Leone A, Flatow U, Van Houtte K, Steeg PS (1993) Transfection of human nm23-H1 into the human MDA-MB-435 breast carcinoma cell line: effects on tumor metastatic potential, colonization and enzymatic activity. *Oncogene* 8: 2325–2333.
66. Kantor JD, McCormick B, Steeg PS, Zetter BR (1993) Inhibition of cell motility after *nm23* transfection of human and murine tumor cells. *Cancer Res* 53: 1971–1973.

67. Howlett AR, Petersen OW, Steeg PS, Bissell MJ (1994) A novel function for nm23-H1 gene: overexpression in human breast carcinoma cells leads to the formation of basement membrane and growth arrest. *J Nat Cancer Inst* 86: 1838–1844.
68. Baba H, Urano T, Okada K, Furukawa K, Nakayama E, Tanaka H, Iwasaki K, Shiku H (1995) Two isotypes of murine nm23/nucleoside diphosphate kinase, nm-23-M1 and nm23-M2, are involved in metastatic suppression of a murine melanoma line. *Cancer Res* 55: 1977–1981.
69. Xu J, Liu LZ, Deng XF, Timmons L, Hersperger E, Steeg PS, Veron M, Shearn A (1996) The enzymatic activity of *Drosophila* AWD/NDP Kinase is necessary but not sufficient for its biological function. *Dev Biol* 177: 544–557.
70. Horejsi V, Vlcek C (1991) Novel structurally distinct family of leukocyte surface glycoproteins including CD9, CD37, CD53 and CD63. *FEBS Lett* 288: 1–4.
71. Wright MD, Tomlinson MG (1994) The ins and outs of the transmembrane 4 superfamily. *Immunol Today* 15: 588–594.
72. Nelson DL, Ledbetter SA, Corbo L, Victoria MF, Ramirez-Solis R, Webster TD, Ledbetter DH, Caskey CT (1989) Alu polymerase chain reaction: a method for rapid isolation of human-specific sequences from complex DNA sources. *Proc Natl Acad Sci USA* 86: 6686–6690.
73. Dong JT, Suzuki H, Pin SS, Bova S, Schalken JA, Isaacs WB, Barrett JC, Isaacs JT (1996) Down-regulation of KAI1 metastasis suppressor gene during the progression of human prostatic cancer infrequently involves gene mutation or allelic loss. *Cancer Res* 56: 4387–4390.
74. Adachi M, Taki T, Leki Y, Huang CL, Higashiyama M, Miyake M (1996) Correlation of KAI1/CD82 gene expression with good prognosis in patients with non-small cell lung cancer. *Cancer Res* 56: 1751–1755.
75. Guo X, Friess H, Graber HU, Kashiwagi M, Zimmermann A, Korc M, Buchler MW (1996) KAI1 expression is up-regulated in early pancreatic cancer and decreased in the presence of metastases. *Cancer Res* 56: 4876–4880.
76. Gaugitsch HW, Hofer E, Huber NE, Schnabl E, Baumruker T (1991) A new superfamily of lymphoid and melanoma cell proteins with extensive homology to *Schistosoma mansoni* antigen Sm23. *Eur J Immunol* 21: 377–383.
77. Gil ML, Vita N, Lebel-Binay S, Miloux B, Chalon P, Kaghad M, Marchiol-Fournigault C, Conjeaud H, Caput D, Ferrara P et al. (1992) A member of the tetra spans transmemembrane protein superfamily is recognized by a monoclonal antibody raised against an HLA class 1-deficient, lymphokine-activated killer-susceptible, B lymphocyte line. *J Immunol* 148: 2826–2833.
78. Imai T, Fukudome K, Takagi S, Nagira M, Furuse M, Fukuhara N, Nishimura M, Hinuma Y, Yoshie O (1992) C33 antigen recognized by monoclonal antibodies inhibitory to human T cell leukemia virus type 1-induced syncytium formation is a member of a new family of transmembrane proteins including CD9, CD37, CD53, and CD63. *J Immunol* 149: 2879–2886.
79. Metzelaar MJ, Wijngaard PLJ, Peters PJ, Sixma JJ, Nieuwenhuis HK, Clevers HC (1991) CD63 antigen. A novel lysosomal membrane glycoprotein, cloned by screening procedure for intracellular antigens in eukaryotic cells. *J Biol Chem* 266: 3239–3245.
80. Azorsa DO, Hyman JA, Hildreth JEK (1991) CD63/Ptgp-40: a platelet activation antigen identical to the stage-specific, melanoma-associated antigen ME491. *Blood* 78: 280–284.
81. Hotta H, Hara I, Miyamoto H, Homma M (1991) Overexpression of the human melanoma-associated antigen ME491 partially suppresses in vivo malignant phenotype of H-*ras*-transformed NIH3T3 cells in athymic nude mice. *Melanoma Res* 1: 125–132.
82. Radford KJ, Mallesch J, Hersey P (1995) Suppression of human melanoma cell growth and metastasis by the melanoma-associated antigen CD63 (ME491). *Int J Cancer* 62: 631–635.
83. Ikeyama S, Koyama M, Yamaoko M, Sasada R, Miyake M (1993) Suppression of cell motility and metastasis by transfection with human motility-related protein (MRP-1/CD9) DNA. *J Exp Med* 177: 1231–1237.
84. Miyake M, Koyama M, Seno M, Ikeyama S (1991) Identification of the motility-related protein MRP-1), recognized by monoclonal antibody M31-15, which inhibits cell motility. *J Exp Med* 174: 1347–1354.
85. Jennings LK, Fox CF, Kouns WC, Mckay CP, Ballou LR, Schultz HE (1990) The activation of human platelets mediated by anti-human platelet p24/CD9 monoclonal antibodies. *J Biol Chem* 265: 3815–3821.
86. Miyake M, Nakano K, Ieki Y, Adachi M, Huang CL, Itoi S, Koh T, Taki T (1995) Motility related protein 1 (MRP-1/CD9) expression: inverse correlation with metastases in breast cancer. *Cancer Res* 55: 4127–4131.
87. Schreck R, Rieber P, Baeuerle PA (1991) Reactive oxygen intermediates as apparently widely used messingersin the activation of NF-kappaB transcription factor and HIV-1. *EMBO J* 10: 2247–2258.
88. Bravard A, Sabatier L, Hoffschir F, Ricoul M, Luccioni C, Dutrillaux B (1992) SOD2: A new type of tumor suppressor gene? *Int J Cancer* 51: 476–480.
89. Safford SE, Oberley TD, Urano M, St Clair DK (1994) Suppression of fibrosarcoma metastasis by elevated expression of manganese superoxide dismutase. *Cancer Res* 54: 4261–4265.
90. Church SL, Grant JW, Meese EU, Trent JM (1992) Sublocalization of the gene encoding manganese superoxide dismutase (MnSOD/SOD2) to 6q25 by fluorescence in situ hybridization and somatic cell hybrid mapping. *Genomics* 14: 823–825.
91. Miele ME, McGary CT, Welch DR (1995) SOD2 (MnSOD) does not suppress tumorigenicity or metastasis of human melanoma C8161 cells. *Anti-Cancer Res* 15(5B): 2065–2070.

92. Takeichi M (1990) Cadherins: a molecular family important in selective cell-cell adhesion. *Annu Rev Biochem* 59: 237–252.
93. Morton RA, Ewing CM, Nagafuchi A, Tsukita S, Isaacs WB (1993) Reduction in E-cadherin levels and deletion of the α-catenin gene in human prostate cancer. *Cancer Res* 53: 3585–3590.
94. Umbas R, Isaacs WB, Bringuier PP, Schaafsma HE, Karthaus HFM, Oosterhof GON, Debruyne FMJ, Schalken JA (1994) Decreased E-cadherin expression is associated with poor prognosis in patient with prostate cancer. *Cancer Res* 54: 3929–3933.
95. Kinsella AR, Lepts GC, Hill CL, Jones M (1994) Reduced E-cadherin expression correlates with increased invasiveness in colorectal carcinoma cell lines. *Clin Exp Metastasis* 12: 335–342.
96. Miyaki M, Tanaka K, Kikuchi-Yanoshita R, Muraoka M, Konishi M, Takeichi M (1995) Increased cell-substratum adhesion, and decreased gelatinase secretion and cell growth, induced by E-cadherin transfection of human colon carcinoma cells. *Oncogene* 11: 2547–2552.
97. Caulin C, Lopez-Barcons L, Gonzales-Garrigues M, Navarro P, Lozano E, Rodrigo I, Gamallo C, Cano A, Fabra A, Quintanilla M (1996) Suppression of the metastatic phenotype of a mouse skin carcinoma cell line independent of E-cadherin expression and correlated with reduced Ha-ras oncogene products. *Mol Carcinogen* 15: 104–114.
98. Graff JR, Herman JG, Lapidus RG, Chopra H, Xu R, Jarrad DF, Isaacs WB, Pitha PM, Davidson NE, Baylin SE (1995) E-cadherin expression is silenced by DNA hypermethylation in human breast and prostate carcinomas. *Cancer Res* 55: 5195–5199.
99. Yoshimura M, Nishikawa A, Ihara Y, Taniguchi S, Taniguchi N (1995) Introduction of the beta1-4 N-acetylglucosaminyltransferase (GnT-III) gene was reported to suppress metastasis in highly metastatic B16-hm murine melanoma cells. *Proc Natl Acad Sci USA* 92: 8754–8758.
100. Yoshimura M, Ihara Y, Matsuzawa Y, Taniguchi N (1996) Aberrant glycosylation of E-cadherin enhances cell-cell binding to suppress metastasis. *J Biol Chem* 271: 13811–13815.
101. Sigurdsson ST, Eckstein F (1995) Structure-function relationships of hammerhead ribozymes: from understanding to applications. *Trends Biotechnol* 13: 286–289.
102. Castanotto D, Rossi JJ, Sarver N (1994) Antisense catalytic RNAs as therapeutic agents. *Adv Pharmacol* 25: 289–317.
103. Hua J, Muschel RJ (1996) Inhibition of matrix metalloproteinase 9 expression by a ribozyme blocks metastasis in a rat sarcoma model system. *Cancer Res* 56: 5279–5284.
104. Melandsomo GM, Hovig E, Skrede M, Engebraaten O, Florenes VA, Myklebost O, Grigorian M, Lukanidin E, Scanlon KJ, Fodstad O (1996) Reversal of the *in vivo* metastatic phenotype of human tumor cells by an anti-*CAPL* (*mts1*) ribozyme. *Cancer Res* 56: 5490–5498.
105. Schafer BW, Heizmann CW (1996) The S100 family of EF-hand calcium-binding proteins: functions and pathology. *Trends Biochem Sci* 21: 134–140.
106. Heierhorst J, Kobe B, Feil SC, Parker MW, Benian GM, Weiss K, Kemp BE (1966) Ca^{2+}/S100 regulation of giant protein kinases. *Nature* 380: 636–639.
107. Yamamoto H, Irie A, Fukushima Y, Ohnishi T, Arita N, Hayakawa T, Sekiguchi K (1996) Abrogation of lung metastasis of human fibrosarcoma cells by ribozyme mediated suppression of integrin alpha6 subunit expression. *Int J Cancer* 65: 519–524.
108. Shaw LM, Chao C, Wewer UM, Mercurio AM (1996) Function of the integrin α6β1 in metastatic breast carcinoma cells assessed by expression of a dominant-negative receptor. *Cancer Res* 56: 959–963.

Molecular Aspects of Cancer and its Therapy
A. Mackiewicz and P.B. Sehgal (eds)
© 1998 Birkhäuser Verlag Basel/Switzerland

Cytokines in breast cancer cell dyshesion*

I. Tamm, T. Kikuchi, I. Cardinale, J.S. Murphy and J.G. Krueger

The Rockefeller University, 1230 York Avenue, New York, NY 10021, USA

Introduction

While the evidence for the genetic basis of cancer is mounting [reviewed in 1–3], at the same time it is becoming apparent that growth factors and cytokines may play critical roles in determining the phenotypic expression of cancer [4–6]. Interleukin-6 (IL-6) decreases intercellular and substratum adhesiveness in lines of human ductal breast carcinoma cells [7–12]. Dyshesiveness is a cardinal pathological feature of breast carcinoma [13]. Ductal breast carcinoma cells are morphologically heterogeneous not only within the same tumor, but also in sublines originating from the same line of tumor cells. In the Ro subline of the ZR-75-1 cells IL-6 converts cuboidal/polygonal cells to stellate cells with long processes [7]. The morphologically altered ZR-75-1-Ro cells separate from each other and display enhanced directional motility although their proliferation is suppressed. No evidence was obtained of growth factor-inducible cell-cell separation with transforming growth factor-α (TGF-α), TGF-β_1, epidermal growth factor (EGF), or insulin-like growth factor (IGF-1) [9]. Colonies of ZR-75-1-Ro cells formed in the presence of acidic fibroblast growth factor (aFGF) or basic fibroblast growth factor (bFGF) (10 or 100 ng/ml) did however show some evidence of cell-cell separation.

A distinctive response of human ductal breast carcinoma cells to IL-6 has recently been described [11, 12]. The Tx subline of ZR-75-1 cells is characterized by angular/fusiform morphology [11, 12]. In response to IL-6 most of the ZR-75-1-Tx cells round up while only some become fibroblastoid. Many of the rounded cells detach from the substratum. These spherical cells continue to divide, as do cells that remain adherent [11]. The detached spherical cells commonly lack pseudopodia and do not translocate directionally. The distinctive IL-6 induced phenotypic changes in the Ro and Tx sublines of ZR-75-1 cells are reversible upon incubation of the cells in IL-6 free medium for several days [7, 11].

The FGF family of growth factors consists of at least seven members which act upon a wide variety of cells (reviewed in [14–16]). Besides stimulating proliferation, they are capable of inducing or inhibiting differentiation. FGFs show neurotrophic and angiogenic activities and play important roles in development. aFGF activates, *via* the tyrosine phosphorylation activities of its receptor, a number of signal transduction pathways [reviewed in 14], including the protein kinase C pathway [17–21].

---

* This review represents a synthesis of two manuscripts left unfinished by the late Dr. Igor Tamm.

ZR-75-1-Tx breast carcinoma cells treated with aFGF for 1 to 3 days lose their predominantly angular/fusiform shape and become polygonal/cuboidal/spherical. Cells displaying the altered morphology commonly form clusters. A small fraction of the aFGF-treated cells detaches from the substratum. The cell-detaching effect of IL-6 and aFGF together exceeds the sum of the effects of each agent used alone. Through cooperative interaction with aFGF even very low concentrations of IL-6 suffice to produce a marked antimorphogenetic effect. Furthermore, low concentrations of aFGF markedly enhance IL-6 action. The sensitivity of the actions of aFGF and IL-6 to kinase inhibitors is consistent with a requirement for protein tyrosine kinase function in the actions. Protein kinase C activation by phorbol esters modulates dyshesive effects of IL-6 and aFGF, as well as development of the actin-cytoskeleton and integrin-mediated focal adhesions.

Antimorphogenetic action of *E. coli*-derived human recombinant IL-6 in ZR-75-1-Tx breast carcinoma cells

Baculovirus-derived IL-6 was used in previous studies that characterized the action of this cytokine in ZR-75-1-Tx cells, including its interaction with aFGF under serum-free conditions [11, 12]. Figure 1 documents the dose dependence of the morphological changes induced by *E. coli*-derived IL-6 in cultures of ZR-75-1-Tx cells treated for 2 days. ZR-75-1-Tx cells not treated with IL-6 are epithelioid but pleiomorphic with angularity of the outline a predominant feature (Fig. 1A). At 0.04 ng/ml, IL-6 caused only localized rounding involving small numbers of cells (Fig. 1D); at 0.2 ng/ml cell rounding is moderate with numerous singlets present (Fig. 1C); and at 1 ng/ml more than half the cells have rounded (Fig. 1B). Some rounded cells remained attached to the culture surface, while others completely detached and were free-floating in the medium. As illustrated in Figure 2, after a 3-day exposure of ZR-75-1-Tx cells to IL-6 the number of detached cells in the culture medium was dependent on IL-6 concentration in the range from 0.008 to 5 ng/ml. Increasing the concentration beyond 5 ng/ml did not increase the effect.

Figure 3 (panel B) shows that IL-6 induced cell detachment was evident within 1 day from the beginning of treatment, and increased with time as indicated by a comparison of numbers of nonadherent cells in IL-6-treated vs control cultures. Taken together, the photomicrographic and cell enumeration data show that the nonadherent cells represent only a fraction of the rounded cells observed by microscopic examination of cultures, as noted previously [11]. IL-6 had no effect on the total number of cells in the culture (Fig. 3C), which indicates that the population sizes of control and IL-6-treated cells were comparable at all times. Due to IL-6 induced cell detachment, the number of adherent cells in IL-6 treated cultures was lower than in control cultures (Fig. 3A).

Expressing nonadherent cells as percentages of total cells present gives a measure of the kinetics of the IL-6-induced detachment. For the cultures shown in Figure 3 in controls on days 1, 2, and 3 these were 1.5, 2.1 and 1.0%, whereas in IL-6 treated cultures they were 10.7, 11.6 and 22.0%, respectively. On the sixth day of incubation, when the total counts had reached 2.4×10^5 cells/cm^2 for control and 3.0×10^5 cells/cm^2 for IL-6 treated cultures, the respective percentages of nonadherent cells had decreased to 0.1 and 11.0%. Time-lapse cinemicrographic observations indicated that on prolonged incubation a fraction of the detached, rounded IL-6-treated cells readhered to the substratum.

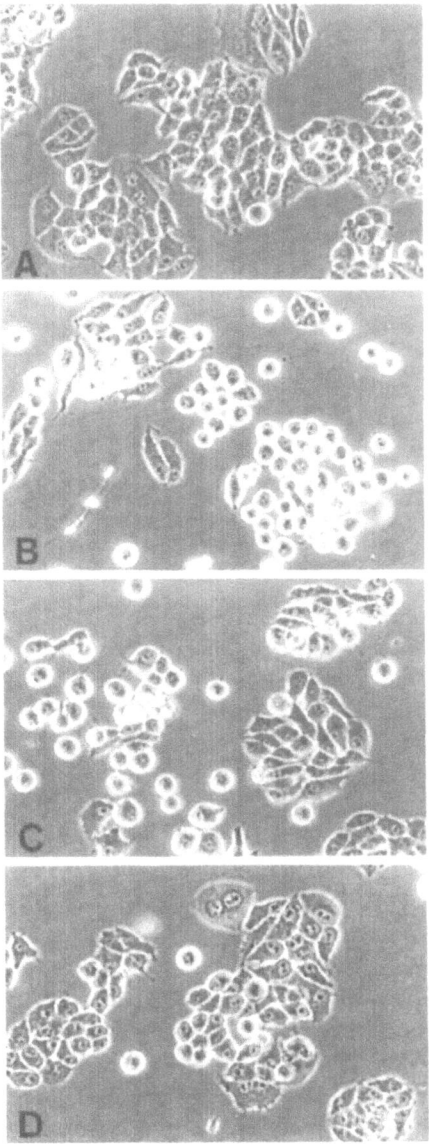

Figure 1. Rounding of ZR-75-1-Tx breast carcinoma cells as a function of IL-6 concentration. Cultures were photographed 2 days after the beginning of treatment. Two cultures were used per variable. (A) Control; (B) IL-6 (1 ng/ml); (C) IL-6 (0.2 ng/ml); (D) IL-6 (0.04 ng/ml). Final magnification ×164.

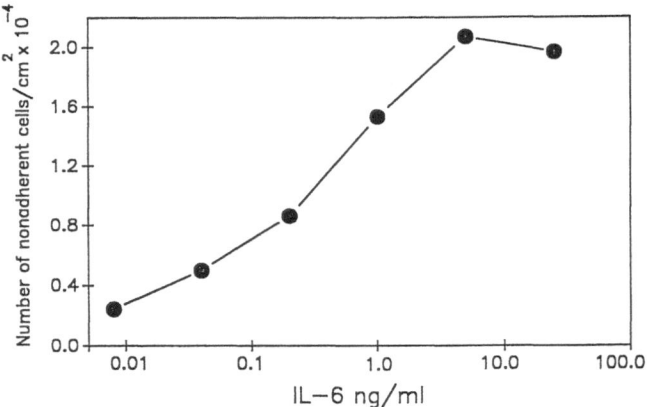

Figure 2. Number of detached ZR-75-1-Tx cells as a function of IL-6 concentration. Coulter counts were done on supernatant media 3 days after the beginning of treatment with IL-6. Two cultures were used per variable. The number of nonadherent cells in control cultures was 0.138×10^4 cells/cm^2. The mean of the coefficients of variation for the seven pairs of determinations was 1.55% and the range was from 0 to 3.48%.

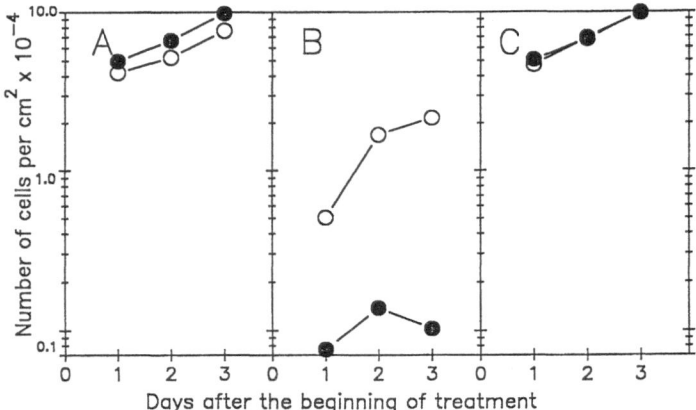

Figure 3. IL-6 does not affect the proliferation rate of ZR-75-1-Tx cells. Nonadherent and adherent cells were enumerated in a hemocytometer. Three cultures were used per variable. (A) Adherent cells; (B) Nonadherent cells; (C) Total. Control ●——●; IL-6 (5 ng/ml) ○——○.

Relationship between time of preincubation and IL-6 induced cell detachment

The extent of IL-6 induced cell detachment is dependent on the interval of time between seeding of cultures and beginning of treatment. Table 1 shows that with a 1-day preincubation before addition of IL-6, the cell-detaching effect of 2-day treatment with IL-6 is close to three times greater than with a 3-day preincubation. This is consistent with the possibility that formation of a more extensive extracellular matrix (ECM) in 3 days *vs* 1 day permits firmer attachment of cells.

Table 1. Prolonged preincubation decreases the response of ZR-75-1-Tx cells to the cell-detaching effect of IL-6

Exp.	Preincubation, days	Control		IL-6, 15 ng/ml	
		Total number of cells/cm$^2 \times 10^{-4}$	Nonadherent cells, % of total	Total number of cells/cm$^2 \times 10^{-4}$	Nonadherent cells, % of total
A	1	5.7	2.3	7.0	24
B	1	4.05	1.2	4.7	23
C	1	8.28	0.7	7.53	15
D	3	14.5	0.2	11.3	7.3
E	3	13.3	0.5	14.6	7.7
F	3	19.8	0.26	20.7	6.9

ZR-75-1-Tx cells were seeded in 25 cm^2 flasks at a density of 2×10^4 cells/cm^2 in 4 ml of medium. Two or three flasks were used per variable. After incubation for 1 or 3 days, the medium was changed and the cultures treated for 2 days. Nonadherent and adherent cells were counted in a hemocytometer.

Antimorphogenetic action of aFGF in ZR-75-1-Tx cells

Figure 4 shows that aFGF markedly alters the morphological characteristics and distribution of ZR-75-1-Tx cells in culture. The changes caused by aFGF (Fig. 4) are clearly different from those caused by IL-6 (Fig. 1). In cultures treated with aFGF at 4 ng/ml many cells are distributed in clusters in which the shape of the cells varies from round to angular. As discussed above, cells treated with IL-6 are more dispersed and the shape tends to be more uniformly spherical. Figure 4 illustrates the dose dependence of the aFGF effect in the range 0.16 to 4 ng/ml. As the concentration of aFGF is increased the changes in individual cells become more marked and an increasing proportion of the cells displays a markedly altered phenotype (Fig. 4). At 20 ng/ml the effects of aFGF are similar in extent and kind to those observed at 4 ng/ml. Even at 0.03 ng/ml aFGF causes the appearance of some clusters of rounded cell.

Figure 5 shows that aFGF (20 ng/ml) did not enhance or suppress the proliferation of ZR-75-1-Tx cells over a 3-day period. In a series of nine experiments in which treatment with aFGF (20 ng/ml) was for 2 days, the mean ratio of total cell yields, aFGF/Control was 0.95 ± 0.15.

An evaluation of the extent of cell rounding seen in photomicrographs of cultures of ZR-75-1-Tx cells (e.g., Fig. 4C) relative to detachment of cells determined by enumeration (e.g., Fig. 5)

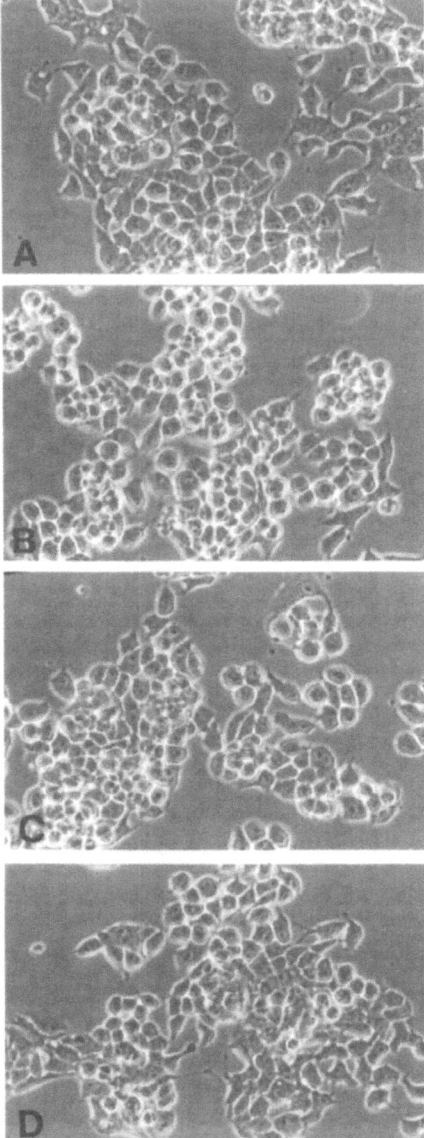

Figure 4. Rounding of ZR-75-1-Tx cells as a function of aFGF concentration. Cultures were photographed 2 days after the beginning of treatment. Two cultures were used per variable. (A) Control with heparin (10 μg/ml), which was also present in B–E; (B) aFGF (20 ng/ml); (C) aFGF (4 ng/ml); (D) aFGF (0.8 ng/ml); (E) aFGF (0.16 ng/ml). Final magnification ×164.

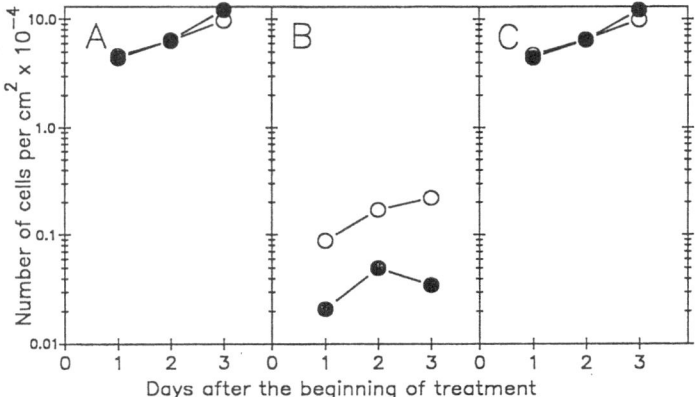

Figure 5. aFGF does not affect the proliferation rate of ZR-75-1-Tx cells. Nonadherent and adherent cells were enumerated in a hemocytometer. Three cultures were used per variable. (A) Adherent cells; (B) Non-adherent cells; (C) Total. Control ●—●; aFGF (20 ng/ml) ○—○.

indicates that the nonadherent cells in aFGF treated cultures represent only a very small fraction of the cells that have rounded. A direct comparison in seven experiments of the cell-detaching activity of IL-6 and aFGF at the maximally effective concentrations of each (5 and 20 ng/ml, respectively) showed that on the average, IL-6 is capable of exerting a 3 to 7-fold greater effect than aFGF after 2 days of treatment.

Presence of heparin was essential for aFGF activity [22]. In ZR-75-1-Tx cells 10 µg/ml of heparin was sufficient to obtain maximal effectiveness of aFGF. Heparin did not *per se* alter the morphological characteristics of ZR-75-1-Tx cells, nor did it affect the antimorphogenetic action of IL-6.

Cooperative interaction of IL-6 and aFGF

Interaction of IL-6 and aFGF occurred at maximally effective concentrations of each as well as at lower concentrations. IL-6 at 5 ng/ml caused marked cell rounding and cell-cell separation, with only patches of epithelioid cells remaining (Fig. 6B). Some fibroblastoid cells are also present. After treatment with aFGF (20 ng/ml) the majority of the cells are morphologically altered, but large cellular aggregates persist (Fig. 6C). Cells are round, ovoid, cuboidal, elongated or angular in shape. Some singlets are also present. The combination of aFGF + IL-6 caused very marked cell rounding with many spherical singlets in evidence and some elongated fibroblastoid cells; only a few epithelioid cells remained in the culture (Fig. 6D). Thus, although IL-6 at 5 ng/ml is

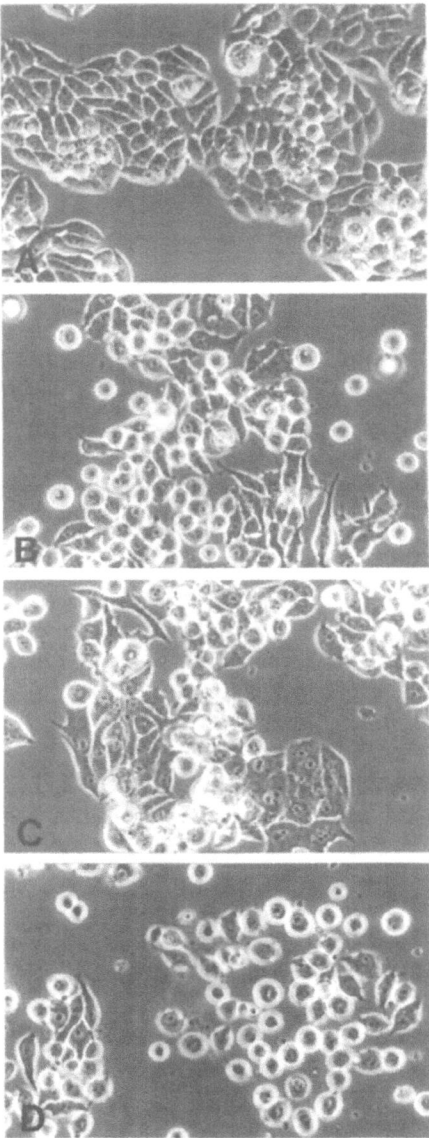

Figure 6. Extensive cell-cell separation and cell rounding in ZR-75-1-Tx cultures treated with IL-6 + aFGF. ZR-75-1-Tx cells were incubated for 3 days before medium change and beginning of treatment. The cultures were photographed 2 days after the beginning of treatment. Two cultures were used per variable. (A) Control; (B) IL-6 (5 ng/ml); (C) aFGF, (20 ng/ml); (D) IL-6 (5 ng/ml) + aFGF (20 ng/ml). Final magnification ×164.

markedly antimorphogenetic, an even greater effect is obtained when both IL-6, and aFGF (20 ng/ml) are present. This is further demonstrated by cell enumeration (Tab. 2, Experiment A). The size of the fraction of nonadherent cells in cultures treated with both IL-6 and aFGF (32.7%) is 2.3 times greater than the arithmetic sum of these fractions (14%) in cultures treated with IL-6 or aFGF alone. All nonadherent cells were viable. Table 2, Experiment B shows results obtained with aFGF at 4 ng/ml. The nonadherent cell fraction in IL-6 + aFGF treated cultures was 2 times greater than the arithmetic sum of these fractions in groups treated with each cytokine alone.

Colony formation assays show (Tab. 3) that nonadherent cells from ZR-75-1-Tx cell cultures that had been treated with IL-6 or aFGF alone or with the combination of IL-6 and aFGF are capable of forming colonies, albeit possibly to varying degrees. It should be emphasized that except for occasional dead cells scattered among the different groups, the nonadherent cells were viable by erythrosin B exclusion. Detached cells from IL-6 treated cultures appear to have a somewhat higher plating efficiency than cells from control cultures, whereas cells from aFGF treated cultures may have a somewhat lower plating efficiency. Furthermore, combining IL-6 and aFGF treatments results in clear suppression of plating efficiency. As for the low (12%) plating efficiency of the detached control ZR-75-1-Tx cells, it is of interest that the plating efficiency of the Ro subline of ZR-75-1 cells [11] used in earlier studies was also low (12%) [7]. For comparison, the plating efficiency of the T-47D line of ductal breast carcinoma cells was 36% [7].

In another colony assay using samples of nonadherent ZR-75-1-Tx cells from Experiment A, Table 2, the medium was replaced with fresh medium after 3 days of incubation of colony assay

Table 2. Cooperative interaction of IL-6 and aFGF in causing detachment of ZR-75-1-Tx cells

Exp.	Group	Number of cells per cm$^2 \times 10^{-4}$			
		Adherent	Nonadherent	Total	Nonadherent, % Total
A	Control	2.9	0	2.90	0
	IL-6, 5 ng/ml	2.4	0.310	2.71	11.4
	aFGF, 20 ng/ml	3.1	0.083	3.18	2.6
	IL-6, 5 ng/ml + aFGF, 20 ng/ml	2.0	0.960	2.94	32.7
B	Control	4.5	0.02	4.49	0.45
	IL-6, 5 ng/ml	3.4	0.46	3.86	12.0
	aFGF, 4 ng/ml	4.6	0.22	4.83	4.6
	IL-6, 5 ng/ml + aFGF, 4 ng/ml	3.6	1.85	5.45	33.9

ZR-75-1-Tx cells were seeded in 75 cm^2 flasks at a density of 2×10^4 cells/cm^2. In Experiment A, four flasks each were used for control or aFGF-treated cultures and two flasks for IL-6 or IL-6 + aFGF-treated cultures. After incubation for 1 day the medium was changed and the cultures treated for 2 days. Nonadherent and adherent cells were counted in a hemocytometer. The nonadherent cells in the pooled supernatants were collected by centrifugation. In Experiment B, two flasks each were used for control and IL-6 treated cultures and one flask each for aFGF or IL-6 + aFGF treated cultures.

Table 3. Colony-forming efficiency of cytokine-treated ZR-75-1-Tx cells

Cytokine	Number of colonies±S.D.	Colony-forming efficiency, %
Control	47±8.9	12
IL-6, ng/ml	65±13	16
aFGF, 4 ng/ml	39±6.7	9.8
IL-6, 5 ng/ml + aFGF, 4 ng/ml	28±12	7

The nonadherent cells are from the same experiment as in Table 2, Experiment B. Six-well plates were seeded with 400 cells/well in 2 ml of control medium, three wells per variable except six wells were seeded with IL-6 treated cells. The plates were incubated for 12 days and stained with DiffQuik. Groups of 10 or more cells were counted as colonies.

plates. Under these conditions, an average of 3 times more colonies formed. However, in terms of the number of colonies formed, the relative order was similar, i.e., IL-6 > aFGF > IL-6 + aFGF. These results show that aFGF induced phenotypic changes are reversible and that a significant fraction of the many cells that detach in response to the combined action of IL-6 and aFGF reattaches and continues to proliferate when the cytokines are removed.

Lack of effect of TGF-α, TGF-β_1, bFGF, KGF, EGF, and IGF-1 on ZR-75-1-Tx cell morphology

The following growth factors, used at the stated concentrations, caused little detectable cell disjunction or rounding: TGF-α (25 to 100 µg/ml); TGF-β_1 (2 to 50 ng/ml); bFGF (30 to 90 ng/ml); keratinocyte growth factor (KGF) (1 to 100 ng/ml); EGF (12 to 75 ng/ml); and IGF-1 (12 to 75 ng/ml).

Inhibition of IL-6 and aFGF effects by inhibitors of protein tyrosine kinases and protein kinase C (PKC)

Figure 7 shows that the protein tyrosine kinase (PTK) inhibitor herbimycin, when used at a concentration of 0.15 µM, partially suppressed either IL-6 or aFGF induced disjunction and rounding of ZR-75-1-Tx cells (Fig. 7, B vs E and C vs F, respectively). The very marked antimorphogenetic effect of combined treatment with IL-6 and aFGF was also suppressed by herbimycin (20 µM). Genistein, a second PTK inhibitor, had only borderline effects in the concentration range from 30 to 100 µM when used against IL-6, aFGF, or IL-6 + aFGF. Tyrphostin A23 at concentrations up to 10 µM had minimal inhibitory effects on IL-6 induced cell rounding and did not suppress aFGF induced cell rounding.

Staurosporine is a protein kinase inhibitor with some selectivity for PKC and PTK when used at low concentration [23, 24]. Figure 8 shows that 10 nM staurosporine inhibited IL-6 or aFGF

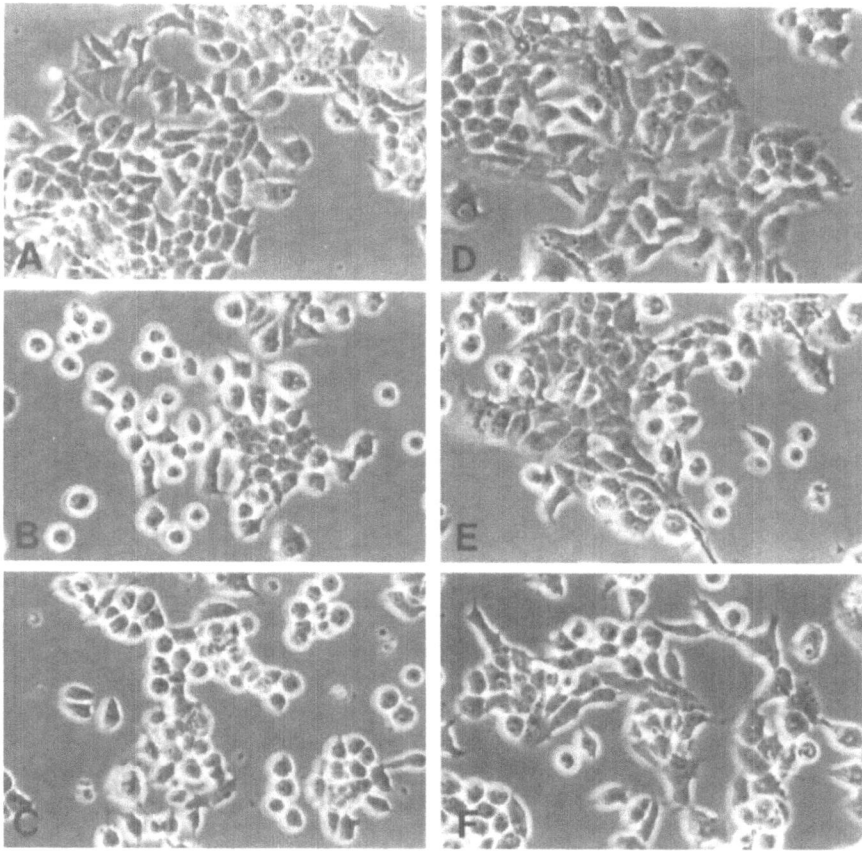

Figure 7. Inhibition of IL-6, aFGF- or aFGF + IL-6 induced cell rounding by herbimycin. ZR-75-1-Tx cells were seeded at a density of 2×10^4 cells/ cm^2 in 6-well plates in 2 ml of growth medium. The following day the medium was changed and treatment begun. Two days later cultures were photographed. (A) Control; (B) IL-6 (5 ng/ml); (C) aFGF (20 ng/ml); (D) Herbimycin (0.15 μM); (E) IL-6 (5 ng/ml) + herbimycin (0.15 μM); and (F) aFGF (20 ng/ml) + herbimycin (0.15 μM). Final magnification ×164.

induced cell rounding. Staurosporine also inhibited the massive cell rounding induced by combined treatment with IL-6 (5 ng/ml) and aFGF (20 ng/ml).

Chelerythrine, a selective PKC inhibitor used at concentrations up to 1 μM showed only borderline effects on IL-6 or aFGF induced cell rounding.

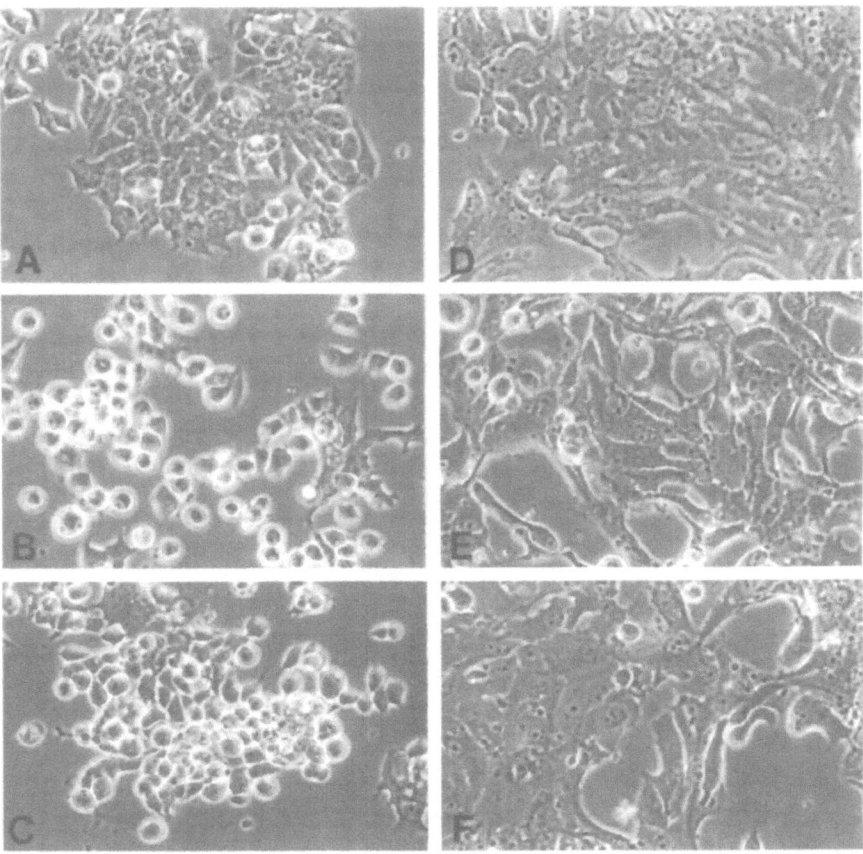

Figure 8. Inhibition of IL-6 or aFGF induced rounding of ZR-75-1-Tx cells by staurosporine. The cultures were photographed 3 days after the beginning of treatment. Two cultures were used per variable. (A) Control; (B) IL-6 (5 ng/ml); (C) aFGF (20 ng/ml); (D) Staurosporine (10 nM); (E) IL-6 (5 ng/ml) + staurosporine (10 nM); (F) aFGF (20 ng/ml) + staurosporine (10 nM). Final magnification: ×164.

Protein kinase C activation by TPA by itself causes little rounding or detachment of ZR-75-1-Tx cells, but it enhances IL-6 actions

The predominant morphologic effect of 12-o-tetradecanoyl phorbol-13-acetate (TPA) (5 nM) is to cause flattening of ZR-75-1-Tx cells (compare Fig. 9, A and E) although rare rounded cells are also present. TPA, however, increases IL-6 induced (5 ng/ml) rounding of ZR-75-1-Tx cells (compare Fig. 9, B and F).

Enumeration of adherent and nonadherent cells showed (see Tab. 4) that whereas TPA (5 nM) caused only a 2.6-fold increase, IL-6 (5 ng/ml) caused a 37-fold increase in the percentage of nonadherent cells after 3 days of treatment. The combination of IL-6 and TPA caused a 52-fold increase. It can also be seen in Table 4 that after 3-day treatment the total number of cells was

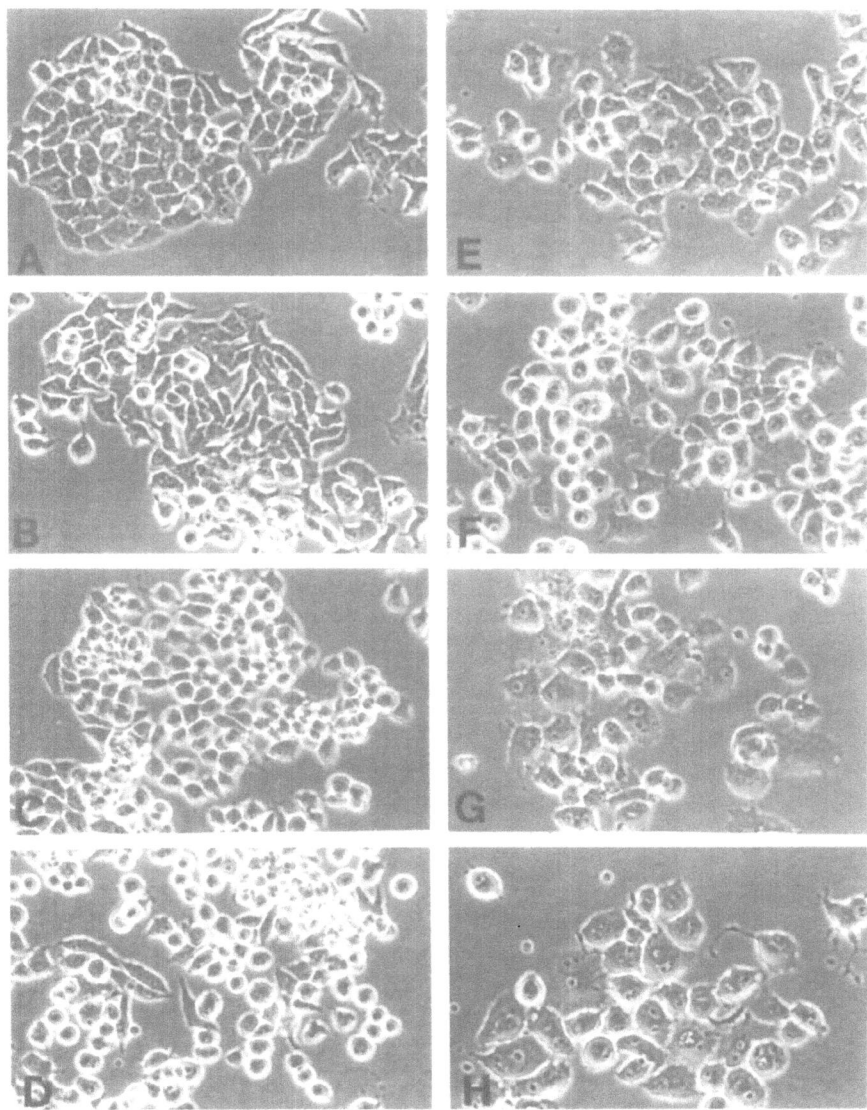

Figure 9. TPA inhibits aFGF-induced ZR-75-1-Tx cell rounding while producing a distinct phenotype. The cultures were photographed 2 days after the beginning of treatment. A-D on left (no TPA) are controls for E-H on right (TPA present in all). (A) No additions; (B) IL-6 (0.2 ng/ml); (C) aFGF (20 ng/ml); (D) IL-6 (0.2 ng/ml) + aFGF (20 ng/ml); (E) TPA (5 nM); (F) TPA (5 nM) + IL-6 (0.2 ng/ml); (G) TPA (5 nM) + aFGF (20 ng/ml); (H) TPA (5 nM) + aFGF (20 ng/ml) + IL-6 (0.2 ng/ml). Final magnification: ×164.

Table 4. TPA by itself causes little detachment of ZR-75-1-Tx cells

Group	Number of cells per $cm^2 \times 10^{-4}$			
	Adherent	Nonadherent	Total	Nonadherent, % of total $\pm$ S.D.
Control	21.4	0.07	21.5	0.33±0.095
IL-6, 5 ng/ml	22.1	3.04	22.1	12.10±0.734
TPA, 5 nM	23.6	0.20	23.8	0.87±0.206
IL-6, 5 ng/ml + TPA, 5 nM	19.1	3.84	22.9	17.26±4.30

ZR-75-1-Tx cells were seeded in 75 cm^2 flasks at a density of 4×10^4 cells/cm^2 in 12 ml of medium (0.16 ml/cm^2). Three flasks were used per variable. After incubation for 3 days, the medium was changed and the cultures were treated as indicated for 2 days. Nonadherent and adherent cells were counted in a hemocytometer.

similar in control, IL-6, TPA, and IL-6 + TPA groups, indicating that ZR-75-1-Tx cell proliferation was not affected by the treatments. In contrast, the proliferation of the ZR-75-1-Ro subline cells was suppressed by IL-6 [7], but enhanced by TPA [9]. Thus, the Ro and Tx sublines of ZR-75-1 cell differ both in cell adhesiveness and cell growth parameters.

Protein kinase C activation by TPA causes enlargement and inhibits detachment of ZR-75-1-Tx cells treated with aFGF alone or with aFGF + IL-6

The interaction of TPA with aFGF or aFGF + IL-6 differs strikingly from its interaction with IL-6. In Figure 9 the controls for TPA (cf. A-D on the left) illustrate the distinctive cellular phenotypes produced by IL-6 (0.2 ng/ml) (B) and aFGF (20 ng/ml) (C), and the marked enhancement of the IL-6 induced phenotype by aFGF (D).

Figure 9 (F) documents further the considerable enhancement of the IL-6 induced phenotype by TPA (5 nM). In contrast, TPA blocks the morphological changes induced by aFGF or by aFGF + IL-6, and in both cases produces a new phenotype characterized by marked cellular flattening and enlargement and presence of processes. The results suggest that TPA interacts negatively with aFGF but in a complex way (compare Figs 9D and H).

Table 5 shows that TPA inhibits detachment of ZR-75-1-Tx cells treated with IL-6 + aFGF. In addition, the results are consistent with microscopic observations showing fewer cells in cultures exposed to IL-6 + aFGF + TPA and presence of debris, some of which may represent fragments of cellular processes. Overall, the antagonism between TPA and aFGF is reminiscent of the antagonism between phorbol esters and EGF in breast cancer cells [25].

Table 5. TPA inhibits detachment of ZR-75-1-Tx cells treated with a combination of IL-6 and aFGF

Group	Number of cells per $cm^2 \times 10^{-4}$			
	Adherent	Non-adherent	Total	Non-adherent, % of Total±S.D.
Control	7.11	0.04	7.2	0.6±
IL-6, 0.2 ng/ml	5.33	0.27	5.6	4.8±
IL-6, 0.2 ng/ml +aFGF, 20 ng/ml	6.81	0.73	7.5	9.7±
IL-6, 0.2 ng/ml + TPA, 5 nM	5.65	0.37	6.0	6.2±
IL-6, 0.2 ng/ml + aFGF, 20 ng/ml + TPA, 5 nM	3.47	0.05	3.5	1.3±

ZR-75-1-Tx cells were seeded in 75 cm^2 flasks at a density of 2×10^4 cells/cm^2 in 10 ml of medium (0.12 ml/cm^2). Two flasks were used per variable. After incubation for 1 day, the medium was changed and the cultures were treated as indicated for 2 days. Nonadherent and adherent cells were counted in a hemocytometer.

TPA-induced cytoskeletal changes increases focal adhesions and actin fibers

As striking morphological or adhesive changes are produced in ZR-75-1-Tx cells by various combinations of IL-6, aFGF or TPA, these agents produce commensurate alterations in cell-substratum adhesions and cytoskeleton architecture. Figure 10 displays micrographs of cell-substratum contacts in living ZR-75-1-Tx cells and in these cells treated with IL-6 or TPA as visualized by interference reflection microscopy [26, 27]. In control cultures (Fig. 10A), cell-substrate adhesions appeared as dark-colored streaks or smaller round puncta, distributed over the entire ventral cell surface. IL-6 treated cells showed reduced numbers of streak-like adhesions and small, round punctate adhesions predominated (Fig. 10B). In contrast, cells treated with TPA displayed a remarkable increase in streak-like focal adhesions and in most cells there was also a spatial reorganization of focal adhesions to the peripheral cytoplasmic edge (Fig. 10C).

To gain further insight into the nature of focal adhesion and cytoskeletal reorganizations in cytokine or TPA treated ZR-75-1-Tx cells, interference reflection microscopy on fixed cells was combined with fluorescence visualization of the F-actin cytoskeleton and cellular phosphotyrosine (Figs 11 and 12). Paired micrographs of cell-substratum adhesions and the F-actin cytoskeleton in control or treated ZR-75-1-Tx cells are shown in Figure 11. Control cells contained few, if any, well-formed F-actin stress fibers (Figs 11A and 12A), with F-actin organized in the cortical cytoplasm at the cell periphery or diffusely present throughout the ventral cell surface (in contact with the substratum). Control cells displayed a number of small, dark colored punctate adhesions (focal adhesions) or more diffuse areas of grey colored adhesions (close contacts) (Fig. 11A'). In cells treated with low concentrations of IL-6, a diffuse F-actin cytoskeleton and small, punctate focal adhesions were observed. A remarkable change in the F-actin cytoskeleton

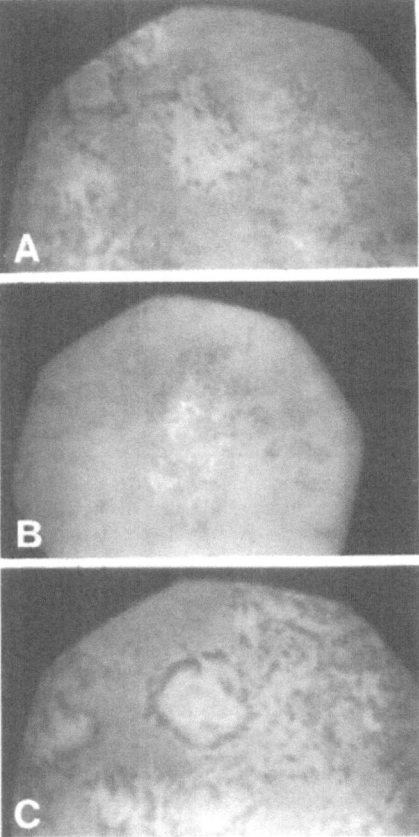

Figure 10. Cell-substratum adhesions in living ZR-75-1-Tx cells as viewed by interference-reflection microscopy. (A) Control, (B) IL-6 (0.2 ng/ml), (C) TPA (5 nM). Magnification approx. ×1500 for all micrographs.

was brought about by addition of TPA to these cells, either alone or in the combination IL-6/aFGF. As illustrated in Figures 11C/C', TPA treated ZR-75-1-Tx cells developed numerous F-actin containing stress fibers that also terminated in long, streak-like focal adhesions. The size of TPA-treated cells was also much larger than those in control or IL-6 treated cultures. The inclusion of aFGF or IL-6 with TPA did not alter the remarkable effect of TPA on formation of actin stress fibers and increased number of focal adhesions (Figs 11D/D').

Figure 12 displays micrographs of F-actin organization and phosphotyrosine localization in control or TPA/cytokine treated cells. Control cultures displayed a number of small phospho-tyrosine-containing puncta in the ventral cell surface (Fig. 12A'), corresponding to punctate-adhesions visualized by interference-reflection microscopy. In cells treated with TPA as a single agent, or in combination with aFGF/IL-6, a large increase in the number/size of phosphotyrosine-containing adhesions (Fig. 12B') was evident and most phosphotyrosine streaks colocalized with

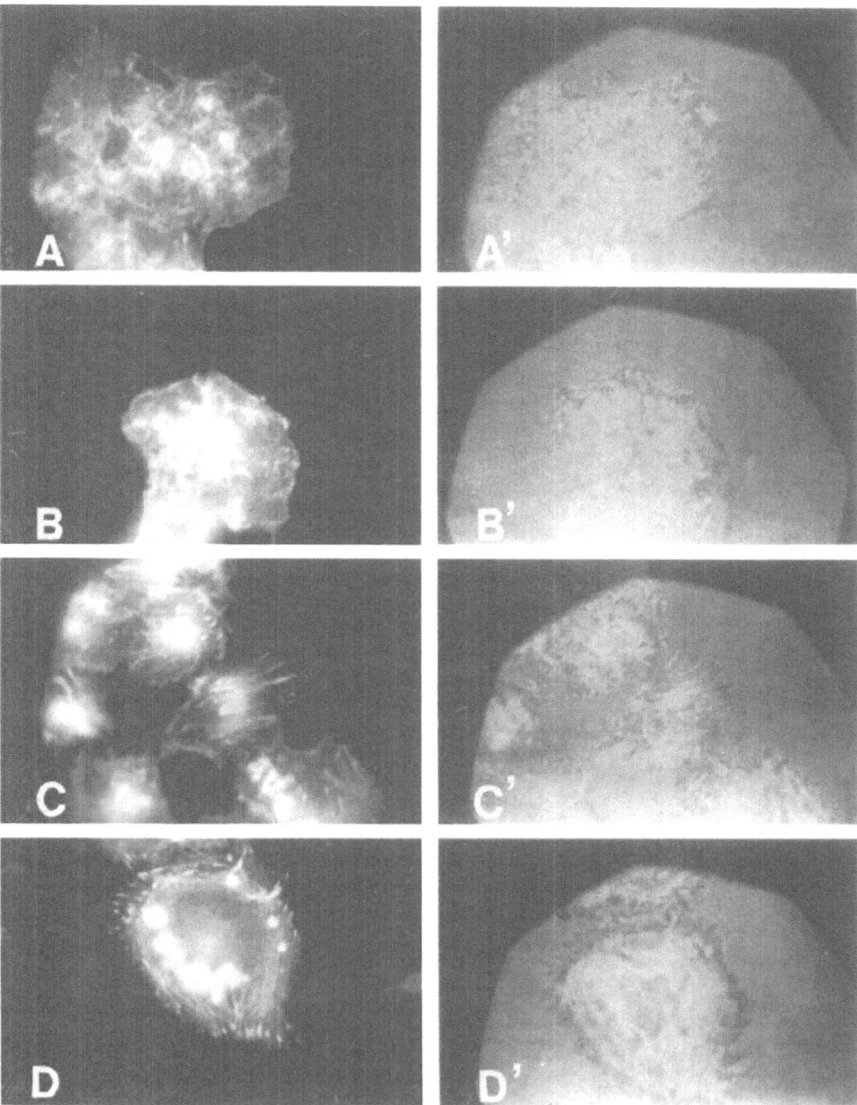

Figure 11. Colocalization of cell-substratum adhesions and the F-actin cytoskeleton in fixed ZR-75-1-Tx cells. (A) Control, (B) IL-6 (0.2 ng/ml), (C) TPA (5 nM), (D) TPA (5 nM) + IL-6 (0.2 ng/ml) + aFGF (20 ng/ml). Micrographs depicting the F-actin cytoskeleton (A-D) are paired with interference-reflection micrographs from the same cells (A'-D'). Magnification approx. ×1500 for all micrographs.

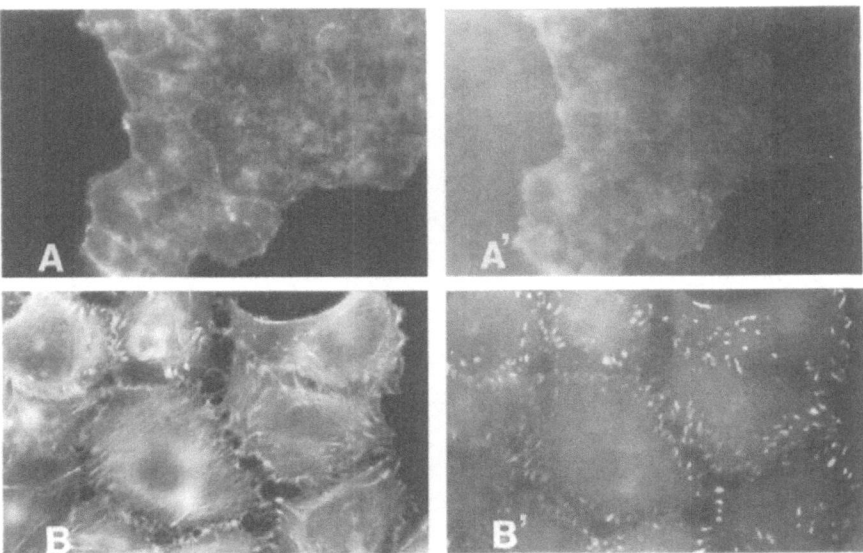

Figure 12. Colocalization of F-actin and phosphotyrosine in ZR-75-1-Tx cells. (A) Control, (B) aFGF (20 ng/ml) + TPAX (5 nM). The F-actin cytoskeleton is depicted in A,B; while phosphotyrosine localization in the same cells is depicted in A', B'. Magnification approx. × 1500 for all micrographs.

termini of actin stress fibers (Fig. 12B). The effect of TPA to increase cell size, induce formation of F-actin stress fibers, and increase phosphotyrosine-containing focal adhesions was the predominant phenotype irrespective of inclusion aFGF or IL-6.

Cytokines in breast cancer metastasis: A model

The special interest of the cell adhesion disruptive actions of IL-6 and aFGF in human ductal breast carcinoma cells arises from the fact that infiltrating carcinomas of this type are characterized by disordered cell adherence [13]. We must consider that in the dyshesion observed in these tumors disjunction-inducing cytokines or growth factors such as IL-6 and aFGF may play a role, but that their action is conditioned on the genetic make-up of the cells.

Based on available information (reviewed in [2]) it is reasonable to assume that cell lines derived from metastatic lesions of human ductal breast carcinomas initially comprise multiple genetic variants. Upon culture further variants probably arise. Striking phenotypic differences among human ductal breast carcinoma ZR-75-1 cell sublines from different laboratories and from the American Type Culture Collection have been previously reported [11]. The subline of ZR-75-1 cells maintained in C.K. Osborne's laboratory [25] permitted detection of a novel form of dyshesion-inducing activity of IL-6 [11]. When exposed to IL-6 these cells, designated the Tx subline, were found to lose junctions both to neighbors and the substratum and to round up.

ZR-75-1-Tx cells treated with aFGF also undergo morphological changes, but these are different from those induced by IL-6. Although aFGF, like IL-6, causes ZR-75-1-Tx cells to lose their epithelioid phenotype without becoming fibroblastoid, the rounding caused by aFGF is less complete than that caused by IL-6. Morphologically altered aFGF-treated cells tend to remain in clusters as compared to the morphologically altered IL-6 treated cells that disperse more extensively. The cell detachment response is about 3 times greater with IL-6 than with aFGF when each is used at the maximally effective concentration.

Of special interest is the finding of cooperative interaction between aFGF and IL-6. aFGF, even at very low concentrations such as 0.016 ng/ml, increases IL-6 induced disruption of cell adhesion. With aFGF present, very low concentrations of IL-6 are sufficient to cause marked antimorphogenetic effects. These findings are consistent with the fact that IL-6 and aFGF belong to two different families of cytokines/growth factors and differ in signal transduction pathways they use. The precise mechanism underlying the cooperative interaction remains to be clarified.

Cytokine-induced tyrosine phosphorylation

In view of the role of protein tyrosine kinases in the transduction of IL-6 or aFGF signals it would be expected that appropriate inhibitors selective for such enzymes would suppress IL-6 or aFGF induced cell rounding and detachment. The findings with PTK inhibitors that IL-6 or aFGF induced cell rounding can be partially suppressed by 0.15 μM herbimycin are consistent with this expectation. Herbimycin (0.20 μM) had a marked inhibitory effect on the extensive cell rounding induced by combined treatment with IL-6 and aFGF. Genistein (56 or 100 μM) had only a slight inhibitory effect on cell rounding induced by IL-6, aFGF, or IL-6 + aFGF. The selective PKC inhibitor chelerythrine, used at concentrations up to 1 μM, only showed a borderline inhibitory effect. However, 10 to 15 nM staurosporine had a marked inhibitory effect on IL-6 or aFGF induced cell rounding. The effectiveness of staurosporine in this experimental system probably relates primarily to its ability to inhibit PTK.

It will be important to determine the respective mediating roles of the JAK-TYK kinases used by IL-6 receptors, and of the FGF receptor kinases and the nature of effector molecules and their targets in breast carcinoma cells. Recently 25 different protein kinases were isolated from breast carcinoma cells using PCR cloning techniques based on consensus sequences in the kinase domain [28]. These included three novel putative tyrosine kinases and two cell cycle associated serine/threonine kinases. Analysis of the levels of expression of all of these kinases in a panel of human breast carcinomas revealed different expression profiles in different primary breast carcinomas [28]. Identification of the specific targets for tyrosine kinase function will be important for the understanding of the respective mechanisms of action of IL-6 and aFGF in breast carcinoma cells.

Modulation of cancer cell phenotypes and metastatic behaviour

Present evidence suggests that aFGF can modulate cellular morphology, migration, adhesion, and ultimately, metastatic potential in some types of carcinoma cells. Exogenous aFGF induces cell dispersion and epithelial to mesenchymal transformation of rat NBT-II bladder carcinoma cells in subconfluent cultures [29–32]. Increased autocrine production of aFGF in these cells, using human aFGF expression vector constructs, produces similar effects on cellular behaviour, independent of aFGF secretion into medium [33]. Thus aFGF might serve as a critical cytokine, altering behaviour of cancer cells, whether supplied as an exogenous ligand (e.g., from paracrine production by other cells), or by increased endogenous production. However, not all NBT-II clones are sensitive to the effect of aFGF, which provides at least one explanation for the heterogeneous behaviour of particular cell clones in tumors. Although the mechanisms through which aFGF modifies the behaviour of NBT-II cells are not fully known, it is clear that increased aFGF production can confer increased tumorigenicity or more rapid development of metastases in NBT-II cell-derived tumors in experimental models [33, 34]. Similar results have been obtained with aFGF in the partially transformed Rat-1 cells [35]. Important cellular effects of aFGF that could accelerate tumor invasiveness or metastasis could be (a) coupled disruption of intercellular cohesion and increased cellular migration and (b) induction of anchorage-independent growth, as observed in SV40-transformed kidney epithelial cells [36].

In the ZR-75-1-Tx line of human breast cancer epithelial cells, aFGF clearly has effects on both intercellular cohesion of tumor cells and on substratum-dependent proliferation (Fig. 13). Acquisition of cellular dyshesion is a cardinal sign of benign to malignant progression of ductal tumors in humans [13] and the ability of the cells to proliferate without attachment to basement membranes (analogous to substratum-independent proliferation) could be important for lymphatic metastasis, which is characteristic for breast carcinomas. Although aFGF has been previously identified as a likely progression factor for tumor cell growth and metastatic conversion in other types of epithelial cells, our studies indicate that, in ZR-75-1-Tx cells, IL-6 is even more potent than aFGF in producing antimorphogenetic effects. In particular, the cooperative interaction between IL-6 and aFGF in producing antimorphogenetic effects provides a means by which very low concentrations of exogenously or endogenously supplied cytokines can reversibly modify cellular properties related to particular cancer phenotypes. The distinct responsiveness of different ZR-75-1 cell populations (Ro vs Tx lines) to IL-6 and aFGF [7, 9, 11, 12] also provides insight as to how cellular variability could favor different mechanisms of tumor spread. Depending on acquisition of particular mutations, different cells within a tumor might be stimulated towards increased local invasiveness (migration) or increased distant metastasis (loss of substratum requirement for growth) in response to variably produced tissue-derived cytokines such as IL-6 and aFGF (Fig. 13).

The potential contributions of IL-6, aFGF, and PKC activation to the biology of ductal breast carcinoma are diagrammed in Figure 13. This model proposes that both genetic and epigenetic factors contribute to the range and type of cellular alterations in the carcinoma. A cardinal feature of intraductal breast carcinoma is loss of cohesion between adjacent ductal epithelial cells such that detached or loosely adherent epithelial cells appear in the lumen of duct carcinomas. The dyshesion of carcinoma cells is readily evident in cytological smears prepared from direct biopsy

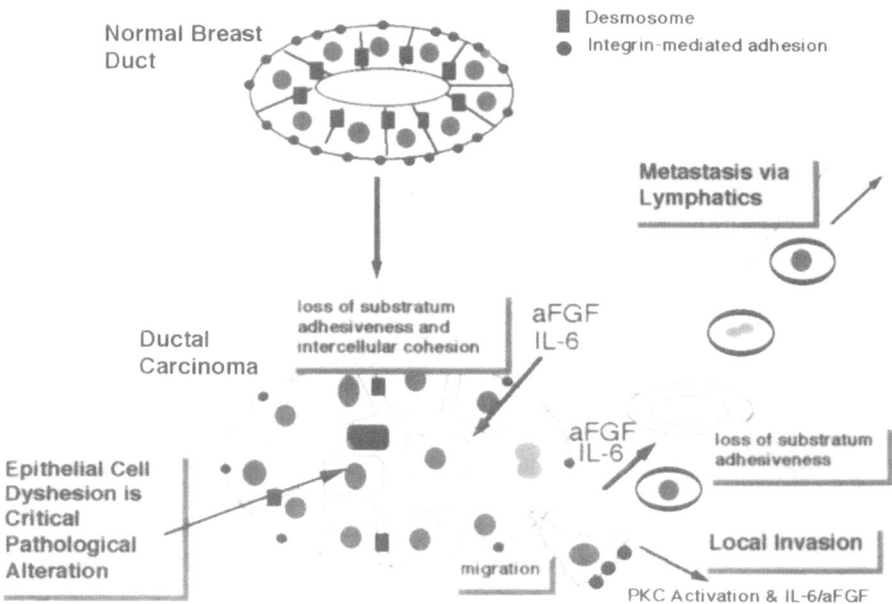

Figure 13. Model for cytokine-induced effects on invasiveness and metastasis of breast carcinoma cells. Please refer to text for detailed description.

specimens and is, in fact, one of the most important alterations that distinguishes normal ductal epithelial cells from their cancerous counterparts [13]. Following *in situ* transformation to ductal carcinoma, malignant ductal carcinomas are characterized by either local invasiveness (particularly as typified by scirrhous carcinomas) or distant metastasis *via* lymphatics. Specifically, the cell rounding and (reversible) detachment produced by IL-6, aFGF, or a synergistic combination of these two cytokines, could alter adhesiveness of ductal carcinomas so as to produce detached, free-floating cells that could easily traverse lymphatics and, at distant sites with reduced cytokine levels, could then reattach and set up a metastatic tumor focus. Continued proliferation of completely detached ductal carcinoma cells at distant sites might be the basis of malignant effusions within pleural or peritoneal spaces. In contrast, the PKC activation by other pathways might enhance the development of actin-based contractile systems and enhanced binding of cells to extracellular matrix (*via* integrin-focal adhesion complexes) that would promote local tumor invasiveness. Hence, localized exposure of genetically altered tumor cells to distinct cytokines could directly alter the type and extent of malignant behaviour of ductal carcinoma cells.

References

1. Varmus H, Weinberg RA (1992) Genes and the Biology of Cancer. Scientific American Library, New York, NY.
2. Leslie KO, Howard P (1992) Oncogenes and antioncogenes in human breast carcinoma. *Pathol Ann* 27: 321–342.
3. Walker RA, Varley JM (1993) The molecular pathology of human breast cancer. *Cancer Surv* 16: 31–57.
4. Stoker M, Gherardi E (1991) Regulation of cell movement: the mitogenic cytokines. *Biochim Biophys Acta* 1072: 81–102.
5. Aaronson SA (1991) Growth factors and cancer. *Science* 254: 1146–1153.
6. Dickson RB, Johnson MD, El-Ashry D, Shi YE, Bano M, Zugmaier G, Ziff D, Lippman ME, Chrysogelos S (1993) Breast cancer: influence of endocrine hormones, growth factors and genetic alterations. *In*: SS Yang, HR Warner (eds). *The underlying molecular, cellular and immunological factors in cancer and aging*. New Youk, Plenum Press, 119–141.
7. Tamm I, Cardinale I, Krueger J, Murphy JS, May LT, Sehgal PB (1989) Interleukin-6 decreases cell-cell association and increases motility of ductal breast carcinoma cells. *J Exp Med* 170: 1649–1669.
8. Chen L, Shulman LM, Revel M (1991) IL-6 receptors and sensitivity to growth inhibition by IL-6 in clones of human breast carcinoma cells. *J Biol Regulat Homeost Agent* 5: 125–136.
9. Tamm I, Cardinale I, Sehgal PB (1991) Interleukin-6 and 12-*O*-tetradecanoyl phorbol-13-acetate act synergistically in inducing cell-cell separation and migration of human breast carcinoma cells. *Cytokine* 3: 212–223.
10. Tamm I, Cardinale I, Murphy JS (1991) Decreased adherence of interleukin-6-treated breast carcinoma cells can lead to separation from neighbors after mitosis. *Proc Natl Acad Sci USA* 88: 4414–4418.
11. Tamm I, Kikuchi T, Cardinale I, Krueger JG (1994a) Cell adhesion-disrupting action of interleukin-6 in human ductal breast carcinoma cells. *Proc Natl Acad Sci USA* 91: 3329–3333.
12. Tamm I, Cardinale I, Kikuchi T, Krueger JG (1994b) E-cadherin distribution in interleukin-6-induced cell-cell separation of ductal breast carcinoma cells. *Proc Natl Acad Sci USA* 91: 4338–4342.
13. Kline TS, Kline IK (1989) Common Breast Carcinomas. *In*: TS Kline and IK Kline: *Breast: Guides to Clinical Aspiration Biopsy*. Igaku-Shoin, New York, pp 85–119.
14. Jaye M, Schlesinger J, Dionne CA (1992) Fibroblast growth factor receptor tyrosine kinases: molecular analysis and signal transduction. *Biochim Biophys Acta* 1135: 185–199.
15. Basilico C, Moscatelli D (1992) The FGF family of growth factors and oncogenes. *Adv Cancer Res* 59: 115–165.
16. Johnson DE, Williams LT (1993) Structural and functional diversity in the FGF receptor multigene family. *Adv Cancer Res* 60: 1–41.
17. Tsuda T, Kaibuchi K, Kawahara Y, Fukuzaki H, Takai Y (1985) Induction of protein kinase C activation and Ca^{2+} mobilization by fibroblast growth factor in Swiss 3T3 cells. *FEBS Lett* 191: 205–210.
18. Kaibuchi K, Tsuda T, Kikuchi A, Tanimoto T, Yamashita T, Takai Y (1986) Possible involvement of protein kinase C and calcium ion growth factor-induced expression of c-*myc* oncogene in Swiss 3T3 fibroblasts. *J Biol Chem* 261: 1187–1192.
19. Magnaldo I, L'Allemain G, Chambard JC, Moenner M, Barritault D, Pouyssegur J (1986) The mitogenic signaling pathway of fibroblast growth factor is not mediated through polyphosphoinositide hydrolysis and protein kinase C activation in hamster fibroblasts. *J Biol Chem* 261: 16916–16922.
20. Malcolm W, Cantley L (1988) Phosphoinositide metabolism and the control of cell proliferation. *Biochim Biophys Acta* 948: 327–344.
21. Rhee SG, Suh P-G, Ryu S-H, Lee SY (1989) Studies of inositol phospholipid-specific phospholipase C. *Science* 244: 546–550.
22. Gospodarowicz D, Chang J (1986) Heparin protects basic and acidic FGF from inactivation. *J Cell Physiol* 128: 475–484.
23. Tamaoki T, Nomoto H, Takahashi I, Kato Y, Morimoto M, Tomita T (1986) Staurosporine, a potent inhibitor of phospholipid/Ca^{++} dependent protein kinase. *Biochem Biophys Res Commun* 135: 397–402.
24. Jones KT, Sharpe GR (1994) Staurosporine, a non-specific PKC inhibitor, induces keratinocyte differentiation and raises intracellular calcium, but Ro31-8220, a specific inhibitor, does not. *J Cell Physiol* 159: 324–330.
25. Osborne CK, Hamilton B, Nover M, Ziegler J (1981) Antagonism between epidermal growth factor and phorbol ester tumor promoters in human breast cancer cells. *J Clin Invest* 67: 943–951.
26. Izzard CS, Lochner LR (1976) Formation of cell-to-substrate contacts during fibroblast motility: an interference-reflexion study. *J Cell Sci* 42: 81–116.
27. Tamm I, Kikuchi T, Krueger J, Murphy JS (1992) Dissociation between early loss of actin fibres and subsequent cell death in serum-deprived quiescent Balb/c-3T3 cells. *Cell Signal* 4: 675–686.
28. Cance WG, Craven RJ, Weiner TM, Liu ET (1993) Novel protein kinases expressed in human breast cancer. *Int J Cancer* 54: 571–577.

29. Boyer B, Tucker GC, Vallés AM, Franke WW, Thiery JP (1989) Rearrangements of desmosomal and cytoskeletal proteins during the transition from epithelial to fibroblastoid organization in cultured rat bladder carcinoma cells. *J Cell Biol* 109: 1495–1509.
30. Vallés AM, Boyer B, Badet J, Tucker D, Barritault D, Thiery JP (1990) Acidic growth factor is modulator of epithelial plasticity in a rat bladder carcinoma cell line. *Proc Natl Acad Sci USA* 87: 1124–1128.
31. Vallés AM, Tucker GC, Thiery J, Boyer B (1990) Alternative patterns of mitogenesis and cell scattering induced by acidic FGF as a function of cell density in a rat bladder carcinoma cell line. *Cell Regul* 1: 975–988.
32. Boyer B, Thiery JP (1993) Cyclic AMP distinguishes between two functions of aFGF in rat bladder carcinoma cell line. *J Cell Biol* 120: 767–776.
33. Jouanneau J, Gavrilovic J, Caruelle D, Jaye M, Moens G, Caruelle J-P, Thiery JP (1991) Secreted or non-secreted forms of acidic fibroblast growth factor produced by transfected epithelial cells influence cell morphology, motility, and invasive potential. *Proc Natl Acad Sci USA* 88: 2893–2897.
34. Jouanneau J, Moens G, Bourgeois Y, Poupon MF, Thiery JP (1994) A minority of carcinoma cells producing acidic fibroblast growth factor induces a community effect for tumor progression. *Proc Natl Acad Sci USA* 91: 286–290.
35. Takahashi JB, Hoshimaru M, Jaye M, Kikuchi H, Hatanaka M (1992) Possible activity of acidic fibroblast growth factor as a progression factor rather than a transforming factor. *Biochem Biophys Res Commun* 189: 398–405.
36. Zhang G, Stevens JL (1991) Altered growth regulation of rat kidney proximal tubule epithelial cells transformed *in vitro* by SV40 viral DNA: fibroblast growth factors (heparin-binding growth factors) are potent inducers of anchorage-independent growth. *Mol Carcinogen* 4: 220–230.

Molecular Aspects of Cancer and its Therapy
A. Mackiewicz and P.B. Sehgal (eds)
© 1998 Birkhäuser Verlag Basel/Switzerland

Clinical relevance of genetic alterations in lung cancer

E. Jassem[1] and J. Jassem[2]

[1]Department of Pneumonology, Medical University of Gdansk, Debinki 7, PL-80-211 Gdansk, Poland
[2]Department of Oncology and Radiotherapy, Medical University of Gdansk, Debinki 7, PL-80-211 Gdansk, Poland

Introduction

Lung cancer is the most common human malignancy in the world and its incidence is increasing. Each year there are almost one million deaths due to lung cancer worldwide, accounting for 40% of all cancer deaths in men and 20% in women. Surgery remains the mainstay of lung cancer treatment. Detection of lung cancer, however, usually occurs late in the course of disease, and in most cases, by the time of presentation the tumour is not amenable to curative resection. Thus, the vast majority of patients are managed with radiation, chemotherapy or a combination of the two. Despite the continued refinement of radiotherapy techniques and progress in pharmacotherapy, in patients to whom these modalities are applied the 5-year survival rates are still only 5–10%.

Molecular studies within the last two decades clearly demonstrated that the majority of malignancies arise due to mutations in dominant and recessive oncogenes. Both small cell lung cancer (SCLC) and non-small cell lung cancer (NSCLC) are among the tumours with a particularly high rate of molecular abnormalities. It is hoped that increasing knowledge of these alterations will permit their use in clinical care and treatment. This review will address selected molecular changes in lung cancer with particular attention to their potential application in the clinic.

Molecular characteristics of lung cancer

Genetic susceptibility to lung cancer

The development of lung cancer is considered a multistep genetic process, initiated in the majority of cases by carcinogens present in cigarette smoke. Clinically apparent tumours are preceded by a series of morphological changes in the bronchial epithelium, including hyperplasia/metaplasia, mild, moderate and severe dysplasia, *carcinoma in situ* and invasion characterized by migration of cancer cells through the basal membrane.

Even the early phase of promotion of carcinogenesis is accompanied by genetic instability. Mutagens from cigarette smoke (e.g., polycyclic aromatic hydrocarbons and quinones) come into close contact with bronchial epithelium, interact with DNA and produce mutagenic DNA adducts [1, 2]. It was demonstrated in experimental systems that the level of adduct formation correlates with carcinogenicity of particular agents [3]. Normally, smoking-induced adducts are eliminated by the nucleotide excision repair pathway [4]. When this process is impaired, the transcription of essential genes may be altered by the accumulated adducts [5]. Most tobacco-related genotoxic agents require metabolic activation by enzymes of the cytochrome P450 superfamily (e.g., CYP1A1) before they interact with DNA. Other enzyme systems, including glutathione S-transferase M1 (GSTM1) as well as T1- and N-acetyltransferase, detoxify these carcinogenic metabolites [6]. The ability to activate *vs.* detoxify inhaled carcinogens varies substantially from individual to individual [7]. It is presumed that the balance between expression of enzymes involved in both processes may be associated with individual risk of lung cancer among smokers. For example, subjects with *CYP1A1* genotype combined with functional *GSTM1* are relatively resistant to tobacco-related lung cancers whereas those with a *CYP1A1* and *GTSM1*(-) combination are highly susceptible [8, 9].

Loss of heterozygosity (LOH)

The earliest cytogenetic changes accompanying carcinogenesis in the bronchial epithelium are deletions in chromosomes 3p, 9p and 17p [10]. LOH, the loss of one allele of the recessive tumour suppressor gene, is a marker of these deletions. One of the genes involved in this process has recently been identified as the *FHIT* gene (fragile histidine triad gene). This gene, deleted in the early stages of carcinogenesis, spans the FRA3B site at 3p14.2. *FHIT* is composed of 10 exons and demonstrates splicing errors in a proportion of lung cancers [11, 12]. Recently, however, the role of *FHIT* in cancerogenesis has been questioned [13]. Another recessive gene, $p16^{INK4}$, was identified on the 9p21 chromosome. The most extensively studied early molecular abnormality is mutation in the *p53* gene located at 17p13. In lung cancer, LOH in this region is particularly common [14 15].

Another location of LOH, relatively common in large cell lung carcinoma, is chromosome 12 [16]. In NSCLC, particularly adenocarcinomas, LOH was also demonstrated in chromosome 17q [17]. Other allelic losses in lung cancer were localized at 5q [18, 19], 8p, 11p [20], 11q [21], 13q and 18q [19, 22]. Also observed was the opposite phenomenon - overrepresentation of DNA. This alteration was found at 3q, 5q, 7p and 8q [23, 24].

Recent studies demonstrated that hypermethylation of CpG islands may play a role in the loss of transcription in suppressor genes [25, 26]. It suggests that other mechanisms, in addition to allelic loss or point mutation leading to gene inactivation, may be relevant.

Microsatellite instability

The human genome contains several hundred thousand repetitive noncoding motifs of up to six base pairs [27]. These repetitions (microsatellites) are highly polymorphic as a consequence of frequent germline mutations. The normal cell contains a DNA mismatch repair system which maintains the rates of spontaneous mutation at low levels [28]. Several mismatch repairing genes have been identified including *MSH2* [29], *MLH1* [30] and *PMS2* [31]. Mutations in these genes, found in a number of human malignancies, result in a defect of the mismatch repair system, and in consequence a high rate of microsatellite instability. Destabilization of microsatellites can be seen as a change in the length of microsatellite sequences – expansions or contractions. Both SCLC and NSCLC are among the malignancies in which microsatellite instability are relatively frequent events [32, 33]. The most frequent localization of the unstable replications of tandem repeats is chromosome 3p or 2p [32, 34, 35]. Microsatellite alterations in SCLC patients were found not only in tumour samples but also in plasma DNA [33].

Telomerase dysregulation

Telomeres are tandem repeats of simple DNA sequence (TTAGGG), which are located at the ends of the chromosomes. Their function is to control the proper length of chromosomes as well as to stabilize and protect chromosomal DNA against either the activity of nucleases or binding to other chromosomes. Telomeres are also most probably involved in cellular senescence [36, 37]. The length of telometric repeats in normal cells is known to shorten progressively with each cell division. Every DNA replication is accompanied by the development of a short 8–12 bp gap generated by the removal of the RNA primer [38]. In telomeric regions this loss cannot be completely maintained by DNA polymerase, and thus 50 to 200 nucleotides are lost with each cell division. There is a critical threshold value of chromosomal shortening after which apoptosis ensues. The number of cell cycle repeats depends on the activity of telomerase, the reverse transcriptase enzyme that synthesizes telomeric DNA. High activity of this enzyme keeps telomeres long (e.g., in germ cells) allowing them to divide 'indefinitely'. In adult somatic cells the activity of telomerase is suppressed. It has been suggested that the synthesis of telomeric specific sequences at the chromosomal ends is required to sustain indefinite proliferation [39].

Recently, telomerase expression was found in most human cancers including lung cancer [40]. Most probably cancer cells require activation of this enzyme to overcome cellular senescence and to attain immortality. Some studies suggested that dysregulation of telomerase occurs early in the pathogenesis of lung cancers, and that intense expression of this enzyme in advanced epithelial changes (like carcinoma *in situ*) may indicate imminent invasion [41, 42]. On the other hand, abnormal shortening of telomeric repeats was demonstrated in lung cancer samples, and frequently this abnormality was related to alterations in both *p53* and retinoblastoma *(Rb)* genes [43]. It was therefore assumed that inactivation of these genes may promote cell divisions causing shortening of telomeres. The exact functional aspects of these changes in carcinogenesis remain to be elucidated.

Mutations of protooncogenes and tumour suppressor genes

Two groups of gene mutations are usually involved in carcinogenesis of lung cancer: activation of protooncogenes and inhibition of tumour suppressor genes. Protooncogenes are the normal dominant genes important for cell proliferation and differentiation. Their abnormal activation, e.g., by gene mutation or amplification (they are then called 'oncogenes'), leads to unregulated growth and malignant transformation. The most extensively studied oncogenes are the *ras* family genes

(K-*ras*, N-*ras* and H-*ras*), *myc* family genes (c-*myc*, N-*myc*, L-*myc*) and *HER*-2/neu (c-*erb*B-2) genes. Protein encoded by *ras* genes acts in the intracell signal transduction pathway from cell surface to the nucleus. When mutated, *ras* loses the ability to become inactivated and may stimulate uncontrolled growth autonomously. In lung cancer point mutations of the *ras* family genes most frequently involve K-*ras* [44]. This mutation is most common in adenocarcinoma, less so in other NSCLC types and absent in SCLC [45, 46]. K-*ras* mutations are very rare among non-smokers, and it may be assumed that mutations of this gene are directly caused by exposure to carcinogens in tobacco smoke [47]. The most frequent sites of K-*ras* mutations are codons 12, 13 and 61 [48].

c-*myc*, the most extensively studied of the *myc*-related genes, transcriptionally controls the expression of different groups of genes. Its alteration results in cellular imbalance in the expression of genes that control both proliferation and apoptosis [49, 50]. The *myc* family dysregulation (amplification and increased expression), was seen most frequently in SCLC [51].

The c-*erb*B-1 and c-*erb*B-2 oncogenes, which encode epidermal growth factor receptor (EGFR), are highly expressed in the majority of NSCLC samples and cell lines [52, 53, 54].

A frequent molecular abnormality in oncogenesis is the dysregulation of apoptosis, 'programmed cell death'. Of the protooncogenes involved in the apoptotic dysregulation in cancer, the best known is *bcl*-2. Bcl-2 protein is present in intracellular membranes, such as the outer mitochondrial membrane, nuclear envelope and parts of the endoplasmic reticulum [55]. Lung cancer, particularly SCLC, is among the malignancies that demonstrated overexpression of this oncoprotein [56, 57].

Tumour suppressor genes are inactivated when both alleles are mutated, thus the intact gene is a 'recessive oncogene'. The best known tumour suppressor genes involved in lung cancer pathogenesis are *p53, Rb* and *p16*. The *p53* gene is located on the short arm of chromosome 17 (17p13), consists of 11 exons and encodes a 393 amino acid nuclear phosphoprotein [58]. This gene acts as a checkpoint protein preventing the transmission of DNA abnormalities to daughter cells. Normally, if DNA damage occurs, products of *p53* either stop a cell cycle between phase G1 and S, or direct injured cell to apoptosis. *p53* may act as a transcriptional activator or as a transcriptional repressor of other genes involved in cell cycle arrest [59, 60]. It stimulates the transcription of genes involved in the inhibition of cell growth, or suppresses the function of genes promoting cell proliferation. Alterations in the *p53* pathway (mutation or epigenetic inactivation) result in impairment of these processes and an increased likelihood of neoplastic transformation and/or malignant progression.

Like *p53*, the *Rb* suppressor gene plays an essential role in the regulation of the cell cycle at the G1 checkpoint. Activation of the *Rb* gene, however, results in an alternative pathway of cell cycle arrest: binding and sequestration of transcription factors which promote cell cycling [61]. Phosphorylation of *Rb* gene by the CDK4 (cyclin-dependent kinase) causes the release of bound transcription factors that then stimulate cell division. The product of the gene *p16* inhibits CDK4, thus the absence of *p16* allows uncontrolled CDK4 phosphorylation of Rb and transcription activation [62]. It is likely that *p53* may become activated in response to *Rb* loss and *vice versa* [63].

Potential clinical applications

Potential clinical applications of molecular genetics in oncology include:
* screening and early detection
* prognosis and prediction of response to treatment
* monitoring and management of premalignant lesions
* gene therapy

In lung cancer molecular markers might additionally be used in the monitoring of 'high risk' groups (e.g., patients with severe dysplasia), evaluation of tumour aggressiveness and prediction of response or resistance to chemotherapy and radiation.

Screening and early detection

The real benefit of screening is expressed in decreased mortality. In view of the low efficacy of chest radiography and/or sputum cytology as screening methods, a number of other assays, including molecular markers, have been investigated. Growing understanding of carcinogenesis has revealed that a clinically evident lung tumour is a late event. Indeed, genetic alterations similar to those found in lung cancer were detected not only in precancerous disorders [64–66] but also in nonmaligant bronchial epithelium of current and former smokers [67–69].

Genetic assays potentially useful in early diagnosis include:
* molecular analysis of the sputum and/or broncho-alveolar lavage fluid
* molecular analysis of bronchial biopsy specimens
* analysis of serum markers.

Mao et al. [70] demonstrated retrospectively a high proportion of *ras* and *p53* mutations in cytologically negative sputum of patients who subsequently developed adenocarcinoma of the lung. In many instances mutations in the sputum were the same as those found in tumours. Vahakangas et al. [71] found an increased rate of mutations in both K-*ras* and *p53* genes in the screened high risk group of uranium mine workers. Recently Miozzo et al. [72] demonstrated the feasibility of assessing microsatellite alterations in sputum from NSCLC patients. In that study a comparison of preoperative sputum samples with tumour tissue showed the same pattern of instability in three out of five cases.

BAL (broncho-alveolar lavage) is a simple diagnostic procedure involving the introduction of a fiberoscope into the bronchial tree, the application of 120–200 ml of saline and careful aspiration of saline mixed with broncho-alveolar fluid containing cells from distant parts of the respiratory tract. Mills and co-authors [73] found K-*ras* codon 12 mutations in BAL fluid samples, which otherwise were considered cytologically negative.

Endoscopic procedures, especially if combined with LIFE (lung imaging fluorescence endoscopy), allow the early detection of bronchial lesions which may be biopsied and assayed for genetic alterations [74]. The widely accepted concept of 'field cancerization', the process frequently detected in heavy smokers, suggests multicentric regional carcinogenic activity in the entire bronchial tree. Miozzo et al. [72] demonstrated microsatellite instability in one-third of NSCLC, but a similar rate of this alteration was also found in phenotypically normal bronchial

mucosa taken far away from the neoplastic lesions. The relatively high rate of microsatellite instability in bronchial samples provides support for the potential use of this assay as a genetic marker
for the early diagnosis of lung cancer. Other attractive targets for early detection studies are telomeres and telomerase [41].

Another potential tool for tumour detection is analysis of serum markers. These assays may
use antibodies against altered proteins e.g., p53 [75, 76], or microsatellite instability in plasma
DNA [33], to mention only a few possibilities.

Prognosis and prediction of response to treatment

A number of studies investigated the prognostic value of genetic abnormalities in lung cancer. In
some series, mutations of the *ras* family in NSCLC, particularly in adenocarcinoma, were found
to be associated with poor prognosis [77–81]. Other studies, however, did not demonstrate such
a correlation [82–84]. Expression of c-*erb*B-2 was found to be related to shortened survival in
adenocarcinoma [85, 86] but not in squamous cell carcinoma [87]. In the study of Harpole et al.
[88] including 271 stage I NSCLC patients, c-*erb*B-2 expression had a significant impact on survival. Of the two studies addressing the prognostic value of c-*erb*B-1 [87, 89], one [87] showed a
negative impact of this alteration.

The prognostic value of *p53* mutations seems to be controversial. Some authors reported shortened survival in carriers of these mutations [90, 91], whereas others did not find such a
correlation [92–95], or demonstrated the positive prognostic impact of these events [96]. No
correlation was found between the presence of anti-p53 serum antibodies and prognosis in SCLC
patients [97]. The differences between the results obtained in particular series may in part have
been due to different techniques of *p53* determination polymerase chain reaction-single strain
conformation polymorphism (PCR-SSCP, sequencing, immunohistochemistry) and the exons
studied. The recent study of de Anta et al. [98], using 152 NSCLC patients managed with curative
surgery, showed the negative prognostic influence of *p53* 'null' mutations but not of missense
mutations. This observation suggests that the knowledge of *p53* status, both with respect to the
presence of mutations and to their influence on normal gene expression, may be required to
predict the course of lung cancer accurately.

Some studies suggested shortened survival in lung cancer patients whose tumours carried
c-*myc* amplification [51, 99]. Moreover, a higher metastatic potential of tumours with L-*myc* polymorphism was demonstrated [100, 101]. Shortened survival was also found in patients with lung
cancers showing aberrant expression of the $p16^{INK4}$ protein [102].

In a series of 515 stage I NSCLC patients managed with definitive surgery, Pastorino et al.
[103] evaluated a panel of immunocytochemical markers: precursors and blood group A antigens,
EGFR (epidermal growth factor receptor), p185 HER2, 67LR (the monomeric lamin receptor
associated with invasiveness and metastatic potential), Bcl-2 and p53, as well as the extent of
blood vessel formation and vascular patterns. No impact on prognosis either for any individual
test or for a panel of tests used was observed. Another study [104] investigating a combination of
tests including Rb, p53 and K-ras expression however, showed a decreased survival in adenocarcinoma patients carrying a Rb-/p53+ pattern of expression. Of the three studies evaluating

expression of Bcl-2 [56, 105, 106], two [56, 105] demonstrated increased survival in patients with Bcl-2-positive tumours but in one of them [56] this correlation was significant only for patients with squamous cell carcinoma. Recently Pifarre et al. [32] demonstrated a strong correlation between microsatellite instability and shortened survival in early-stage NSCLC patients managed with surgery.

The predictive value of genetic markers for response to chemotherapy and radiation has been investigated only occasionally. As mentioned earlier, the cytostatic effects of some drugs and irradiation are mediated by activation of endogenous cellular pathways for apoptotic cell death [107]. The *p53* gene is required for induction of apoptosis and loss of its function may contribute to treatment failures in cancer patients by rendering malignant cells more resistant to both cyto-toxic agents and irradiation [108]. Patients with advanced NSCLC carrying this mutation were found to have poor response to paclitaxel [109] and cisplatin-based chemotherapy [110]. On the other hand, no correlation between *in vivo* [83] or *in vitro* [111] chemotherapy resistance and *ras* mutations was demonstrated. Funa et al. [112] reported a high level of chemoresistance in SCLCs with increased expression of N-*myc* oncogenes. Another molecular mechanism of resistance to chemotherapy includes loss of DNA mismatch repair due to the lack of either MSH2 or MSH1 activity. This alteration was found to induce resistance to platinum derivatives [113].

The importance of unaffected *p53* genes for radiation-induced apoptosis was first demon-strated in an experimental model [108]. Subsequently, the Langendijk et al. study [114] con-firmed the correlation between *p53* status and survival after radiotherapy.

Monitoring and management of premalignant lesions

The identification of genetic events accompanying premalignant stages of lung cancer make altered genes and their products potential targets for monitoring and molecular preventive strate-gies. Carcinogenesis does not occur in all premalignant lesions, therefore their optimal manage-ment remains a clinical dilemma. Apart from stopping smoking, which seems to be a crucial requirement, metaplastic and dysplastic lesions can probably simply be sequentially monitored by radiology, sputum cytology and bronchial sampling. Molecular methods, due to their high sensi-tivity, might aid in this process. Therapeutic interventions in high risk groups include photo-dynamic therapy and chemoprevention [115]. These procedures also require monitoring, which could include genetic assays. Finally, premalignant lesions may be approached with gene therapy. An attractive route of gene delivery in premalignant lesions, which are widely dispersed in the bronchial tree, is the aerosolized application of encapsulated liposomal vectors [116].

Gene therapy

The development of gene transfer technology with either transfection or functional deletion of a gene has raised the possibility of using these methods as a therapeutic tool. Despite the multi-plicity of molecular abnormalities in lung cancer, correction of a single genetic defect was found to produce a potentially advantageous therapeutic effect [117, 118]. Strictly speaking, cancer gene therapy includes inactivation of oncogenes or replacement of defective tumour suppressor genes. Frequently, however, alternative approaches, like the use of genes inducing immunity, protection of bone marrow during chemotherapy by transducing drug-resistance genes into marrow stem cells, or the use of expression vector constructs that bring about the conversion of inactive pro-drugs into active drugs, have been attempted [119].

The most common method of inactivating mutated oncogenes is an antisense technique. This procedure involves introduction into the cell of a gene construct or oligonucleotide that has a base sequence complementary to the normal DNA sequence targeted for inhibition. The antisense fragment binds and inhibits the sense sequence by base pairing. Protein synthesis may be inhibited at the levels of mRNA splicing, RNA transport or translation. Another strategy, the replacement of a nonfunctioning copy of the tumour suppressor gene, e.g *p53*, with a functioning copy, is expected to restore normal growth and proliferation pathways.

A critical problem in the direct correction of genetic abnormalities in cancer cells is the safe and effective delivery of genetic constructs to the target cells. Most gene transfer protocols use retroviruses as delivery vehicles [119]. More recent studies employed other viral or non-viral vectors and naked DNA. Although spectacular progress has been made in the ability to transfer genes successfully to cells, many obstacles have to be surpassed before the implementation of this technology in clinical care.

The current experience in gene therapy of lung cancer is scarce and limited to patients with advanced incurable tumours. Both strategies (inactivation of oncogenes and the replacement of defective suppressor genes) were tested in a series of phase I studies [119]. Early observations suggest the feasibility and acceptable toxicity of this approach. Anecdotal tumour responses [117, 120] have also been reported which however should be validated in further clinical research.

This review outlines the possible clinical applications of molecular pathology in lung cancer. Although at present there is insufficient scientific basis for standard use of molecular methods in the clinic, it is highly probable that their role will increase. Hopefully, more precise identification of the genetic events responsible for malignant transformation and differentiation will aid the estimation of the risk carried by particular mutagens. Screening with the use of genotyping will allow identification of premalignant molecular abnormalities and high-risk individuals in whom the application of specific preventive measures could significantly decrease the risk of cancer. Molecular markers for drug resistance may also prove useful in predicting response to specific therapies and in selection of patients for adjuvant treatment. The final step in this process would be the elaboration of effective therapeutic strategies with molecular targets.

References

1. Ryberg D, Hewer A, Phillips DH, Haugen A (1994) Different susceptibility to smoking-induced DNA damage among male and female lung cancer patients. *Cancer Res* 54: 5801–5803.
2. Denissenko MF, Pao A, Tang M, Pfeifer GP (1996) Preferential formation of benzo(a)pyrene adducts at lung cancer mutational hot spots in p53. *Science* 274: 430–432.
3. Yuspa SH, Pirier MC (1988) Chemical carcinogenesis: from animal models to molecular models in one decade. *Adv Cancer Res* 50: 25–70.
4. Tang MS, Pierce JR, Doisy RP, Nazimiec ME, MacLeod MC (1992) Differences and similarities in the repair of benzo[a]pyrene diol epoxide isomers induced DNA adducts by *uvrA, uvrB, uvrC* gene products. *Biochemistry* 32: 8429–8436.

5. Chen RH, Maher VM, Brouwer J, van de Putte P, McCormick JJ (1992) Preferential repair and strand-specific repair of benzo[a]pyrene diol epoxide adducts in *HPRT* gene of diploid human fibroblasts. *Proc Natl Acad Sci USA* 89: 5413−5417.
6. Seidegard J, Vorachek WR, Pero WR, Pearson WR (1988) Hereditary differences in the expression of the human glutathione transferase active on *trans*-stilbene oxide are due to a gene deletion. *Proc Natl Acad Sci USA* 85: 7293−7297.
7. Spivack SD, Fasco MJ, Walker VE, Kaminsky LS (1997) The molecular epidemiology of lung cancer. *Crit Rev Toxicol* 27: 319−365.
8. Hayashi S-I, Watanabe J, Kawajiri K (1992) High susceptibility to lung cancer analyzed in terms of combined genotypes of P450Ia1 and Mu-class glutathione S-transferase genes. *Jpn J Cancer Res* 83: 866−870.
9. Goto I, Yoneda S, Yamamoto M, Kawajiri K (1996) Prognostic significance of germ line polymorphism of the *CYP1A1* and glutathione S-transferase genes in patients with non-small cell lung cancer. *Cancer Res* 56: 3725−3730.
10. Todd S, Franklin WA, Varella-Garcia M, Kennedy T, Hilliker CE, Hahner L, Anderson M, Wiest JS, Drabkin HA, Gemmill RM (1997) Homozygous deletions of human chromosome 3p in lung tumors. *Cancer Res* 57: 1344−1352.
11. Sozzi G, Veronese ML, Negrini M, Baffa R, Cotticelli MG, Inoue H, Tornielli S, Pilotti S, Degregorio L, Pastorino U et al. (1996) The FHIT gene 3p14.2 is abnormal in lung cancer. *Cell* 85: 17−26.
12. Fong KM, Biesterveld EJ, Virmani A, Wistuba I, Sekido Y, Bader SA, Ahmadian M, Ong ST, Rassool FV, Zimmerman PV et al. (1997) *FHIT* and FRA3B 3p14.2 allele loss are common in lung cancer and preneoplastic bronchial lesions and are associated with cancer-related *FHIT* cDNA splicing aberrations. *Cancer Res* 57: 2256−2267.
13. Gayther SA, Barski P, Batley SJ, Li L, de Foy KAF, Cohen SN, Ponder BAJ, Caldas C (1997) Aberrant splicing of the *TSG101* and *FHIT* genes occurs frequently in multiple malignancies and in normal tissue and mimics alterations previously described in tumours. *Oncogene* 15: 2119−2127.
14. Sundaresan V, Ganly P, Hasleton P, Rudd R, Sinha G, Bleehan NM, Rabbits P (1992) p53 and chromosome 3 abnormalities, characteristic of malignant lung tumors, are detectable in preinvasive lesions of the bronchus. *Oncogene* 7: 1989−1897.
15. Ridanpää M, Anttila S, Husgafvel-Pursiainen K (1995) Detection of loss of heterozygosity in the p53 tumor suppressor gene using a PCR-based assay. *Pathol Res Pract* 191: 399−402.
16. Takeuchi S, Mori N, Koike M, Slater J, Park S, Miller CW, Miyoshi I, Koeffler HP (1996) Frequent loss of heterozygosity in region of the *KIP1* locus in non-small cell lung cancer: evidence for a new tumor suppressor gene on the short arm of chromosome 12. *Cancer Res* 56: 738−740.
17. Fong KM, Kida Y, Zimmerman PV, Ikenaga M, Smith PJ (1995) Loss of heterozygosity frequently affects chromosome 17q in non-small cell lung cancer. *Cancer Res* 55: 4268−4272.
18. Miura I, Graziano SL, Cheng JQ, Doyle LA, Testa JR (1992) Chromosome alterations in human small cell lung cancer: frequent involvement of 5q. *Cancer Res* 52: 1322−1328.
19. Fong K, Zimmerman PV, Smith P (1995) Tumor progression and loss of heterozygosity at 5q and 18q in non-small cell lung cancer. *Cancer Res* 55: 220−223.
20. Tran YK, Newsham IF (1996) High-density marker analysis of 11p15.5 in non-small cell lung carcinomas reveals allelic deletion of one shared and one distinct region when compared to breast carcinomas. *Cancer Res* 56: 2916−2921.
21. Rasio D, Negrini M, Maneneti G, Draggani TA, Croce CM (1995) Loss of heterozygosity at chromosome 11q in lung adenocarcinoma: identification of three independent regions. *Cancer Res* 55: 3988−3991.
22. Uchida K, Nagatake M, Osada H, Yatabe Y, Kondo M, Mitsudomi T, Masuda A, Takahashi T, Takahashi T (1997) Somatic *in vivo* alterations of the *JV18-1* gene at 18q21 in human lung cancers. *Cancer Res* 57: 5583−5585.
23. Balsara BR, Sonoda G, du Manoir S, Siegfried JM, Gabrielson E, Testa JR (1997) Comparative genomic hybridization analysis detects frequent, often high-level overrepresentation of DNA sequences at 3q, 5p, 7p, and 8q in human non-small cell lung cancer. *Cancer Res* 57: 2116−2120.
24. Brass N, Ukena I, Remberger K, Mack U, Sybrecht GW, Meese EU (1996) DNA amplification on chromosome 3q26.1-q26.3 in squamous cell carcinoma of the lung detected by reverse chromosome painting. *Eur J Cancer* 32A: 1205−1208.
25. Merlo A, Herman JG, Mao L, Lee DJ, Gabrielson E, Burger PC, Baylin SB, Sidransky D (1995) 5′ CpG island methylation is associated with transcriptional silencing of the tumour suppressor p16/CDKN2/MTS1 gene in human cancers. *Nature Med* 1: 686−692.
26. Nagatake M, Osada H, Kondo M, Uchida K, Mishio M, Shimokata K, Takahashi T, Takahashi T (1996) Aberrant hypermethylation at the *bcl*-2 locus at 18q21 in human lung cancers. *Cancer Res* 56: 1886−1891.
27. Hearne CM, Ghosh S, Todd JA (1992) Microsatellites for linkage analysis of genetic traits. *Trends Genet* 8: 288−294.
28. Modrich P, Lahue R (1996) Mismatch repair in replication fidelity, genetic recombination and cancer biology. *Annu Rev Biochem* 65: 101−133.

29. Fishel R, Lescoe MK, Rao MR, Copeland NG, Jenkins NA, Garber J, Kane M, Kolodner R (1993) The human mutator gene homolog MSH2 and its association with hereditary nonpolyposis colon cancer. *Cell* 75: 1027–1038.
30. Bronner CE, Baker SM, Morrison PT, Warren G, Smith LG, Lescoe MK, Kane M, Earabino C, Lipford J, Lindblom A et al. (1994) Mutation in the DNA mismatch repair gene homologue hMLH1 is associated with hereditary nonpolyposis colon cancer. *Nature* 368: 258–261.
31. Risinger JI, Umar A, Barrett JC, Kunkel TA (1995) A hPMS2 mutant cell line is defective in strand-specific mismatch repair. *J Biol Chem* 270: 18183–18186.
32. Pifarre A, Rosell R, Monzo M, De Anta JM, Moreno I, Sanchez JJ, Ariza A, Mate JL, Martinez E, Sanchez M (1997) Prognostic value of replication errors on chromosomes 2p and 3p in non-small cell lung cancer. *Brit J Cancer* 75: 184–189.
33. Chen XQ, Stroun M, Magnenat J-L, Nicod JL, Lederrey C, Anker P (1996) Microsatellite alterations in plasma DNA of small cell lung cancer patients. *Nature Med* 2: 1033–1035.
34. Merlo A, Mabry M, Gabrielson E, Vollmer R, Baylin SB, Sidransky D (1994) Frequent microsatellite instability in primary small cell lung cancer. *Cancer Res* 54: 2098–2101.
35. Shridhar V, Siegfried J, Hunt J, Alonso MDM, Smith DI (1994) Genetic instability of microsatellite sequences in many non-small cell lung carcinomas. *Cancer Res* 54: 2084–2087.
36. Counter CM, Avilion AA, LeFeuvre CE (1992) Telomere shortening associated with chromosome instability is arrested in immortal cells which express telomerase activity. *EMBO J* 11: 1921–1929.
37. Kim NW, Piatyszek MA, Prowse KR, Harley CB, West MD, Ho PL, Coviello GM, Wright WE, Wienrich SL, Shay J (1994) Specific association of human telomerase activity with immortal cells and cancer. *Science* 266: 2011–2015.
38. Zakian VA (1995) Telomeres: beginning to understand the end. *Science* 270: 1601–1607.
39. Shay JW, Werbin H, Wright WE (1994) Telomere shortening may contribute to aging and cancer. *Mol Cell Differ* 2: 1–21.
40. Shirotani Y, Hiyama K, Ishioka S (1994) Alterations in length of telomeric repeats in lung cancer. *Lung Cancer* 11: 29–41.
41. Shay JW, Gazdar AF (1997) Telomerase in the early detection of cancer. *J Clin Pathol* 50: 106–109.
42. Yashima K, Litzky LA, Kaiser L, Rogers T, Lam S, Witsuba II, Milchgrub S, Srivastava S, Piatyszek MA, Shay JW et al. (1997) Telomerase expression in respiratory epithelium during multistage pathogenesis of lung carcinomas. *Cancer Res* 57: 2373–2377.
43. Hiyama K, Ishioka S, Shirotani Y, Inai K, Hiyama E, Murakami I, Isobe T, Inamizu T, Yamakido M (1995) Alterations in telomeric repeat length in lung cancer are associated with loss of heterozygosity in p53 and Rb. *Oncogene* 10: 937–944.
44. Rosell R, Monzo M, Molina F, Martinez E, Piffare A, Moreno I, Mate JL, de Anta JM, Sanchez M, Font A (1995) K-ras genotypes and prognosis in non-small cell lung cancer. *Ann Oncol* 6 (Suppl. 3): 15–20.
45. Rodenhuis S, van de Wetering ML, Mooi WJ, Evers SG, van Zandwijk N, Bos JL (1987) Mutational activation of the K-*ras* oncogene: a possible pathogenetic factor in adenocarcinoma of the lung. *N Engl J Med* 317: 929–935.
46. Mitsudomi T, Steinberg SM, Oie H, Mulshine JL, Phelps R, Viallet J, Pass H, Minna JD, Gazdar AF (1991) *ras* gene mutation in non-small cell lung cancers are associated with shortened survival irrespective of treatment. *Cancer Res* 51: 4999–5002.
47. Rodenhuis S (1992) *ras* in human tumors. *Semin Cancer Biol* 3: 241–247.
48. Slebos RJC, Hruban RH, Dalesio O, Mooi WJ, Offerhaus GJA, Rodenhuis S (1991) Relationship between K-*ras* oncogene activation and smoking in adenocarcinoma of the lung. *J Nat Cancer Inst* 83: 1024–1027.
49. Amati B, Land H (1994) Myc-Max-Mad: a transcription factor network controlling cell cycle progression, differentiation and death. *Curr Opin Genet Dev* 4: 102–108.
50. Harrington EA, Fanidi A, Evan GI (1994) Oncogenes and cell death. *Curr Opin Genet Dev* 4: 120–129.
51. Brooks B, Battey J, Nau M, Gazdar A, Minna J (1987) Amplification and expression of the *myc* gene in small-cell lung cancer. *Adv. Viral Oncol* 7: 155–172.
52. Sherwin SA, Minna JD, Gazdar AFTodaro GJ (1981) Expression of epidermal growth factor and nerve growth factor receptors and soft agar growth factor production by lung cancer cells. *Cancer Res* 41: 3538–3542.
53. Cerny T, Barnes D, Haselton PS, Barber PV, Healy K, Gullick W, Thatcher N (1986) Expression of epidermal growth factor receptors in human lung tumors. *Brit J Cancer* 54: 265–269.
54. Tateishi M, Ishida T, Mitsudomi T, Kaneko S, Sugimachi K (1990) Immunohistochemical evidence of autocrine growth factors in adenocarcinoma of the human lung. *Cancer Res* 50: 7077–7080.
55. Jacobson MD, Burna JF, King MP, Miyashita T, Reed JC, Raff MC (1993) Bcl-2 blocks apoptosis in cells lacking mitochondrial DNA. *Nature* 361: 365–369.
56. Pezella F, Turley H, Kuzu I, Tungekar MF, Dunnill MS, Pierce CB, Harris A, Gatter KC, Mason DY (1993) *bcl-2* protein in non-small cell lung carcinoma. *N Engl J Med* 329: 690–694.
57. Higashiyama M, Doi O, Kodama K, Yokouchi H, Tateishi R (1995) High prevalence of bcl-2 oncoprotein expression in small cell lung cancer. *Anti-Cancer Res* 15: 503–505.

58. Greenblatt MS, Bennett WP, Hollstein M, Harris CC (1994) Mutations in the *p53* tumor suppressor gene: clues to cancer ethiology and molecular pathogenesis. *Cancer Res* 54: 4855–4878.
59. Chen X, Farmer G, Zhu H, Prywes R, Prives C (1993) Cooperative DNA binding of p53 with TFIID (TBP): a possible mechanism for transcriptional activation. *Genes Dev* 7: 1837–1849.
60. el-Deiry WS, Harper JW, O'Connor PM, Velculescu VE, Canman CE, Jackman J, Pietenpol JA, Burrel M, Hill DE, Wang Y et al. (1994) WAF1/CIP1 is induced in p53-mediated G1 arrest and apoptosis. *Cancer Res* 54: 1169–1174.
61. Weinberg RA (1995) The retinoblastoma protein and cell cycle control. *Cell* 81: 323–330.
62. de Vos S, Miller CW, Takeuchi S, Gombart AF, Cho SK, Koeffler HP (1995) Alterations of CDKN2 (p16) in non-small cell lung cancer. *Gene Chromosome Cancer* 14: 164–170.
63. Moregenbesser SD, Williams BO, Jacks T (1994) p53 dependent apoptosis produced by Rb deficiency in developing mouse lens. *Nature* 371: 72–74.
64. Bennett WP, Colby TV, Travis WD, Borkowski A, Jones RT, Lane DP, Metclaf RA, Samet JM, Takeshima Y, Gu JR et al. (1993) p53 protein accumulates frequently in early bronchial neoplasia. *Cancer Res* 53: 4817–22.
65. Sundaresan V, Ganly P, Hasleton P, Rudd R, Sinha G, Bleehen NM, Rabbitts P (1992) *p53* and chromosome 3 abnormalities, characteristic of malignant lung tumors, are detectable in preinvasive lesions of the bronchus. *Oncogene* 7: 1989–1997.
66. Thiberville L, Payne P, Vielkinds J, LeRiche J, Horsman D, Nouvet G, Palcic B, Lam S (1995) Evidence of cumulative gene losses with progression of premalignant epithelial lesions to carcinoma of the bronchus. *Cancer Res* 55: 5133–5139.
67. Witsuba II, Lam S, Behrens C, Virmani AK, Fong KM, LeRiche J, Samet M, Srivastava S, Minna JD, Gazdar AF (1997) Molecular damage in the bronchial epithelium of current and former smokers. *J Nat Cancer Inst* 89: 1366–1373.
68. Mao L, Lee JS, Kurie JM, Hong Y, Lippman SM, Lee JJ, Ro JY, Broxson A, Yu R, Morice RC et al. (1997) Clonal genetic alterations in the lungs of current and former smokers. *J Nat Cancer Inst* 89: 857–862.
69. Sozzi G, Sard L, De Gregorio L, Marchetti A, Musso K, Buttitta F, Tornielli S, Pellegrini S, Veronese ML, Manenti G et al. (1997) Association between cigarette smoking and *FHIT* gene alterations in lung cancer. *Cancer Res* 57: 2121–2123.
70. Mao L, Hruban RH, Boyle JO, Tockman M, Sidransky D (1994) Detection of oncogene mutations in sputum precedes diagnosis of lung cancer. *Cancer Res* 54: 1634–1637.
71. Vahakangas KH, Samet JM, Metcalf RA, Welsh JA, Bennett WP, Lane DP (1992) Mutations of p53 and *ras* genes in radon-associated lung cancer from uranium miners. *Lancet* 339: 576–80.
72. Miozzo M, Sozzi G, Musso K, Pilotti S, Incarbone M, Pastorino U, Pierotti MA (1996) Microsatellite alterations in bronchial and sputum specimens of lung patients. *Cancer Res* 56: 2285–2288.
73. Mills NE, Fishman CL, Scholes J (1995) Detection of K-ras oncogene mutations in bronchoalveolar lavage fluid for lung cancer diagnosis. *J Nat Cancer Inst* 87: 1056–1060.
74. Lam S, MacAulay C, Palcic B (1993) Detection and localization of early lung cancer by imaging techniques. *Chest* 103: 12–14.
75. Lubin R, Zalcman G, Bouchet L (1995) Serum p53 antibodies as early markers of lung cancer. *Nature Med* 1: 701–702.
76. Jassem E, Bigda J, Jassem J, Rzyman W, Skokowski J, Grodzki T, Stominski JM (1997) Serum p53 auto-antibodies in small cell lung cancer. *Eur Respir J* 10 (Suppl. 25): 263, A1705 (abstract).
77. Slebos RJC, Kibbelaar RE, Dalesio O, Kooistra A, Stam J, Meijer CJLM, Wagenaar SS, Vanderschueren RGJRA, van Zandwijk N, Mooi WJ et al. (1990) K-*ras* oncogene activation as a prognostic marker in adenocarcinoma of the lung. *N Engl J Med* 323: 561–565.
78. Rodenhuis S, Slebos RJC (1992) Clinical significance of *ras* oncogene activation in human lung cancer. *Cancer Res* 52 (Suppl. 1): 2665s–2669s.
79. Harada M, Dosaka-Akita H, Miyamoto H, Kuzumaki N, Kawakami Y (1992) Prognostic significance of the expression of *ras* oncogene product in non-small cell lung cancer. *Cancer* 69: 72–77.
80. Keohavong P, De Michele MAA, Melacrinos AC, Landreneau RJ, Weyant RJ, Sigfried JM (1996) Detection of K-*ras* mutations in lung carcinomas: relationship to prognosis. *Clin Cancer Res* 2: 411–418.
81. Cho JY, Kim JH, Lee YH, Chung KY, Kim SK, Gong SJ, You NC, Chung HC, Roh JK, Kim BS (1997) Correlation between K-*ras* gene mutation and prognosis of patients with non-small cell lung carcinoma. *Cancer* 79: 462–467.
82. Sugio K, Ishida T, Yokoyama H, Inone T, Sugimachi K, Sazazuki T (1992) *ras* gene mutations as a prognostic marker in adenocarcinoma of the human lung without lymph node metastasis. *Cancer Res* 52: 2903–2906.
83. Rodenhuis S, Boerrigter L, Top B, Slebos RJC, Mooi WJ, van't Veer L, Zandwijk N (1997) Mutational activation of K-*ras* oncogene and the effect of chemotherapy in advanced adenocarcinoma of the lung: a prospective study. *J Clin Oncol* 15: 285–291.
84. Keohavong P, Zhu D, Melacrinos AC, De Michele MA, Weyant RJ, Luketich JD, Testa JR, Fedder M, Siegfried JM (1997) Detection of low-fraction K-ras mutations in primary lung tumors using a sensitive method. *Int J Cancer* 74: 162–170.

85. Tateishi M, Ishida T, Mitsudomi T, Kaneko S, Sugimachi K (1991) Prognostic value of c-*erb*B-2 protein expression in human lung adenocarcinoma and squamous cell carcinoma. *Eur J Cancer* 27: 1372–1375.
86. Kern JA, Slebos RJ, Top B, Rodenhuis S, Lager D, Robinson RA, Weiner D, Schwartz DA (1994) C-*erb*B-2 expression and codon 12 K-*ras* mutations both predict shortened survival for patients with pulmonary adenocarcinomas. *J Clin Invest* 93: 516–520.
87. Volm M, Drings P, Wodrich W (1993) Prognostic significance of the expression of c-*fos*, c-*jun* and c-*erb*B-2 oncogene products in human squamous cell carcinomas. *J Cancer Res Clin Oncol* 119: 507–510.
88. Harpole DH, Herndon JE, Wolfe WG, Iglehart JD, Marks JR (1995) A prognostic model of recurrence and death in stage I non-small cell lung cancer utilizing presentation, histopathology and oncoprotein expression. *Cancer Res* 55: 51–56.
89. Scagliotti GV, Leonardo E, Cappia S, Masiero P, Micela M, Gubetta L, Pozzi E (1993) Epidermal growth factor receptor and *neu*-oncogene expression in lung cancer. *Proc Am Soc Clin Oncol* 12: 328 (abstract).
90. Mitsudomi T, Oyama T, Nishida K, Ogami A, Osaki T, Nakanishi R, Surgio K, Yasumoto K, Sugimachi K (1995) p53 nuclear immunostaining and gene mutations in non-small cell lung cancer and their effect on patients survival. *Ann Oncol* 6 (Suppl. 3): S9–S13.
91. Horio Y, Takahashi T, Kuroishi T, Hibi K, Suyama M, Niimi T, Shimokata K, Yamakawa K, Nakamura Y, Ueda R (1993) Prognostic significance of p53 mutations and 3p deletions in primary resected non-small cell lung cancer. *Cancer Res* 53: 1–4.
92. Chiba I, Takahashi T, Nau MM, D'Amico D, Curiel DT, Mitsudomi T, Buchhagen DL, Carbone D, Piantadosi S, Koga H et al. (1990) Mutations in the p53 gene are frequent in primary, resected non-small cell lung cancer. *Oncogene* 5: 1603–1610.
93. Carbone DP, Mitsudomi T, Chiba I, Piantadosi S, Rusch V, Nowak JA, McIntire D, Slamon D, Gazdar A, Minna J (1994) p53 immunostaining positivity is associated with reduced survival and is imperfectly correlated with gene mutations in resected non-small cell lung cancer. *Chest* 106: 377–381.
94. Nishio M, Koshikawa T, Kuroishi T, Suyama M, Uchida K, Takagi Y, Washimi O, Sugiura T, Ariyoshi Y, Takahashi T et al. (1996) Prognostic significance of abnormal p53 accumulation in primary, resected non-small cell lung cancers. *J Clin Oncol* 14: 497–502.
95. McLaren R, Kuzu I, Dunnill M, Harris A, Lane D, Gatter KC (1992) The relationship of p53 immunostaining to survival in carcinoma of the lung. *Brit J Cancer* 66: 735–738.
96. Passlick B, Izbicki JR, Haussinger K, Thettero O, Pantel K (1995) Immunohistochemical detection of p53 protein is not associated with a poor prognosis in non-small-cell lung cancer. *J Thorac Cardiovasc Surg* 109: 1205–1211.
97. Rosenfeld MR, Malats N, Schramm L, Vinolas N, Rosell R, Tora M, Real FX, Posner JB, Dalmau J (1997) Serum anti-p53 antibodies and prognosis of patients with small-cell lung cancer. *J Nat Cancer Inst* 89: 381–385.
98. de Anta JM, Jassem E, Rosell R, Martinez-Roca M, Jassem J, Martinez-Lopez E, Monzo M, Sanchez-Hernandez JJ, Moreno I, Sanchez-Cespedes M (1997) *TPp53* mutational pattern in Spanish and Polish non-small cell lung cancer patients: null mutations are associated with poor prognosis. *Oncogene* 24: 2951–2959.
99. Chiba W, Sawai S, Hanawa T, Ishida H, Matsui T, Kosaba S, Watanabe S, Hatakenaka R, Matsubara Y, Funatsu T et al. (1993) Correlation between DNA content and amplification of oncogenes (c-myc, L-myc, c-erB-2) and correlation with prognosis in 143 cases of resected lung cancer. *Gan Ro Kagaku Ryoho* 20: 824–827.
100. Kawashima K, Nomura S, Hirai H, Fukushi S, Karube T, Takeushi K, Naruke T, Nishimura S (1992) Correlation of L-myc RFLP with metastasis, prognosis and multiple cancer in lung-cancer patients. *Int J Cancer* 50: 557–561.
101. Fong KM, Kida Y, Zimmerman PV, Smith PJ (1996) MYCL genotypes and loss of heterozygosity in non-small cell lung cancer. *Brit J Cancer* 74: 1975–1978.
102. Kratzke RA, Greatens TM, Rubins JB, Maddaus MA, Niewoehner DE, Niehans GA, Geradts J (1996) *Rb* and p16^{INK4a} expression in resected non-small cell lung tumors. *Cancer Res* 56: 3415–3420.
103. Pastorino U, Andreola S, Tagliabue E, Pezzella F, Incarbone M, Sozzi G, Buyse M, Menard S, Pierotti M, Rilke F (1997) Immunocytochemical markers in stage I lung cancer: relevance to prognosis. *J Clin Oncol* 15: 2858–2866.
104. Dosaka-Akita H, Hu S-X, Fujino M, Harada M, Kinoshita I, Xu H-J, Kuzumaki N, Kawakami Y, Benedict WF (1997) Altered retinoblastoma protein expression in non-small cell lung cancer. *Cancer* 79: 1329–1337.
105. Fontanini G, Vignati S, Bigini D, Mussi A, Lucchi M, Angeletti CA, Basolo F, Bevilacqua G (1995) *Bcl*-2 protein: a prognostic factor inversely correlated to p-53 in non-small-cell lung cancer. *Brit J Cancer* 71: 1003–1007.
106. Ritter JH, Dresler CM, Wick MR (1995) Expression of *bcl*-2 protein in stage T1N0M0 non-small cell lung carcinoma. *Hum Pathol* 26: 1227–1232.
107. Lane DP (1993) A death in the life of *p53*. *Nature* 362: 786–787.
108. Lowe SW, Schmitt EM, Smith SW, Osborne BA, Jacks T (1993) p53 is required for radiation induced apoptosis in mouse thymocytes. *Nature* 362: 847–849.

109. Rosell R, Gonzalez-Larriba JS, Alberola V, Molina F, Monzo M, Benito D, Perez JM, de Anta JM (1995) Single-agent paclitaxel by 3-hour infusion in the treatment of non-small cell lung cancer: Links between *p53* and K-*ras* gene status and chemosensitivity. *Sem Oncol* 22 (Suppl. 14): 12–18.
110. Rusch V, Klimstra D, Venkatraman E, Oliver J, Martini N, Gralla R, Kris M, Dmitrovsky E (1995) Aberrant p53 expression predicts clinical resistance to cisplatin-based chemotherapy in locally advanced non-small cell lung cancer. *Cancer Res* 55: 5038–5042.
111. Tsai CM, Chang KT, Perng RP, Mitsudomi T, Chen MH, Kadoyama C, Gazdar AF (1993) Correlation of intrinsic chemoresistance of non-small cell lung cancer cell lines with HER-2/neu gene expression but not with *ras* gene mutations. *J Nat Cancer Inst* 85: 897–901.
112. Funa K, Steinholz L, Nou M, Bergh J (1987) Amplification and expression of N-*myc* in human small cell lung cancer biopsies predict lack of response to chemotherapy and poor prognosis. Am. *J Clin Pathol* 88: 216–220.
113. Fink D, Nebel S, Aebi S, Zheng H, Cenni B, Nehme A, Christen RD, Howell SB (1996) The role of DNA mismatch repair in platinum drug resistance. *Cancer Res* 56: 4881–4886.
114. Langendijk JA, Thunnissen FBJM, Lamers RJS, de Jong JMA, ten Velde GPM, Wouters EFM (1995) The prognostic significance of accumulation of p53 protein in stage III non-small cell lung cancer treated by radiotherapy. *Radiother Oncol* 36: 218–224.
115. Pastorino U (1995) Lung cancer chemoprevention. *Cancer Treat Res* 72: 43–74.
116. Stribling R, Brunette E, Liggitt D, Gaensler K, Debs R (1992) Aerosol gene delivery *in vivo*. *Proc Natl Acad Sci USA* 89: 11277–11281.
117. Roth JA, Nguyen D, Lawrence DD, Kemp BL, Carrasco CH, Ferson DZ, Hong WK, Komaki R, Lee JJ, Nesbitt JC et al. (1996) Retrovirus-mediated wildtype *p53* gene transfer to tumors of patients with lung cancer. *Nature Med* 2: 985–991.
118. Fujiwara T, Cai DW, Georges RN, Mukhopadhyay T, Grimm EA, Roth JA (1994) Therapeutic effect of a retroviral wildtype p53 expression vector in an orthotopic lung cancer model. *J Nat Cancer Inst* 86: 1458–1462.
119. Roth JA, Cristiano RJ (1997) Gene therapy for cancer: what have we done and where are we going? *J Nat Cancer Inst* 89: 21–39.
120. Tursz T, Cesne AL, Baldeyrou P, Gautier E, Opolon P, Schartz C, Pavirani A, Courtney M, Lamy D, Ragot T et al. (1996) Phase I study of a recombinant adenovirus-mediated gene transfer in lung cancer patients. *J Nat Cancer Inst* 88: 1857–1863.

Molecular Aspects of Cancer and its Therapy
A. Mackiewicz and P.B. Sehgal (eds)
© 1998 Birkhäuser Verlag Basel/Switzerland

Recent advances in understanding function and mutations of breast cancer susceptibility genes

A. Jasinska, K. Sobczak, P. Kozłowski, M. Napierała and W.J. Krzyzosiak

Laboratory of Cancer Genetics, Institute of Bioorganic Chemistry, Polish Academy of Sciences, PL-71-604 Poznan, Poland

Introduction

The genetic basis of many hereditary cancer susceptibility syndromes is now well established. In contrast to the diseases that exhibit classic mendelian inheritance and are caused by alterations in single genes, hereditary cancer is more complex. Besides a germline mutation in a cancer-predisposing gene, additional somatic mutations in cancer related genes are required to develop the disease phenotype. The rate at which they are acquired is influenced by environmental factors and the efficiency of cellular protective activities. The inheritance of a single altered cancer-predisposing allele is sufficient to place the carrier at much higher risk of the disease compared with the general population. Thus, cancers with hereditary background are characterized by a much earlier average age of onset, usually occurring 15 to 20 years earlier than sporadic cancers. It is anticipated that most forms of cancer have a hereditary subgroup, which can be as high as 40% in hereditary retinoblastoma. In most adult tumours the estimated hereditary fraction is much smaller, about 10% or less. Inherited cancers give, however, valuable information about genetics of cancer in general.

Depending on the number of different predisposing genes involved, hereditary cancer syndromes can be divided into two groups. The first includes genetically homogenous diseases associated with germline mutations in single genes. Examples are: familial adenomatous polyposis (*APC*), familial retinoblastoma (*Rb*), ataxia telangiectasia (*ATM*), Li-Fraumeni syndrome (*p53*), Von Hippel Lindau disease (*VHL*) and multiple endocrine neoplasia (*RET*). In the second group of syndromes the same phenotype is associated with mutations in one of several predisposing genes. Examples are: hereditary non-polyposis colon cancer (*MSH2, MLH1, PMS1, PMS2*) and hereditary breast/ovarian cancer (*BRCA1, BRCA2...*).

Taking into account cellular functions of the cancer-predisposing genes, and their role in determination of cancer, Vogelstein and Kinzler divided them into two distinct groups, gatekeepers and caretakers [1]. Gatekeeper genes are directly involved in tumour growth regulation. They either inhibit cell growth or promote cell death. It is postulated that each cell type has one or at most only a few active gatekeepers. Inactivation of them leads to very specific tissue distribution of cancer. Examples of gatekeeper genes are *APC, NF1, VHL* and *Rb1*, leading to tumours of colon, Schwan cells, kidney and retina, respectively. Both copies of the gatekeeper gene must be inactivated: this is the rate-limiting step in tumour initiation. As the predisposed individuals inherit one mutant allele of the gatekeeper, they need only one additional somatic mutation in the second allele of the same gene to initiate neoplasia. By contrast, both copies of the gatekeeper gene have to be altered somatically in sporadic tumours. This is much less likely to happen, and it is estimated that carriers of a germline mutation in the gatekeeper gene are at risk of developing cancer at least three orders of magnitude higher than the general population. The function of caretaker genes is to maintain the integrity of the genome [1]. Inactivation of them does not lead directly to tumour initiation but to genetic instability of the entire genome. This results in the increased mutability of all genes, among them the gatekeeper genes. Once the latter become altered, tumour initiation takes place and its progress is more rapid due to the increased rate of mutations. According to the concept of gatekeepers and caretakers, the carriers of the mutant caretaker allele are at risk of developing cancer only 5 to 50 times higher than the general population [1]. This is so because three additional somatic mutations are usually required for tumour initiation: one in the remaining caretaker allele and two in the gatekeeper alleles. The concept of gatekeepers and caretakers implies also that the caretaker genes will rarely be mutated in sporadic tumours as the probability of acquiring four somatic mutations (two in caretaker alleles and two in gatekeeper alleles) is low. The class of caretaker genes include the mismatch repair genes that cause hereditary nonpolyposis colon cancer, and the nucleotide excision repair genes responsible for xeroderma pigmentosum. According to Vogelstein and Kinzler [1], this group probably also includes the *ATM*, *BRCA1* and *BRCA2* genes.

BRCA1 and BRCA2 genes and proteins

In 1990 the first breast cancer-susceptibility gene *BRCA1* was localized to chromosome 17q21 by linkage analysis [2]. A year later, the same locus was shown also to be linked to hereditary ovarian cancer [3]. In 1994 the *BRCA1* gene was isolated by positional cloning [4]. The gene contains 24 exons that span 81 kb of the genomic sequence [4, 5]. It encodes a protein of 1863 amino acids. The exon lengths range from 41 bp to 3426 bp, the longest of which is exon 11 which makes up 61% of the entire translated sequence, while the *BRCA1* introns range from 402 bp to about 9.2 kb [4, 5]. The organization of the *BRCA1* gene including all its exons and introns is shown in Figure 1a. The gene is very rich in Alu repetitive DNA which makes up over 40% of the genomic sequence, whereas other repetitive sequences contribute to less than 5% [5]. Another study revealed that the *BRCA1* genomic region contains a tandem duplication of about 30 kb [6]. This results in two copies of *BRCA1* exons 1 and 2 and two copies of the adjacent 1A1-3B gene fragment, including the 295 bp intragenic region, which separates the two genes located head to head [6–8]. The presence of the duplicated exons has to be taken into account in *BRCA1* mutation analysis. It may also influence regulation of *BRCA1* transcription, translation and function [6].

    Most of the BRCA1 protein shows no significant sequence similarity to other, previously described proteins. The only domain, easily recognized by the predicted amino acid sequence analysis, was the zinc finger motif at the N-terminus, at amino acids 24–64 [4]. Further analysis of human *BRCA1* sequence revealed several other potentially functional motifs which are shown in Figure 2a. They include the granin consensus sequence at amino acids 1214–1223 [9]; the putative leucine zipper at amino acids 1209–1230 [10] which overlaps with the granin consensus

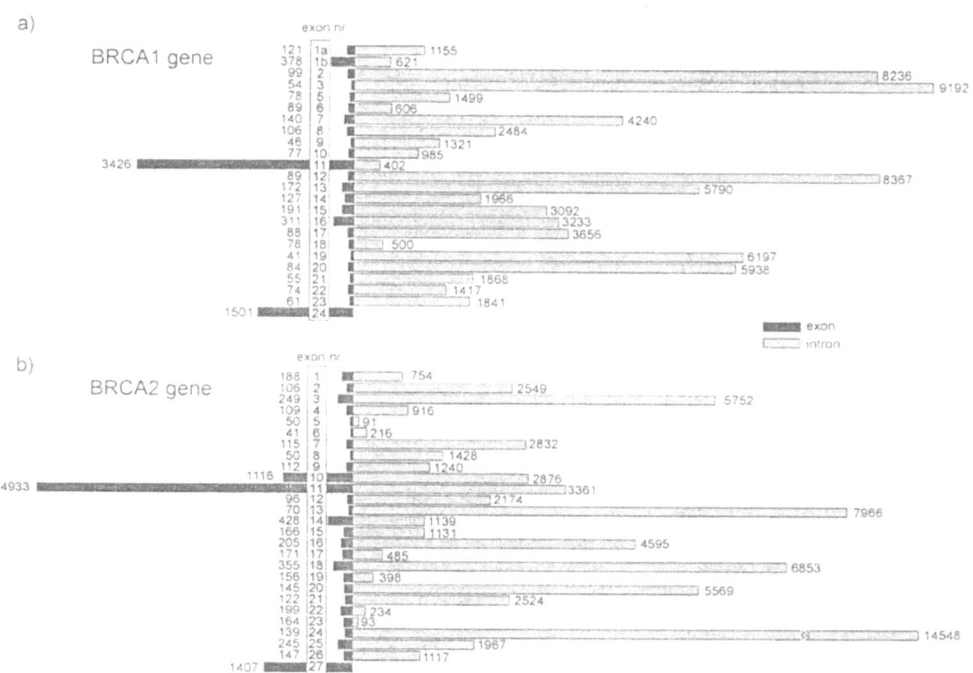

Figure 1. Exon/intron structure of (a) the *BRCA1* and (b) *BRCA2* genes. Dark bars on the left represent exons and light bars on the right – introns. Except for *BRCA2* intron 24 the bar length corresponds to exon or intron length. The lengths of all exons and introns (in bp) are indicated.

sequence; two basic motifs at amino acids 503–508 and 606–615 [11] which could serve as nuclear localization signals; and the transcription activation domain at amino acids 1750–1863 [12].

Important structural and functional domains in proteins can also be identified by comparing sequences of the same gene in different species. The nucleotide sequences of murine and canine *Brca1* were determined and compared with the human sequence [10, 13, 14]. A striking finding of this analysis was a very low level of identity between the sequences, much lower than in the case of proteins encoded by other cancer-predisposing genes. The amino acid sequence of murine Brca1 is only 58% identical to human BRCA1 [10], the canine sequence is 73.8% identical [10], whereas the identity of human and mouse NF1 and NF2 is 98%, WT1 95%, APC and VHL 90%, ATM 84% and TP53 78% [15]. Despite the low level of identity between the complete human, murine and canine sequences, some regions of the proteins are significantly less divergent (Fig. 2a). For example, the amino terminal 120 residues of the gene are more than 80% identical among the three species [10]. The C-terminus is highly conserved, containing a stretch of 67 amino acids which are 85% identical [10]. The granin consensus sequence is also highly maintained [9]. The RING finger motif is, however, the most conserved. Its 40 amino acids are

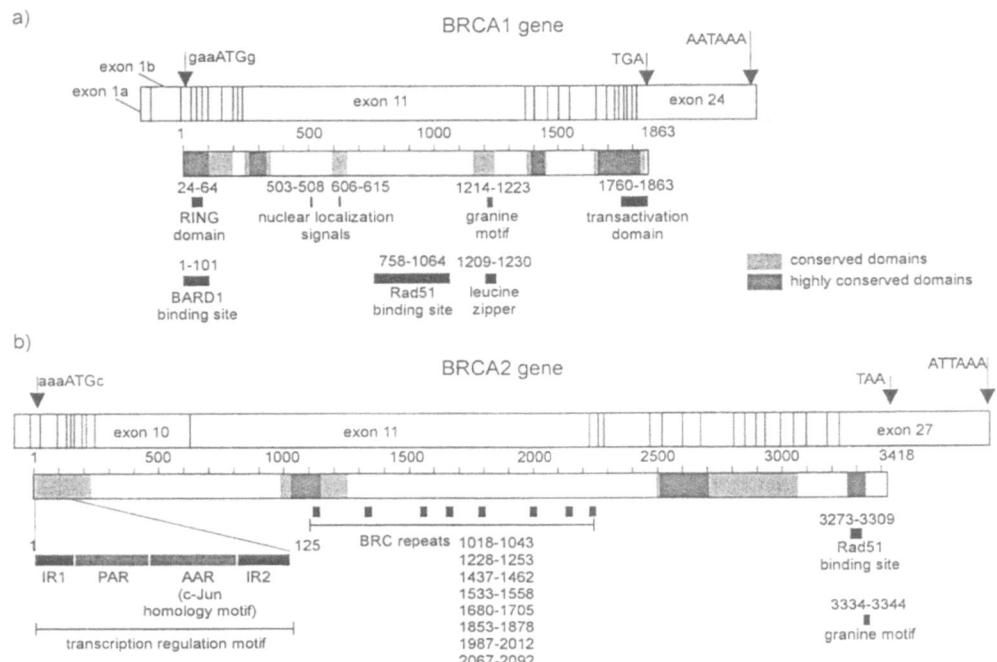

Figure 2. Diagram of the (a) *BRCA1* and (b) *BRCA2* mRNA and protein structure including the conserved regions and putative functional domains.

identical in human and murine sequences, and the canine sequence differs in only one amino acid K55E [10]. Of the basic motifs, the second one, residues 604–614, is perfectly conserved [10].

The *BRCA2* gene was localized by linkage analysis to human chromosome 13q12-13 in 1994 [16], and the following year the gene was identified by positional cloning [17]. The complete sequence of the *BRCA2* gene and protein was reported in 1996 [18]. The gene contains 27 exons distributed over the 84 kb of genomic DNA, and encodes a large protein of 3418 amino acids. The *BRCA2* gene, like *BRCA1*, has a translation start codon in exon 2, and a very large exon 11, spanning 4933 bp, and encoding almost half of the BRCA2 protein [18]. The exon/intron structure of the *BRCA2* gene is shown in Figure 1b. Neither the gene nor the protein was shown to have a significant sequence similarity to other DNA and protein sequences deposited in databases. The exception was the short sequence fragment, known as granin motif, in the BRCA2 C-terminal [9], which is also present in the central part of BRCA1. When the sequence was compared with itself, by dot matrix analysis, the presence of an internal repeat was revealed (Fig. 2b). A segment of exon 11 contained eight repetitive units, composed of 30–80 amino acids, termed the BRC repeats [19]. Later, the murine *Brca2* sequence was determined [15]. The mouse protein is shorter, composed of 3329 amino acids [15]. Although overall identity between the two protein sequences is only 59 % [15], as low as in the case of BRCA1 [10], some parts of the sequence are more conserved (Fig. 2b). For example, the 115 amino acid stretch, residues 2501–2616, is in 92% identical [15]. Among the more conserved regions are the BRC repeats [19]. However, the significance of the granin motif had to be questioned, based on human and murine sequence comparisons. The murine motif further departs from the poorly defined granin consensus in the human *BRCA2* gene.

More recently, it was found that exon 3 of *BRCA2*, residues 60–105, which is within the region highly conserved in human and mouse, shows a significant sequence similarity to the transcription activation domain of *c-Jun* [20]. BRCA2 amino acids 23–105 were shown to activate transcription in yeast and mammalian cells, when fused to a DNA binding domain of a reporter gene. It was shown in these studies that BRCA2 residues 18–60 represent a primary, and residues 60–105 an auxiliary activating region. There are also two inhibitory regions, IR1 and IR2, located on either side of exon 3, which completely mask the activating potential of the BRCA2 protein [20]. This type of transcription regulation is known from several transcription factors.

Information about protein function can also be obtained from analysis of its pattern of expression, cellular localization and specific interactions with other proteins. Both *BRCA1* and *BRCA2* show widespread expression, in testis, brain, eye, ovary, and in mammary gland where they are highly induced on pregnancy. A very similar pattern of expression suggests that these genes may be coordinately regulated [15, 21]. There are also reports on cancer-related changes in *BRCA1* expression. A ten-fold reduction in *BRCA1* mRNA levels was observed in breast tumour specimens relative to normal breast tissue [22]. Furthermore, the decrease of *BRCA1* expression in MCF7 cell lines, mediated by antisense oligonucleotides, increased proliferative potential of the cells [22]. In agreement with the above, a retroviral transfer of the wildtype *BRCA1* gene to breast and ovarian cancer cell lines resulted in inhibition of their growth [23]. A similar effect was observed with MCF7 tumours in nude mice transfected with the wildtype *BRCA1* [23]. Survival of the mice increased significantly after transfection [23].

Several conflicting results were reported concerning the cellular localization of the BRCA1 protein. They suggested nuclear, or nuclear and cytoplasmic, or extracellular localization. Extracellular localization, consistent with granin function [9], was not confirmed by further studies [24]. According to other authors BRCA1 is a 220 kD nuclear phosphoprotein [25] that shows aberrant cytoplasmic localization in breast and ovarian tumour cells [26]. It was also demonstrated that the expression and phoshorylation of BRCA1 is cell cycle dependent [25]. The expression is elevated in the S and M phases and the BRCA1 protein binds to cyclin-dependent kinases associated with cyclins A and D [25]. These observations were confirmed by other authors [27]. They showed that *BRCA1* is poorly expressed in phases G0 and early G1, while high levels of the protein are present in the late G1 and S phases. *BRCA2* expression was also shown to vary according to the cell cycle, and the pattern of its expression was the same as in case of *BRCA1* [15, 21].

The BRCA1 protein interacts *in vivo* with BARD1 (BRCA1-associated RING domain) protein [28]. The N-terminal region of BRCA1 is involved in this interaction. BARD1 also contains the N-terminal RING motif, the C-terminal sequence similarity to BRCA1, and three ankyrin repeats: sequences of 33 amino acids present in several regulatory proteins. In support of functional significance of the BRCA1/BARD1 interaction in tumour suppression is the fact that their complex is disrupted by missense mutations in the conserved BRCA1 N-terminus [28].

Immunostaining of the BRCA1 protein during the S-phase of the cell cycle revealed similar nuclear localization of BRCA1 and human Rad51 protein [29]. These proteins coimmunoprecipitate, which suggests their functional interaction in the mitotic and meiotic cell cycles. It was also demonstrated that BRCA1 residues 758–1064 are alone capable of forming *in vitro* complexes with Rad51 [29] (Fig. 2a). In yeast, rad51 participates in double stranded break repair and meiotic recombination [30]. In human cells, Rad51 interacts *in vivo* also with TP53, which plays a central role in the cellular response to DNA damage [31]. BRCA1 contains a putative TP53 interaction sequence, distinct from the Rad51 interaction site [30]. These facts suggest that *BRCA1* may be a caretaker gene that participates in Rad51 DNA repair function. Very recently, it was demonstrated that the murine Brca2 protein also interacts with Rad51, and the minimum region that showed a strong association with Rad51 was the C-terminal 36 amino acid fragment, residues 3196–3232, which is 95% identical in mouse and human proteins [32] (Fig. 2b). Rad51 uses its N-terminal sequence amino acids 1–43 in this interaction [32]. As Rad51 serves to suppress tumour formation *via* interaction with both BRCA1 and BRCA2, this protein might itself also be the product of a tumour suppressor gene. Human *Rad51* maps to chromosome 15q15.1 which often shows loss of heterozygosity (LOH) in breast tumours [33, 34].

Earlier, murine models proved very helpful in understanding the biology of human diseases, and so mice deficient in the *Brca1* gene were developed. *Brca1* knockout mice, homozygous for the exon 11 deletion, died between the 10th and 13th day of embryonic development, showing a variety of neuroepithelial defects [35]. Other mice, homozygous for the deleted exons 5 and 6, were even more severely affected, and died at day 7.5 of gestation, showing reduced cell proliferation and no signs of mesoderm formation [35]. In contrast, mice heterozygous for the *Brca1* mutation showed no evidence of cancer after one year of age [35]. Similarly, *Brca2*-deficient mice embryos suffer an overall development arrest after 6.5 days of gestation [35]. The homozygous mutant *Brca2* phenotype is similar to the murine *Rad51* mutant phenotype, which again suggests that *Brca2*, *Brca1* and *Rad51* may function in similar pathways [35]. Radiation sensitivity assays show that *Brca2* and Rad51 deficient cells are hypersensitive to radiation, which may have important implications for therapy of the cancers in which defects in these genes are involved [32].

Taken together, the *BRCA1* and *BRCA2* genes show similarity in unusual gene organization, low sequence conservation and expression pattern. The proteins they encode are very large and have the potential to perform several functions. Although they have no apparent sequence similarity, their similar cellular localization, and interaction with the same DNA repair protein, suggest their function in maintaining genome integrity. It is indeed very likely that they belong to the class of caretaker genes.

Mutations in *BRCA1* and *BRCA2* genes

Besides efforts to determine the function of *BRCA* genes, the identification and characterization of their cancer-predisposing mutations became another research priority. An enormous activity in this area began immediately after the *BRCA* genes were isolated. It has been necessary to compile a comprehensive list of mutations in order to develop a reliable genetic test. A detailed knowledge of penetrance and the clinical expression of specific mutations has been required to offer genetic counseling based on a precise cancer risk assessment. In the first period of this research nearly all studies were carried out in breast-ovarian and breast cancer families. According to linkage studies, and early results of mutation analysis, conducted in approximately 200 families with at least four cases of breast cancer, 50% of these families were linked to *BRCA1*, 30% to *BRCA2*, and the rest showed no linkage to either of the genes [36]. This suggested the existence of yet unidentified gene(s) responsible for the substantial fraction of hereditary breast cancer.

The lifelong risks of developing breast and ovarian cancer were estimated from studies of families with multiple affected members. In case of *BRCA1* mutation carriers, the risk figures reported by different authors ranged from 76 to 87% for breast cancer [16, 37–40] and from 32 to 84% for ovarian cancer [16, 38–40]. In case of *BRCA2* mutation carriers, the estimated risk of breast cancer was as high as for *BRCA1* but the risk of ovarian cancer was significantly lower [17]. However, there is a prevailing opinion that these risk figures were overestimated, as they derived from atypical cancer-dense families.

Less biased samples were then subjected to analysis: women with the early onset breast cancer [41–43], unselected females [44–47] and males [48–50] diagnosed with breast cancer, unselected ovarian cancer patients [47, 51–58], men diagnosed with prostate cancer [59] and women attending clinics that evaluate the risk of breast cancer [60]. One of the largest studies of this series [58], aimed at determining the contribution of *BRCA1* mutations to ovarian cancer in the general population, included 374 women diagnosed with epithelial ovarian cancer before the age of 70. It was concluded from these studies that the mutations in *BRCA1* occur in about 5% of all ovarian cancer cases in Great Britain. Similar frequency value was estimated for the U.S. population, based on results from three population-based case-control studies of ovarian cancer [40]. According to the later studies, the *BRCA1* mutations contribute to 5.3% of all ovarian cancers and to 4.2% of all breast cancers in the U.S.

Most population-based studies revealed that a substantial proportion of the mutation carriers had no family history of breast or ovarian cancer. Thus, a striking family history cannot be the sole selection criterion in attempts to identify all carriers of mutations in the *BRCA* genes. Francis Collins explained why the lack of family history among mutation carriers is, in some cases at least, not surprising [61]. Men carrying *BRCA1* mutations have only a moderately increased risk of prostate cancer, and they often do not develop the disease. Therefore women who inherit the mutant *BRCA1* gene paternally will frequently not have an affected first-degree relative.

Present knowledge regarding the frequency and penetrance of mutations in the *BRCA* genes is most advanced for the Ashkenazi Jewish population. A combined frequency of the three most prevalent mutations, 185delAG and 5382insC in *BRCA1* and 6174delT in *BRCA2* exceeds 2% in this genetically distinct population of Jews of eastern European descent [62–64]. In the most comprehensive population-based study that included 5318 Jews, men and women from the Washington D.C. area, many carriers of these mutations were identified by simple tests, and the associated risks of cancer were established [65]. Among 120 mutation carriers, 59 had the 6174delT mutation, 41 carried the 185delAG mutation and in 12 individuals the 5382insC mutation was found [65]. The risks of cancer estimated by comparing cancer histories of relatives of the carriers and noncarriers turned out to be significantly lower than those reported earlier. The risk of breast cancer by the age of 70 was determined to be 56%, of ovarian cancer 16%, and of prostate cancer also 16%, for the three mutations combined [65]. The risks for individual mutations were also evaluated. Although the values obtained were not statistically significant, it was observed that the most prevalent 6174delT mutation in *BRCA2* confers only slightly lower risk of breast cancer than the 185delAG mutation in *BRCA1* [65]. Earlier results suggested much higher risk for the 185delAG mutation carriers [41, 43, 63, 64, 66]. The highest risk of breast cancer, as well as of ovarian cancer, seems to be associated with the presence of the 5382insC mutation [65]. The two mutations in *BRCA1* confer higher risk of prostate cancer than the mutation in *BRCA2* [65]. This largest study so far also showed that a high proportion of the mutation carriers, about 26% had no family history of breast and ovarian cancer [65]. Thus, the risk of cancer among mutation carriers is highly variable. Due to the fact that the risk modifying factors involved are still unknown, the problem of variable penetrance and expression of the specific mutations, between and within families, will not be quickly solved. The identification of genetic and environmental factors that modify the impact of specific mutations in the *BRCA* genes must therefore become another research priority in the coming years.

In the case of other populations and ethnic groups the research is generally less advanced. The data accumulated so far suggest that mutations in the *BRCA* genes are less prevalent, and individual mutations less frequent, than those characteristic for the Ashkenazi Jews. One exception may be the 999del5 mutation in the *BRCA2* gene found in men with breast cancer in Iceland [45, 67]. The large size of *BRCA1* and *BRCA2* does not allow screening the entire genes in thousands of individuals representing the general population, to estimate precisely carrier frequencies and the risks associated with mutations. Despite these difficulties, research is in progress and new mutations are reported not only from the United States, Canada, western and northern Europe and Japan but also from eastern [68, 69] and central Europe [70–72].

For example, in Poland, where breast cancer morbidity is approximately one third of that known for the U.S. population, and about two times lower than the European average, a search for mutations in the *BRCA1* gene was conducted [70]. Participants in that study were from the Poznan region in western Poland where the incidence of breast cancer is the highest in the country. Analysis of the *BRCA1* gene in 122 women with positive, but mostly moderate family history of breast and/or ovarian cancer, 34 unselected breast cancer tissues specimens, and 80 controls revealed three novel mutations, one novel common polymorphism, two new rare sequence variants and an unusually high frequency of the 12 bp insertion/duplication in intron 20. The incidence of *BRCA1* mutations and variants in the analysed groups is shown in Figure 3. The high frequency of the alteration in intron-20 is particularly interesting. In earlier studies this insertion was always associated with a serious medical history of cancer, and was not found in many controls. Only one in five Polish women with this insertion resembled the patients described earlier. We have shown that this insertion does not impair splicing [70].The relation of this intronic alteration to cancer needs therefore to be clarified by further studies. Analysing the small set of tumour samples, we found the Trp > STOP mutation in exon 22, which turned out to be a germline mutation. It occurred in a patient in whose tumour tissue the somatic p53 mutation Pro278Ala had earlier been found. This observation gave new insight into the molecular mechanism of breast tumour development, by showing that during the process of multistep carcinogenesis the *p53* gene mutation can also occur with a background of mutated *BRCA1*. The result of our study suggests that in tissue specimens harboring germline mutations in *BRCA1* or *BRCA2* a systematic search for somatic mutations in other breast cancer-related genes is required.

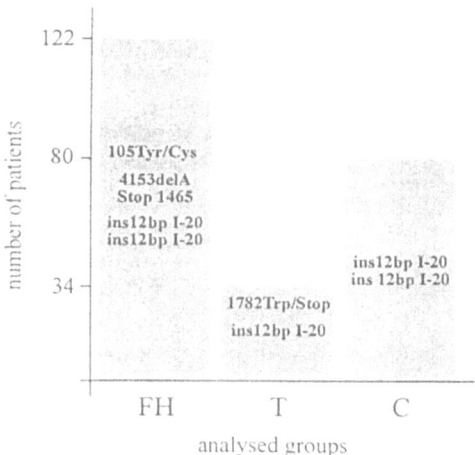

Figure 3. The incidence of *BRCA1* mutations and intronic alteration in the analyzed sample of Polish women with positive family history of breast and/or ovarian cancer (FH), tumor samples (T) and controls (C).

It will help to distinguish between the mutation pathways leading to hereditary and sporadic cancers. Our study also showed that more population-oriented research is needed, involving women with less profound or even no family history of breast and ovarian cancer, to understand better the role and significance of different *BRCA1* variants and mutations.

Genetic susceptibility to breast and ovarian cancer seems not to be entirely determined by mutations in the *BRCA* genes, which are rare but confer a high lifetime risk. Common genetic polymorphisms also contribute to cancer predisposition by modulating the influence of environmental and genetic risk factors [73]. In the *BRCA* genes a number of common polymorphic variants have been described so far, 17 in *BRCA1* and 7 in *BRCA2*. There are also many less frequent polymorphisms and rare sequence variants. It was reasonable to expect that at least some of the polymorphic variants, especially those resulting from missense amino acids substitutions, confer different risks of breast and/or ovarian cancer than other variants. These expectations proved correct, and one study demonstrated a higher predisposition to breast cancer associated with the Leu871Pro polymorphic variant [74]. The opposite, protective effect against breast cancer was shown for the Gln356Arg variant [75]. Residue 356, however, is not located within any functional or highly conserved *BRCA1* domain. This suggests that the Arg 356 allele may not be directly responsible for the protective effect, but is perhaps within some specific, protective haplotype [75].

The Breast Cancer Information Core (BIC) database established in 1995 plays an important role in facilitating research and gives easy access to all published and unpublished mutations [76]. By the end of May 1997 the BIC database contained more than 1000 entries for *BRCA1* and about 150 entries for *BRCA2* (Fig. 4). In case of the *BRCA1* gene this number included 340 distinct mutations, polymorphisms and rare variants. Altogether there were about 660 definite mutations. Among 180 distinct mutations 119 were frameshift, 46 nonsense and 15 missense. Of

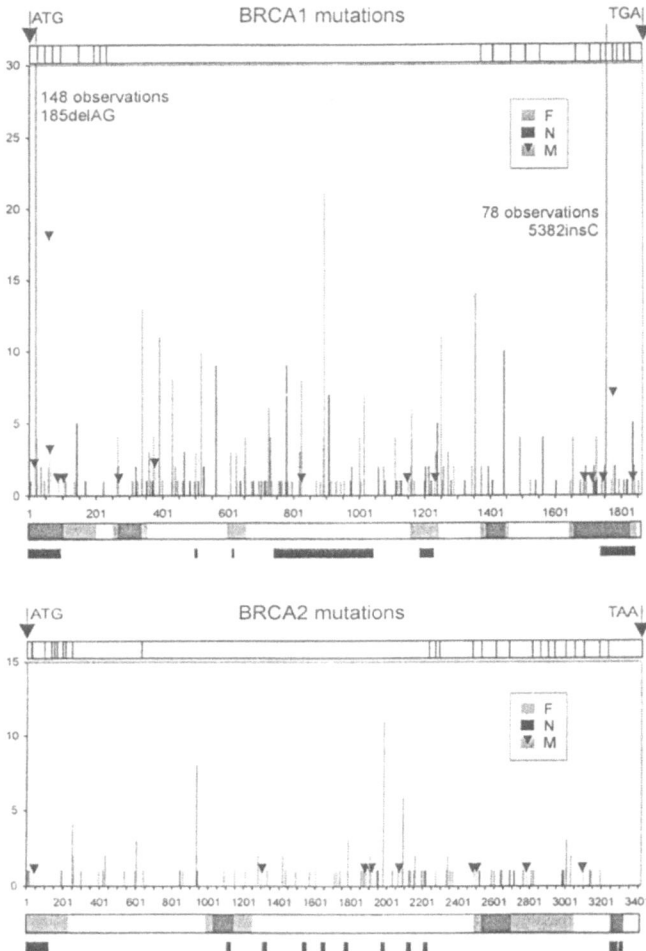

Figure 4. Summary of (a) *BRCA1* and (b) *BRCA2* mutations deposited to the BIC database. Positions of frameshift (black), nonsense (gray) and missense (gray with arrowhead) mutations are shown along the mRNA sequence (top) and protein sequence (bottom). Positions of start and stop codons, conserved and functional domains are also indicated.

the *BRCA2* entries, there were 113 distinct mutations, polymorphisms and rare variants. As in the case of *BRCA1*, the frameshift mutations dominated. There were 76 distinct frameshift mutations, 13 nonsense and 11 missense. The eight most frequent *BRCA1* mutations, repeated more than ten times each, make a total of 315 (48%) of all mutations deposited in the database. Among them there are three mutations which were reported more than 20 times each. They comprise 37% of all *BRCA1* mutations reported to the *BRCA1* BIC database.

From the perspective of genetic testing for breast cancer susceptibility, the spectra of mutations in *BRCA* genes look very complicated (Fig. 4). The distribution of mutations, although uneven in different coding sequence regions, does not allow focusing of the analysis on some exons and omitting others. The exception is the Ashkenazi Jewish population discussed earlier. Of the methods used for mutation detection, direct sequencing gives the best results, but is very expensive. About 80 amplicons from the two *BRCA* genes have to be sequenced in both directions to obtain reliable data. Protein truncation test gives good results as 94% of *BRCA1* mutations and 92% of *BRCA2* mutations identified so far are frameshift or nonsense and lead to truncated proteins. The most popular is, however, the SSCP technique which is simple, rapid and effective in detecting mutations [77]. When SSCP is combined with heteroduplex analysis it is capable of detecting the majority of missense, nonsense and splicing mutations, and perhaps all frameshift mutations. It is amenable to multiplexing and to analysing PCR products amplified from pooled genomic DNA samples [78]. In principle, this approach may be very efficient and cost-effective in large-scale screening of the *BRCA* genes. Future methods will use 'DNA chips' for detecting mutations by hybridization. The first application of this technology in *BRCA1* gene analysis has already been reported [79]. The question remains: when will this technique become widely available?

Acknowledgements
Supported by the grant 6P04B00212 from the Polish Committee for Scientific Research.

References

1. Kinzler KW, Vogelstein B (1997) Gatekeepers and caretakers. *Nature* 386: 761–763.
2. Hall JM, Lee MK, Newman B, Morrow JE, Anderson LA, Huey B, King M-C (1990) Linkage of early-onset familial breast cancer to chromosome 17q21. *Science* 250: 1684–1689.
3. Narod SA, Feunteun J, Lunch HT, Watson P, Conway T, Lynch J, Lenoire GM (1991) Familial breast-ovarian cancer locus on chromosome 17q12-q23. *Lancet* 338: 82–83.
4. Miki Y, Swensen J, Shattuck-Eidens D, Futreal PA, Harshman K, Tavtigian S, Liu Q, Cochran C, Bennett LM, Ding W et al. (1994) A strong candidate for the breast and ovarian cancer susceptibility gene BRCA1. *Science* 266: 66–71.
5. Smith TM, Lee MK, Szabo CI, Jerome N, McEuen M, Taylor M, Hood L, King M-C (1996) Complete genomic sequence and analysis of 117 kb of human DNA containing the gene BRCA1. *Genome Res* 6: 1029–1049.
6. Brown MA, Xu C-F, Nicolai H, Griffiths B, Chambers JA, Black D, Solomon E (1996) The 5' end of the BRCA1 gene lies within a duplicated region of human chromosome 17q21. *Oncogene* 12: 2507–2513.
7. Brown MA, Xu C-F, Nicolai H, Griffiths B, Jones KA, Solomon E, Hosking L, Trowsdale J, Black DM, McFarlane R (1994) Regulation of BRCA1. *Nature* 372: 733.
8. Barker DF, Liu X, Almeida ER (1996) The BRCA1 and 1A1.3B promoters are parallel elements of a genomic duplication at 17q21. *Genomics* 38: 215–222.
9. Jensen RA, Thompson ME, Jetton TL, Szabo CI, van der Meer R, Helou B, Tronick SR, Page DL, King M-C, Holt JT (1996) BRCA1 is secreted and exhibits properties of a granin. *Nat Genet* 12: 303–222.
10. Szabo CI, Wagner LA, Francisco LV, Roach JC, Argonza R, King M-C, Ostrander EA (1996) Human, canine and murine BRCA1 genes: sequence comparison among species. *Hum Mol Genet* 5: 1289–1298.
11. Chen C-F, Li S, Chen Y, Chen P-L, Sharp ZD, Lee W-H (1996) The nuclear localization sequences of the BRCA1 protein interact with the importin-α subunit of the nuclear transport signal receptor. *J Biol Chem* 271: 32863–32868.
12. Monteiro MN, August A, Hanafusa H (1996) Evidence for a transcriptional activation function of BRCA1 C-terminal region. *Proc Natl Acad Sci USA* 93: 13595–13599.
13. Abel KJ, Xu J, Yin G-Y, Lyons RH, Meisler MH, Weber BL (1995) Mouse Brca1: localization, sequence analysis and identification of evolutionary conserved domains. *Hum Mol Genet* 4: 2265–2273.

14. Sharan SK, Wims M, Bradley A (1995) Murine Brca1: sequence and significance for human missense mutations. *Hum Mol Genet* 4: 2275–2278.
15. Connor R, Smith A, Wooster R, Stratton M, Dixon A, Campbell E, Tait T-M, Freeman T, Ashworth A (1997) Cloning, chromosomal mapping and expression pattern of the mouse Brca2 gene. *Hum Mol Genet* 6: 291–300.
16. Wooster R, Neuhausen SL, Mangion J, Quirk Y, Ford D, Collins N, Nguyen K, Seal S, Tran T, Averill D (1994) Localization of a breast cancer susceptibility gene, BRCA2, to chromosome 13q12-13. *Science* 256: 2088–2090.
17. Wooster R, Bignel G, Lancaster J, Swift S, Seal S, Mangion J, Collins N, Gregory S, Gumbs C, Micklem G et al. (1995) Identification of the breast cancer susceptibility gene BRCA2. *Nature* 378: 789–792.
18. Tavtigian SV, Simard J, Rommens Couch F, Shattuck-Eidens D, Neuhausen S, Merajver S, Thorlacius S, Offit K (1996) The complete BRCA2 gene and mutations in chromosome 13q-linked kindreds. *Nat Genet* 12: 333–337.
19. Bingel G, Micklem G, Stratton MR, Ashworth A, Wooster R (1997) The BRC repeats are conserved in mammalian BRCA2 proteins. *Hum Mol Genet* 6: 53–58.
20. Milner J, Ponder B, Hughes-Davies L, Seltmann M, Kouzarides T (1997) Transcriptional activation functions in BRCA2. *Nature* 386: 772–773.
21. Rajan JV, Wang M, Marquis ST, Chodosh LA (1996) Brca2 is coordinately regulated with Brca1 during proliferation and differentiation in mammary epithelial calls. *Proc Natl Acad Sci USA* 93: 13078–13083.
22. Thompson ME, Jensen RA, Obermiller PS, Page DL, Holt JT (1995) Decreased expression of BRCA1 accelerates growth and is often present during sporadic breast cancer progression. *Nat Genet* 9: 444–450.
23. Holt JM, Thompson ME, Szabo C, Robinson-Benion C, Arteaga CL, King M-C, Jensen RA (1996) Growth retardation and tumor inhibition by BRCA1. *Nat Genet* 12: 298–302.
24. Wilson CA, Payton MN, Pekar SK, Zhang K, Pacifi RE, Gudas JL, Thukral S, Calzone FJ, Reese DM, Slamon DI (1996) BRCA1 protein products: antibody specificity. *Nat Genet* 13: 264–265.
25. Chen Y, Farmer AA, Chen C-F, Jones C, Chen P-L, Lee W-H (1996) BRCA1 is a 220-kDa phosphoprotein that is expressed and phosphorylated in a cell cycle-dependent manner. *Cancer Res* 56: 3168–3172.
26. Chen Y, Chen CF, Riley DJ, Allerd DC, Chen PL, Von Hoff D, Osborne CK, Lee WH (1995) Aberrant subcellular localization of BRCA1 in breast cancer. *Science* 270: 789–791.
27. Vaughn JP, Davis PL, Jarboe MD, Huper G, Evans AC, Wiseman RW, Berchuck A, Iglehart JD, Futreal PA, Marks JR (1996) BRCA1 expression is induced before DNA synthesis in both normal and tumor-derived breast cells. *Cell Growth Diff* 7: 711–715.
28. Wu LJ, Wang ZW, Tsan JT, Spillman MA, Phung A, Xu XL, Yang M-HW, Hwang L-Y, Bowcock AM, Baer R (1996) Identification of a RING protein that can interact *in vivo* with BRCA1 gene product. *Nat Genet* 14: 430–440.
29. Scully R, Chen J, Plug A, Xiao Y, Weaver D, Feunteun J, Ashly T, Livingston DM (1997) Association of BRCA1 with Rad51 in mitotic and meiotic cells. *Cell* 88: 265–275.
30. Koonin VF, Altschul SF, Bork P (1996) BRCA1 protein products: functional motifs. *Nat Genet* 13: 266–267.
31. Sturzbecher HW, Donzelmann B, Henning W, Knippschild U, Buchhop S (1996) p53 is linked directly to homologous recombination processes *via* RAD51/RecA protein interaction. *EMBO J* 15: 1992–2002.
32. Sharan S, Morimatsu M, Albrecht U, Lim D-S, Regel E, Dinh C, Sands A, Eichele G, Hasty P, Allan B (1997) Embryonic lethality and radiation hypersensitive mediated by Rad51 in mice lacking BRCA2. *Nature* 386: 804–810.
33. Devilee P, van Vliet M, van Sloun P, Kuipers Dijkshoorn N, Hermans J, Pearson PL, Cornelisse CJ (1991) Allelotype of human breast carcinoma: a second major site for heterozygosity is on chromosome 6q. *Oncogene* 6: 1705–1711.
34. Wick W, Petersen I, Schmutzler RK, Wolfarth B, Lenartz D, Bierhoff E, Hummerich J, Muller DJ, Schramm J, Wiestler OD et al. (1996) Evidence for a novel tumor suppressor gene on chromosome 15 associated with progression to a metastatic stage in breast cancer. *Oncogene* 12: 973–978.
35. Hakem R, de la Pompa JL, Sirard C, Mo R, Woo M, Hakem A, Wakeham A, Potter J, Reitmair A, Billia F et al. (1996) The tumor suppressor gene Brca1 is required for embryonic cellular proliferation in the mouse. *Cell* 85: 1009–1023.
36. Szabo CI, King M-C (1995) Inherited breast and ovarian cancer. *Hum Mol Genet* 4: 1811–1817.
37. Easton DF, Bishop DT, Ford D, Crockford GP (1993) Genetic linkage analysis in familial breast and ovarian cancer: results from 214 families. The Breast Cancer Linkage Consortium. *Am J Hum Genet* 52: 678–701.
38. Ford D, Easton DF, Bishop DT, Narod SA, Goldgar DE, Breast Cancer Linkage Consortium (1994) Risk of cancer in BRCA1-mutation carriers. *Lancet* 343: 692–695.
39. Easton DF, Ford D, Bishop DT (1995) Breast and ovarian cancer incidence in BRCA1-mutation carriers. *Am J Hum Genet* 8: 8–18.
40. Whittemore AS, Gong G, Intyre J (1997) Prevelance and contribution of BRCA1 mutations in breast cancer and ovarian cancer: results from three U.S. population-based case-control studies of ovarian cancer. *Am J Hum Genet* 60: 496–504.

41. FitzGerald MG, MacDonald DJ, Krainer M, Hoover I, O'Neil E, Unsal H, Silva-Arrieto S, Finkelstein DM, Beer-Romero P, Englert C et al. (1996) Germ-line BRCA1 mutations in Jewish and non-Jewish women with early-onset breast cancer. *N Engl J Med* 334: 143–149.

42. Langston AA, Malone KE, Thompson JD, Dailing JR, Ostrander EA (1996) BRCA1 mutations in a population-based sample of young women with breast cancer. *N Engl J Med* 334: 137–142.

43. Krainer M, Silva-Arrieta S, FitzGerald MD, Shimada A, Ishioka C, Kanamaru R, MacDonald DJ, Unsal H, Finkelstein DM, Bowcock A et al. (1997) Differential contribution of BRCA1 and BRCA2 to early-onset breast cancer. *N Engl J Med* 336: 1416–1421.

44. Miki Y, Katagiri T, Kasumi F, Yoshimoto T, Nakamura Y (1996) Mutation analysis in the BRCA2 gene in primary breast cancers. *Nat Genet* 13: 245–247.

45. Johannesdottir G, Gudmundsson J, Bergthorsson JT, Arason A, Agnarsson BA, Eiriksdottir G, Johannsson OT, Borg A, Ingvarsson S, Easton DF et al. (1996) High prevalence of the 999del5 mutation in icelandic breast and ovarian cancer patients. *Cancer Res* 56: 3663–3665.

46. Teng DH, Bogden R, Mitchell J, Baumgard M, Bell R, Berry S, Davis T, Ha PC, Kehrer R, Jammulapati S et al. (1996) Low incidence of BRCA2 mutations in breast carcinoma and other cancers. *Nat Genet* 13: 241–244.

47. Lancaster JM, Wooster R, Mangion J, Phelan CM, Cochran C, Gumbs C, Seal S, Barfoot R, Collins N, Bignell G et al. (1996) BRCA2 mutations in primary breast and ovarian cancers. *Nat Genet* 13: 238–240.

48. Friedman LS, Gayther SA, Kurosaki T, Gordon D, Noble B, Casey G, Ponder BAJ, Anton-Culver H (1997) Mutation analysis of BRCA1 and BRCA2 in a male breast cancer population. *Am J Hum Genet* 60: 313–318.

49. Thorlacius S, Olafsdottir G, Tryggvadottir L, Neuhausen S, Jonasson JG, Tavtigian SV, Tulinius H, Ogmundsdottir HM, Eyfjord JE (1996) A single BRCA2 mutation in male and female breast cancer families from Iceland with varied cancer phenotypes. *Nat Genet* 13: 117–119.

50. Couch FJ, Farid LM, DeShano ML, Tavtigian SV, Calzone K, Campeau L, Peng Y, Bogden B, Chen Q, Neuhausen S et al. (1996) BRCA2 germline mutations in male breast cancer cases and breast cancer families. *Nat Genet* 1: 123–125.

51. Foster KA, Harrington P, Kerr J, Russell P, DiCioccio RA, Scott IV, Jacobs I, Chenevix-Trench G, Ponder BA, Gayther SA (1996) Somatic and germline mutations of the BRCA2 gene in sporadic ovarian cancer. *Cancer Res* 56: 3622–3625.

52. Modan B, Gak E, Sade-Bruchim RB, Hirsh-Yechezkel G, Theodor L, Lubin F, Ben-Baruch G, Beller U, Fishman A, Dgani R et al. (1996) High frequency of BRCA1 185delAG mutation in ovarian cancer in Israel. National Israel Study of Ovarian Cancer. *JAMA* 276: 1823–1825.

53. Shushan A, Abeliovich D, Peretz T, Weinberg N, Paltiel O (1997) BRCA1 mutations in women with ovarian cancer. *JAMA* 277: 963.

54. Merajver SD, Pham TM, Caduff RF, Chen M, Poy EL, Cooney KA, Weber BL, Collins FS, Johnston C, Frank TS (1995) Somatic mutations in the BRCA1 gene in sporadic ovarian tumours. *Nat Genet* 9: 439–443.

55. Matsushima M, Kobayashi K, Emi M, Saito H, Saito J, Suzumori K, Nakamura Y (1995) Mutation analysis of the BRCA1 gene in 76 Japanese ovarian cancer patients: four germline mutations, but no evidence of somatic mutation. *Hum Mol Genet* 4: 1953–1956.

56. Takahashi H, Chiu HC, Bandera CA, Behbakht K, Liu PC, Couch FJ, Weber BL, LiVolsi VA, Furusato M, Rebane BA et al. (1996) Mutations of the BRCA2 gene in ovarian carcinomas. *Cancer Res* 56: 2738–2741.

57. Rubin SC, Benjamin I, Behbakht K, Takahashi H, Morgan MA, LiVolsi VA, Berchuck A, Muto MG, Garber JE, Weber BL et al. (1996) Clinical and pathological features of ovarian cancer in women with germ-line mutations of brca1. *N Engl J Med* 335: 1413–1416.

58. Stratton JF, Gayther SA, Russel P, Dearden J, Gore M, Blake P, Easton D, Ponder BA (1997) Contribution of BRCA1 mutations to ovarian cancer. *N Engl J Med* 336: 1125–1130.

59. Langston AA, Stanford JL, Wicklund KG, Thompson JD, Blazej RG, Ostrander EA (1996) Germ-line BRCA1 mutations in selected men with prostate cancer. *Am J Hum Genet* 58: 881–884.

60. Couch FJ, DeShand ML, Blackwood A, Ganguly A, Rebbeck T, Weber B (1997) BRCA1 mutations in women attending clinics that evaluate the risk of breast cancer. *N Engl J Med* 336: 1409–1415.

61. Collins FS (1996) BRCA1 – lots of mutations, lots of dilemmas. *N Engl J Med* 334: 186–188.

62. Struewing JP, Abelovich D, Perez T, Avishai N, Kaback MM, Collins FS, Brody LC (1995) The carrier frequency of the BRCA1 185delAG mutation is approximately 1 percent in Ashkenazi Jewish individuals. *Nat Genet* 11: 198–200.

63. Roa BB, Boyd AA, Volcik K, Richards CS (1996) Ashkenazi Jewish population frequencies for common mutations in BRCA1 and BRCA2. *Nat Genet* 14: 185–187.

64. Oddoux C, Struewing JP, Clayton CM, Neuhausen S, Brody LC, Kaback M, Haas B, Norton L, Borgen P, Jhanwar S et al. (1996) The carrier frequency of the BRCA2 6174delT mutation among Ashkenazi Jewish individuals is approximately 1%. *Nat Genet* 14: 188–190.

65. Struewing JP, Hartge P, Wacholder S, Baker SM, Berlin M, McAdams M, Timmerman MM, Brody AL, Tucker M (1997) The risk of cancer associated with specific mutations of BRCA1 and BRCA2 among Ashkenazi Jews. *N Engl J Med* 336: 1401–1406.

66. Offit K, Gilewski T, McGuire P, Schluger A, Hampel H, Brown K, Swensen J, Neuhausen S, Skolnick M, Norton L et al. (1996) Germline BRCA1 185delAG mutations in Jewish women with breast cancer. *Lancet* 347: 1643–1645.
67. Thorlacius S, Sigurdsson S, Bjarnadottir H, Olafsdottir G, Jonasson JG, Tryggvadottir L, Tulinius H, Eyfjord JE (1997) Study of a single BRCA2 mutation with high carrier frequency in a small population. *Am J Hum Genet* 60: 1079–1084.
68. Gayther SA, Harrington P, Russell P, Kharkevich G. Garkavtseva RF, Ponder BA (1997) Frequently occurring germ-line mutations of the BRCA1 gene in ovarian cancer families from Russia. *Am J Hum Genet* 60: 1239–1242.
69. Gayther SA, Harrington P, Russell P, Kharkevich G, Garkavtseva RF, Ponder BA (1996) Rapid detection of regionally clustered germ-line BRCA1 mutations by multiplex heteroduplex analysis. UKCCCR Familial Ovarian Cancer Study Group. *Am J Hum Genet* 58: 451–456.
70. Sobczak K, Kozłowski P, Napierała M, Czarny J, Wozniak M, Kapuscinska M, £osko M, Koziczak M, Jasinska A, Powierska J et al. (1997) Novel BRCA1 mutations and more frequent intron-20 alteration found among 236 women from western Poland. *Oncogene* 15: 1773–1779.
71. Ramus SJ, Friedman LS, Gayther SA, Ponder BA, Bobrow L, van der Looji M, Papp J, Olah E (1997) A breast/ovarian cancer patient with germline mutations in both BRCA1 and BRCA2. *Nat Genet* 15: 14–15.
72. Ramus SJ, Kote-Jarai Z, Friedman LS, van der Looij M, Gayther SA, Csokay B, Ponder BA, Olah E (1997) Analysis of BRCA1 and BRCA2 mutations in Hungarian families with breast or breast-ovarian cancer. *Am J Hum Genet* 60: 1242–1246.
73. Dunning AM, Chiano M, Easton D, Ponder BAJ (1996) The potential role of common polymorphism in predisposition to breast and ovarian cancer. *In*: H Müller, RJ Scott, W Weber (eds): *Hereditary Cancer*. Basel: Karger, 22–34.
74. Durocher F, Shattuck-Eidens D, McClure M, Labrie F, Skolnick MH, Goldgar DE, Simard J (1996) Comparison of BRCA1 polymorphisms, rare sequence variants and/or missense mutations in uffeceted and breast/ovarian cancer populations. *Hum Mol Genet* 5: 835–842.
75. Dunning AM, Chiano M, Smith NR, Dearden J, Gore M, Oakes S, Wilson C, Stratton M, Peto J, Easton D et al. (1997) Common BRCA1 variants and susceptibility to breast and ovarian cancer in the general population. *Hum Mol Genet* 6: 285–289.
76. Friend S, Borresen AL, Brody L, Casey G, Devilee P, Gayther S, Goldgar D, Murphy P, Weber BL, Wiseman R (1995) Breast cancer information on the web. *Nat Genet* 11: 238–239.
77. Orita M, Iwahana H, Kanazawa H, Hayashi K, Sekiya T (1989) Detection of polymorphisms of human DNA by gel electrophoresis as single-strand conformation polymorphisms. *Proc Natl Acad Sci USA* 86: 2766–2770.
78. Kozlowski P, Sobczak K, Napierala M, Wozniak M, Czarny J, Wlodzimierz J, Kryzosiak J (1996) PCR-SSCP-HDX analysis of pooled DNA for more rapid detection of germline mutations in large genes. The BRCA1 example. *Nucl Acids Res* 24: 1177–1178.
79. Hacia JG, Brody LC, Chee MS, Fodor SP, Collins FS (1996) Detection of heterozygous mutations in BRCA1 using high density oligonucleotide arrays and two-colour fluorescence analysis. *Nat Genet* 14: 441–447.

Molecular Aspects of Cancer and its Therapy
A. Mackiewicz and P.B. Sehgal (eds)
© 1998 Birkhäuser Verlag Basel/Switzerland

Tumour immunology

A. Maraveyas, D. Hrouda and A.G. Dalgleish

Division of Oncology, Department of Cellular and Molecular Sciences, St. George's Hospital Medical School, Cranmer Terrace, London SW17 ORE, UK

Introduction

The ability to mount the effective antitumour response is the net result of a complicated interplay of factors relating to phenotypes of the tumour and host. Although the subject of tumour immunology is usually narrowed down to the stimulation and response of the cellular and humoral compartments of the lymphocytic response, in addition to the nonspecific effects of neutrophils, complement etc., it must be borne in mind that dissecting the response in this manner leaves out the holistic view of the immune system being part of a healthy host that can react appropriately to stress and disease. Lack of health in other compartments not usually conceived of as being a significant part of the immune system may lead to the inability to mount an effective immune response. The integrity of neurohormonal routes, such as bioactive amines and free-radical mediators is needed in addition to an intact immune system capable of the necessary cytokine-mediated 'cross-talk' for an effective immune response.

There are four main components that will determine the immune competence of a host to a tumour cell: (1) the actual existence of truly specific tumour antigens; (2) the manner in which tumour-associated antigens are presented to the immune system: this dictates the profile of the immune response. Manipulation of these pathways by the tumour leads to the inability of the host to detect and mount a primary response to tumour antigens. We have named this a 'camouflage' type of evasion; (3) the preconditioning of the immune system that is called upon to respond; this feature of the response is directly associated with the non-cancer morbidity/immunogen exposure profile of the host but can also be affected by (4) the sum of counter-actions that tumour cells develop to mediate suppression or evasion of an already activated immune system. This review will look into the latest developments in these four major components governing the immune responses to non-haematological malignancies.

Tumour antigens

Tumour immunotherapy is based on the theory that tumours possess specific antigens which can be recognised by the immune system. Lack of antigens does not seem to be the reason why the immune system fails to detect tumours. The successful treatment of established tumours using whole tumour cell vaccines transfected with cytokines indicates that tumour antigens do exist but that under normal circumstances they are poorly immunogenic [1]. Several tumour-associated antigens have been described in the last few years, the majority relating to melanoma and containing peptide sequences that can be recognised by specific cytotoxic T lymphocytes (Tab. 1).

They include protein antigens that are normally expressed in some adult tissues but have a higher level of expression in some tumours e.g., carcinoembryonic antigen. This antigen is also processed differently in malignant tissues (e.g., colon, breast and lung carcinomas) compared to normal tissues [2], which increases its potential application as a target for immunotherapy. Similarly, mucins such as MUC1 are expressed at higher levels in certain tumours compared to normal tissues [3] and differences in glycosylation allow new tumour-specific epitopes to be uncovered [4]. Organ-specific molecules, such as prostate-specific antigen (PSA) and prostate-specific membrane antigen (PSMA), are also being considered as target molecules, and CTLs within the T cell repertoire which are specific for peptides of these molecules have been isolated [5, 6]. Both of these antigens are found on normal prostate cells and no qualitative differences in the molecules have been found between benign and malignant cells. However, the potential of using dendritic cells loaded with peptides of PSMA has recently been demonstrated in a phase I clinical trial, where a number of patients receiving this therapy showed biochemical evidence of response [7].

Table 1. Peptides recognized by human CD8[+] anti-melanoma T cells

CTL	MHC restriction	Peptide	Parent protein or gene	Tissue distribution
PBL	A1	EADPTGHSY	MAGE-1	melanoma, other tumours, normal testis
PBL	A1	EVDPIGHLY	MAGE-3	melanomas, other tumours, normal testis
PBL	A2	FLWGPRALV	MAGE-3	melanomas, other tumours, normal testis
PBL	A2	MLLAVLYCL	Tyrosinase	melanomas, melanocytes
PBL	A2	YMNGTMSQV	Tyrosinase	melanomas, melanocytes
TIL/PBL	A2	AAGIGILTV	MART-1/Melan-A	melanomas, melanocytes, retinal cells
TIL/PBL	A2	ILTVILGVL	MART-1/Melan A	melanomas, melanocytes, retinal cells
LN	A2	YLEPGPVTA	gp100/Pmel17	melanomas, melanocytes, retinal cells
TIL	A2	LLDGTATLRL	gp100	melanomas, melanocytes, retinal cells melanomas, melanocytes, retinal cells
TIL	A2	KTWGQYWQV	gp100	melanomas, melanocytes, retinal cells
TIL	A2	(T)ITDQVPFSV	gp100	melanomas, melanocytes, retinal cells
TIL	A2	VLYRYGSFSV	gp100	melanomas, melanocytes, retinal cells
PBL	A2	ACDPHSGHFV	CDK4	diverse
TIL	A24	(E)AYGLDFYIL	p15	melanomas, normal tissues
TIL	A24	AFLPWHRLF(L)	Tyrosinase	melanomas, melanocytes
TIL	B44	SEIWRDIDF	Tyrosinase	melanomas, melanocytes
PBL	B44	EEKLIVVLF	MUM-1	autochthonous melanoma
PBL	Cw6	YRPRPRRY	GAGE1,2	melanomas, other tumours, normal testis
PBL	Cw16	SAYGEPRKL	MAGE-1	melanomas, other tumours, normal testis
PBL	Cw16	AARAVFLAL	BAGE	melanomas, other tumours, normal testis

MAGE, BAGE and GAGE are possible oncofetal antigens which are present in some adult tissues such as the testis and the placenta, and have been found to be expressed in melanomas and a number of other tumours. MAGE-1 and MAGE-3, GAGE-1, GAGE-2 are recognised by specific CTLs [8]. Other tumour antigens found in melanomas and recognised by CTLs but not expressed in normal tissues include tyrosinase, MART-1 and gp100. Gangliosides are being considered as potential target antigens in melanoma because normal expression is restricted to the brain, an immunologically privileged site, and neural crest tissues.

Mutated genes may be different antigenic entities to their wildtype counterparts and can therefore represent tumour-specific antigens, in that they are not found in normal adult or fetal tissues. An example of this is the truncated c-*erb*-b3 receptor on glioma cell lines and gliomas [9]. If one assumes sequential steps in tumorigenesis it is very likely that during the cell's lifeevents leading to the completely transformed immortal cell with malignant potential, novel mutated proteins or products of mutated genes will be expressed.

Viral gene products expressed in some tumours are potentially powerful immunogens capable of eliciting T cell and antibody responses, e.g., human papilloma virus (HPV) in cancer of the cervix, Epstein-Barr virus (EBV) in Burkitt's lymphoma, nasopharyngeal carcinoma and some cases of Hodgkin's lymphoma. HPV genes *E6* and *E7* are constitutively expressed in squamous cell carcinoma of the cervix [10, 11]. The advantage of these as target antigens is that their expression in tumour cells is essential for maintenance of the transformed state. They are therefore unlikely to be lost as part of clonal selection, and being of viral origin they should be highly immunogenic and tumour-specific.

According to present immunological dogma we could expect full tolerance of most of the target tumour-associated antigens presently being investigated. Much of the experimental evidence suggests that this tolerance can be broken under certain circumstances, perhaps lending weight to the 'Danger' model, where the immune system is thought to discriminate between dangerous and harmless entities rather than between self and non-self [12]. According to this theory, the absence of costimulatory molecules on normal cells renders lymphocytes tolerant. Recent re-examination of the classical neonatal tolerance experiments suggests that tolerance is not an intrinsic property of the newborn immune system, but tolerance or immunisation could be induced depending on the nature of the antigen-presenting cell [13].

A number of immunotherapy strategies have arisen as a result of the identification of genes that encode tumour antigens, including vaccination with dendritic cells loaded with the antigen, bacteria or recombinant viruses containing tumour antigen genes, naked DNA for antigens, immunodominant peptides and proteins. A number of trials are underway using MART-1 and gp100 vaccination in patients with melanoma [14]. It is now clear that in addition to the first signal involving ligation of the T cell receptor with antigen and class I MHC, a second signal involving either soluble factors such as IL-2 or ligation of cell surface costimulatory molecules is also essential.

'Camouflage' mechanisms of immune evasion (tampering with antigen presentation)

Accessory molecules (costimulatory molecules)

It is now clear that in addition to the first signal involving ligation of the T cell receptor with antigen and class I MHC, a second signal involving either soluble factors such as IL-2 or ligation of cell surface costimulatory molecules is also essential for amplification of the immune response [15]. Receptor ligand pairs imparting a costimulus to antigen-specific stimulation include the adhesion molecules ICAM-1, LFA-1, LFA3-CD, CD40-CD40L, CD5-CD72, CD24-CD24L, as well as B7-1/B7-2 and the CD28/CTLA-4 interaction.

The most important costimulatory pathway appears to involve CD28 /CTLA-4 present on the majority of T cells [16] interacting with the B7 glycoproteins present on dendritic cells, Langerhans cells, activated monocytes and B cells and also on some tumours, in particular some malignant melanomas [17]. *B7-1* and *B7-2* are both members of the immunoglobulin gene super family. B7-2 (CD86) has only 25 % amino acid identity with B7-1 (CD80) but both are high affinity receptors for CTLA-4 and low affinity receptors for CD28 [16]. Dendritic cells are thought to express *B7-1* [18] constitutively although some researchers have shown that dendritic cells need to be activated before they express *B7-1* [19]. *B7-2* is induced in the majority of APCs following the appropriate stimulus and is constitutively expressed on monocytes. B7-1 and B7-2 both interact with CD28 which is expressed on resting lymphocytes (95 % CD4+ve and 50 % of CD8+ve) and expression increases following activation [20].

CTLA4, although only 31 % similar to CD28 at the amino acid level, also interacts with B7-1 and B7-2. Cells must be activated for it to be induced and is not expressed on resting T cells [21–24]. Binding to the CTLA4 receptor directly counters the effects of CD28 on T cell activation. Thus it is a counter-regulatory receptor to CD28 and forms part of the normal homeostatic mechanism, whereby T cell activation returns to baseline once the antigen has been cleared [25]. It has been shown that *in vivo* administration of antibodies to CTLA4 in mice with pre-existing tumours results in tumour rejection and potentiated immune responses against the tumour cells [26]. It has been suggested that a new therapeutic approach might involve administration of cancer vaccines with short term anti-CTLA4 treatment.

Furthermore, it has been shown that binding of the T cell receptor (TCR) to antigen complexed with MHC can result in T cell anergy in the absence of costimulation in both self- and allo-antigen-specific systems [27, 28]. B7 expression on APCs can be downregulated by IL-10, a cytokine released by some tumours, with resulting anergy [29].

Several other important details concerning the mechanism of CD28 signalling have recently emerged. Inhibition of the CD28/B7 interaction does not seem to affect initial T cell proliferation but it does result in late apoptosis of T cells [30, 31]. Subsequent work has shown that CD28 signalling results in upregulation of *bcl-xL* with Fas-dependent protection from cell death [32]. A number of studies have shown that interaction with CD28 plays a role in the differentiation of Th1/Th2 subsets, with a Th1-like cytokine response predominating in the absence of costimulatory signalling [33, 34]. The absence of a costimulatory molecule could explain why tumour cells are not rejected by immune surveillance, and why tumour vaccine protocols can induce immune responses that can see the parental tumour. A number of studies have shown that tumour cells transfected with *B-7* are rapidly rejected and the immune response to them is able to prevent a challenge with parental cells.

Transfection of *B7.1* into immunogenic tumours renders them incapable of growing in syngeneic immunocompetent animals, but this is not the case in nonimmunogenic tumours such as MCA102 and B16 [35]. Chen et al. demonstrated in murine melanoma expressing viral antigens that B7+ cells were able to induce a response against established micrometastases, which indicates that the B7 molecule was able to reverse a state of anergy, or that the CTLs were not anergic. The immune responses were antigen- and MHC-specific and mediated through CD8+ cells (and not CD4 or NK cells) [36]. In another study in murine melanoma, transfection of *B7-1* induced an immune response resulting in CD8+ mediated rejection of the tumour without the involvement of CD4+ cells [37]. Similar findings were subsequently reported when *B7-2* was transfected into immunogenic mouse mastocytoma cells, but there was no tumour regression or antitumour immunity when the experiment was repeated in a nonimmunogenic MCA102 fibrosarcoma [38]. A further cautionary note arises from a study in K1735 murine melanoma, a mildly immunogenic tumour, which showed that the expression of transfected *B7.1* or *B7.2* resulted in less protective immunity than that elicited by the parental K1735 cells [39]. The fact that B7 expression is not required in target cells suggests that the antitumour effect is induced by enhancing the cytolytic effector stage. Becker and coworkers showed that B16- melanoma is able to induce unresponsiveness in an autologous CD4+ clone. Thus it is possible that tumours can actively re-anergise the immune response to their own antigens [40].

Human tumour cells of melanoma, ovarian cancer and myelo-monocytoic leukaemia origin transfected to express B7 have been found to stimulate strong proliferative and cytotoxic responses in allogenic T cells [41]. As with animal models, the effector CTLs were able to recognise both transfected and untransfected tumour cells. Additionally B7+ cells were able to induce cytotoxic responses by CD4 depleted T cells, which suggests that B7 is able to induce a cytotoxic response in the absence of CD4 and other APCs. Another study using *B7-1* transfected B16 murine melanoma showed that in addition to CD8+ cells, NK cells were also required for *in vivo* rejection of tumours but CD4+ cells were not essential [42].

The hypothesis that B7-1+ tumour cells can provide both signals one and two directly to activate naive CTL has been challenged by an elegant study in murine colorectal carcinoma using a parent into F1 bone marrow chimeras, which showed that although B7-1+ tumour vaccines resulted in some degree of direct presentation to CD8+ T cells, the dominant mechanism of CTL priming was through uptake and presentation of tumour antigens by bone marrow derived APCs [43].

The co-transfection of cytokine genes into the cells, or the addition of exogenous cytokines, has also been considered as there appears to be synergy between, for example B7.1 and IL-12. Vaccines consisting of a combined application of B7.1 and IL-12 transfected cells have been shown to slow or abrogate growth of even nonimmunogenic distant wildtype tumours [44]. The major cytokine groupings are divided into Th1 and Th2. Th1 cytokines, including γIFN and IL-2, are thought to be involved in inducing cell-mediated immunity; and Th2 cytokines, including IL-4, IL-5 and IL-6, are involved in mainly humoral-mediated immunity. Th1 responses are enhanced by IL-12 and it may be that IL-12 enhances costimulatory pathways. IL-10, a downregulator of costimulatory molecules, is known to enhance Th2 responses. B7 and IL-12 cooperate in the induction of proliferation of mouse T helper clones and their resultant production of γIFN [45].

Th1 cells did not proliferate to stimulation with the APCs transfected with FcR+ with or without B7+ plus anti-CD3 monoclonal antibody in the absence of IL-12. However, the addition of IL-12 resulted in a very pronounced proliferation of T cells and γIFN production. In contrast naive T cells proliferated well to stimulation in the absence of IL-12. The anti-Th1 activity of IL-10 is probably due to its ability to inhibit the APC function of splenic and peripheral blood monocytes and macrophages by inhibiting to the costimulatory pathways, a defect overcome by IL-12.

No trials of *ex vivo* gene therapy strategies using transfected B7-1 or B7-2 expressing tumour vaccines in human melanoma have yet been reported. *In vivo* gene therapy, using vectors that will be able to deliver and express B7-1 and B7-2 on the surface of tumour tissue, is a technically more difficult strategy for a number of reasons including the need for a tissue-specific promoter (e.g., tyrosinase) so that the gene is only expressed in target cells, as well as an effective way of delivering it. Retroviral vectors are unable to deliver such genes to the majority of tumour cells, but a bystander effect, where uninfected cells are also killed, may mean that 100% transfection of target cells is unnecessary.

MHC class I and CTL recognition

One of the major events associated with tumor proliferation, invasion and metastasis is alteration of the HLA class I phenotype of the tumour. Given our current understanding of the function of HLA, the most probable explanation is that this state confers a selection advantage to tumour cells. Certainly, in experimental systems it has been shown that both *in vitro* [46] and *in vivo* [47] MHC-loss mutants can be generated under selection pressures from CTLs. Events at different levels in the HLA expression pathway can lead to loss or downregulation of MHC class I e.g., (a) mutations in HLA and related genes (*b2m* gene and heavy chain gene) or the promoter regions; (b) defects in the transcription and translation pathways due to abnormal methylation of the DNA; (c) deficient peptide transport into the ER due to *TAP* gene down-regulation or mutation and (d) defective glycosylation of the class I molecule. Recent evidence is however emerging that even this mechanism of evasion needs to be finely balanced. Total loss of HLA, a frequent finding (9 to 52%), through interference for example with the β-microglobulin synthesis or transport, may not be the most effective method of evading the immune system. This may expose these tumour variants to NK cell attack since these cells lyse HLA class I deficient targets [47, 48]. Recognition activation and lysis by the NK cells requires only a few hours. The experimental evidence tends to favour a modulatory function of HLA through killer-cell inhibitory receptors (KIR) on NK cells. The process of characterising the components and diversity of this modulatory pathway is under way. Some of these receptors belong to the immunoglobulin superfamily (Ig-SF) [49] while others bear a C-type lectin domain (e.g CD94) [50]. Hence we can deduce that the maximum loss of HLA not inducing NK attack is the tumour phenotype that will be selected by the environmental pressures of the immune system. 'Half-way house' phenotypes characterised by HLA haplotype loss (rare), HLA locus loss (19%), HLA allelic loss (15 to 51%) or combinations of the above, are more likely to exhibit the survival advantage needed for the tumour cells to proliferate and invade [51]. Recent observations of downregulation of HLA class I in cervical carcinoma metastases to lymph nodes, compared to the primary, support these hypotheses [52]. However, the matter is far from clear, as some cells with total MHC class I loss are still capable of evading NK cell destruction. It is possible that other, hitherto unrecognised, regulatory receptors of NK activity exist on the tumour cells.

MHC class II and tumour antigen recognition

Although some of the studies report that CD4 help can be bypassed, most of them clearly show that the afferent arm of the immune system is defective, as opposed to the effector arm. When tumours are transfected with MHC class II they can induce an effective antitumour response, which can prevent a challenge with parental or wildtype cells from taking [54, 55]. Class II molecules can occasionally make the tumour more aggressive, perhaps because anergy is induced when MHC class II is expressed in a tumour cell that is devoid of any costimulatory molecules. MHC class II molecules with truncated cytoplasmic tails do not induce antitumour immunity against murine sarcoma cells, but this can be overcome by supertransfecting with *B7-1*. It appears that CD4+ T cell activation in this system requires the delivery of both an antigen-specific signal *via* three class II heterodimers, and a costimulatory signal *via* B7 [56, 57].

The hypothesis that MHC class II expressing tumour cells may function as APCs for tumour peptides does not at first appear to be consistent with the finding that class II molecules usually present exogenous, and not endogenous, peptides. However, tumour cells may in fact present their own peptides on class II because the invariant chain Ii, which normally prevents the interaction with endogenous peptides, appears to be absent in tumour cells. When tumour cells are transfected with Ii they are no longer immunogenic in autologous mice [58].

Heat shock proteins

Heat shock (or better named stress) proteins [59] are thought to represent a prevailing response of mammalian cells to adverse environmental stress, be it physical (thermo-, cryo-, radio-), chemical, nutrient or oxygen deprivation. They are ubiquitous and highly conserved, and are thought to represent an inducible protective response to exogenous stressful insults. Three major subgroups have been reported: (a) The major HSPs, (b) the glucose regulated SPs (GRPs) and (c) the low molecular weight HSPs [59]. Classically they were believed to be located intracellularly, associated to the ribonucleus or intracellular membranes, and were thought to function mainly as chaperones. Both the finding that major HSPs can be found on the cell membrane surface [60], and the observation that antitumour immunity can be elicited in murine models by the injection of purified HSPs from syngeneic tumours and not from normal tissues, suggests that this class of ubiquitous proteins may have antigen-presenting functions. It has been shown that numerous peptides can be bound noncovalently to various HSPs [61–63]. Peptides eluted from these preparations do not elicit immunity by themselves. Two interesting properties of these molecules have emerged: there seems to be no requirement for the use of adjuvants, and the response elicited is an MHC class I-restricted type of response. It has also been shown that depletion of CD8+ or macrophages, but not CD4+, T cells during the priming phase abrogates the immunity elicited by puri-ied HSP from tumours. During the post-priming effector phase however, all three components are mandatory for an efficient immune response to be maintained [61]. This immune profile was found to be distinct from that achieved by the inoculation of the whole syngeneic irradiated cells from which the HSP preparation had been obtained. In this case the depletion of CD4+ cells abrogated the immune response [61]. The above data seem to indicate that HSPs may have the capability to induce a preferential cytotoxic CD8+ type of profile which characterises a Th1 type of response.

Apart from the postulate that HSPs purified from tumour cells have small antigenic peptides conformationally bound to them, it has also been shown that larger proteins such as P53 [63], and maybe even MUC1, may form complexes with HSPs [64]. The significance of this finding is not yet clear, but seems to be associated with the development of humoral type of responses against the complexed protein [63].

Preconditioning of host

Th1 cytokine profile vs Th2 cytokine profile

Studies in murine models (and also in humans) have demonstrated that there exist at least two distinct Th subsets based on cytokine activation profiles and a preferential production of IgG isotypes [66, 67]. The so-called Th1 profile is characterised by a preferential production of IL-2, IFN-γ, TNF-β, IL-12 and stimulation of IgG2a antibody production (murine models) [66, 67]; the Th2 profile is associated with production of IL-4, IL-5, IL-6, IL-10 and IL-13 and provides stimulation for the secretion of IgG1 and IgE antibody isotypes [68, 69]. These populations of T cells regulate each other reciprocally through their respective cytokines. It has been clearly shown that differential activation of one or the other subset is an important determinant of the protective or pathological outcome of infectious and immunological diseases [70]. Many factors have been shown to be involved in the regulation of Th1 and Th2 subsets: the importance of the genetic background of the host, the type of antigen-presenting cells, the form and dose of antigen employed, the route of administration and so on [69, 70]. Moreover, evidence is accruing that the balance of these subpopulations of T cells plays an important role in tumour immunosurveillance and in the ability of a tumour vaccine to induce an appropriate immune response [69, 71]. Although the mechanisms which govern the preferential activation of a Th subset have yet to be characterised, it is becoming clear that the existence of cancer in the host seems to predispose the overall response towards a Th2 type of profile. We have recently shown that surrogate markers in the form of PBLC-activation profiles for IL-2 and IFN-γ, and more recently IL-4, can be studied prospectively for cancer patients undergoing nonspecific immunotherapy [B. Baban, *submitted*]. The hope is that assays of this sort will clarify the type of immunosuppression found in these patients over the evolution of their disease, and will also provide a tool to rationalise immunotherapy treatments. Of great practical interest would be the development of an immune staging system, which could be the combination of clinical and surrogate immunological parameters to predict response of a host to an immunotherapy protocol. This could also help identify a subset of patients who would not benefit from immunotherapy, as there seem to be rare but well-documented instances where nonspecific immunotherapy has led to apparent acceleration of under-lying disease [72].

T cells signal transduction dysfunction

Abnormalities in signal transduction in activated T cells, both in preclinical models and patients, have been clearly demonstrated. The mechanism through which this dysfunction is mediated is far from clear, but some interesting observations have been made. Decreased levels of the ζ chain of the TCR/CD3 complex is a recurring theme; furthermore, altered patterns of protein tyrosine phosphorylation by PTKs p56lck and p59fyn have been reported [73, 74]. Tumour-infiltrating lymphocytes from renal cell carcinomas [75], colorectal cancers [75] and PBLCs from patients with head and neck squamous carcinomas and patients with colon cancer metastases to the liver have been shown to be deficient in CD3 ζ chain when compared to PBLCs from healthy controls [76]. The mechanism that leads to diminution or disappearance of the CD3 ζ chain is unclear but importantly there are indications that this state seems to be reversible [77].

Antibodies

Antibodies against tumour-associated antigens have been found in many circumstances, but the actual role of humoral antitumour responses is not yet clear. A number of diverse functions have both been shown and postulated: for example (a) direct cytotoxicity through ADCC functions [78], (b) maintenance of dormancy by negative signalling [79], (c) propagation of anti-idiotypic cascades with a net affect of signalling for cell cycle arrest or even induction of apoptosis [80, 81]. Humoral responses have been detected against a number of tumour-associated antigens such as MUC-1 [82], tumour suppressor gene products such as P53 [83] and gangliosides [84–86].

One of the practical aspects of these humoral responses at present seems to be that of a 'marker' function. For example, induction of anti-GM2 IgM antibodies [87], and in some cases IgG antibodies [86], in patients with melanoma receiving a vaccine, has been found to predict a favourable response. Despite the fact that association of antibody responses with antitumour manifestations in cases of established tumour is not clear-cut, two recent postulates are worthy of mention. One is the protective function of pre-existing humoral responses, which may be medi-ated through the ability of antibodies to maintain negative signalling which accounts for tumour latency or dormancy [80]. This is one of the proposed mechanisms to explain the efficacy of an antiglycolipid antibody (M17-1A, 'Panorex') as an adjuvant treatment for Dukes C colorectal cancer [88]. Second, the possibility of using antibodies as tumour markers has been proposed. This would establish a possible screening potential: *P53* mutations represent the most common earliest genetic change in lung cancer, and on the strength of this, high-risk populations for lung cancer could be screened using P53 antibodies [89, 90].

'Counter-attack' mechanisms of immune evasion

It has become evident that the concept of a passive tumour population, simply developing evasive action against a constant attack from a competent immune system, is only part of the events underlying tumour escape mechanisms. Recent experimental evidence supports a more active immunosuppressive role for malignant cells. Some of the possible mechanisms are as follows.

Induction of tolerance through antigen overload

The host immune system may be overwhelmed by an overload of continuously shed TAAs, with a net result of induction of tolerance. This would be proportionate to the tumour size, explaining in one sense progressive deterioration of the immune status of the host with progression of the cancer [91]. Such suppression may be reversed by removing the growing neoplasm. For example, when serum samples were analysed for antitumour antibodies in patients undergoing surgery for sarcoma, successful resection of tumour was associated with a four-fold rise in antitumour antibody titre. It has also been shown that circulating TAA-antibody complexes may reduce the ability of circulating antibodies to mediate complement-dependent ADCC [92].

Production of soluble factors (cytokines) inducing immunoparesis

Tumour-infiltrating lymphocytes proliferate less readily in response to IL-2 or mitogens. CD4 T cells are more abundant in TIL subpopulations, possibly furthering immunosuppression through propagation of local Th2 response cytokines. Cell suspensions from melanomas derived from patients have been shown to manufacture immunosuppressant cytokines (IL-10) [93]. Even more interestingly, growth factors such as TGF-β [94], and VEGF [95], a growth factor ubiquitously expressed by cancer cells, has been shown to have a profound immunosuppressant effect on APCs, perturbing adequate antigen presentation. These mechanisms may be operative both at a systemic level and in paracrine/autocrine type of loops affecting the immediate tumour surroundings and milieu.

Immune escape through apoptosis machinery

Fas is a member of the tumour necrosis factor (TNF)/nerve growth factor receptor superfamily [96]. It is expressed by a number of cells including B and T lymphocytes, liver, heart, kidney [97], and some tumour cells [98, 99]. FasL is a 45 kDa type II transmembrane protein of the TNF family, and is widely expressed by activated CTLs and NK cells [96]. Upon activation CTLs express FasL on their surface, and when this comes in contact with Fas expressed by tumour cells (target cells), it induces rapid and dominant death through an apoptotic pathway of the Fas-expressing cell. Once these activated T cells have accomplished their task they undergo Fas/FasL-mediated apoptosis due to co-expression of Fas, thus limiting the accumulation of

CTLs [100, 101]. In lymphoproliferative (lpr) and generalised lymphoproliferative disease (gld) mice which express mutant Fas and FasL respectively, both mutations lead to an accumulation of activated T cells and the onset of accelerated autoimmune diseases resembling nephritis and vasculitis [102].

Considering that both circulating activated T cells and NK cells express FasL, it was not surprising that early investigations identified a number of lymphoproliferative malignancies as being FasL positive. Recently a number of groups have identified the expression of FasL on tumours of non-lymphoid origin, including colon cancer [45] hepatocellular carcinoma [103], and melanoma [98]. It is thought that FasL expression by tumour cells leads to the induction of apoptosis of normal cells at the tumour site as well as the destruction en masse of Fas positive tumour-infiltrating T cells and NK cells [103]. In addition to constitutive expression of FasL on these tumour cells, a soluble albeit truncated (sFasL, a 26 kDa glycoprotein) proteolytic fragment retaining full activity (apoptotic) has been detected in patients' sera. This soluble form is possibly related to the occurrence of tolerisation in some patients [104].

It is becoming apparent that Fas may not be the only surface receptor mediating apoptosis. The TRAIL ligand for which a receptor was recently identified [105], and the TRAMP receptor, for which a ligand has yet to be identified and which is found to be abundant on lymphocytes and thymocytes [106], seem to be alternative routes. Whether they are relevant in tumour immunology is currently unknown.

Conclusion

Characterisation of the immunosuppressive mechanisms evolved and substances produced by tumours, working at the level of both the tumour milieu and the host's immune system, has progressed rapidly. These processes are not mutually exclusive and probably operate at one time or another as the tumour progresses through different stages. Current applications of the above include the use of autologous and allogeneic whole cell vaccines with cytokine and costimulatory molecule cDNA transfer, dendritic cells pulsed with cell membranes, proteins, peptides or even transfected with cDNA, naked DNA vaccines using either enhancement molecules (e.g., HLA-B7 or tumour antigens), or tumour-associated gangliosides and mucins, in addition to a growing number of adjuvants to co-administer with the above. It is conceivable that combinations of these immunostimulatory tumour vaccines, coupled with strategies aimed at inhibiting tumour evasion/suppression factors, will work in some but not other situations, and that a repertoire of new vaccine/immunotherapies will evolve for different tumours over the next few years.

References

1. Dranoff G, Jaffee E, Lazenby A et al. (1993) Vaccination with irradiated tumor cells engineered to secrete murine granulocyte-macrophage colony-stimulating factor stimulates poten, specific and long-lasting anti-tumor immunity. *Proc Natl Acad Sci USA* 90: 3539–3543.
2. Muraro R, Wunderlich D, Thor A et al. (1985) Definition by monoclonal antibody of a repertoire of epitopes on carcino-embryonic antigen differentially expressed in human colon carcinomas *versus* adult tissues. *Cancer Res* 45: 5769–5780.

3. Zotter S, Hageman PC, Lossnitzer A et al. (1988) Monoclonal antibodies to epithelial sialomucins recognize epitopes at different cellular sites in adenolymphomas of the parotid gland. *Int J Cancer Suppl* 3: 38–44.
4. Finn OJ, Jerome KR, Henderson RA et al. (1995) MUC-1 epithelial tumor mucin-based immunity and cancer vaccines. *Immunol Rev* 145: 61–89.
5. Tjoa B, Boynton A, Kenny G (1996) Presentation of prostate tumor antigens by dendritic cells stimulates T-cell proliferation and cytotoxicity. *Prostate* 28: 65–69.
6. Correale P, Walmsley K, Nieroda C et al. (1997) *In vitro* generation of human cytotoxic T lymphocytes specific for peptides derived from prostate-specific antigen. *J Nat Cancer Inst* 89: 293–300.
7. Murphy G, Tjoa B, Ragde H, Kenny G, Boynton A (1996) Phase I clinical trial: T-cell therapy for prostate cancer using autologous dendritic cells pulsed with HLA-A0201-specific peptides from prostate-specific membrane antigen. *Prostate* 29: 371–380.
8. van der Bruggen P, Bastin J, Gajewski T (1994) A peptide encoded by human gene MAGE 3 and presented by HLA-A2 induces cytolytic T lymphocytes that recognise tumor cells expressing MAGE-3. *Eur J Immunol* 24: 3038–43.
9. Hills D, Rowlinson-Busza G, Gullick WJ (1995) Specific targeting of a mutant, activated EGF receptor found in glioblastoma using a monoclonal antibody. *Int J Cancer* 63: 537–543.
10. Smottkin D, Wettstein FO (1986) Transcription of HPV16 early genes in a cervical cancer derived cell line and the identification of the E7 protein. *Proc Natl Acad Sci USA* 83: 4680–4686.
11. Baker CJ, Phelps WC, Lindgren V, Braun MJ, Gonda MA, Howley PM (1987) Structural and transcriptional analysis of HPV16 sequences in cervical carcinoma cell lines. *J Virol* 61: 962–970.
12. Matzinger P (1994) Tolerance. *Annu Rev Immunol* 12: 991–1045.
13. Ridge JP, Fuchs EJ, Matzinger P (1996) Neonatal tolerance revisited: turning on newborn T cells with dendritic cells. *Science* 271: 1723–1725.
14. Rosenberg SA (1996) Development of cancer immunotherapies based on the identification of the genes encoding cancer regression antigens. *J Nat Cancer Inst* 88: 1635–1644.
15. Janeway CA, Bottomley K (1994) Signals and sign for lymphocyte responses. *Cell* 76: 275–85.
16. Linsley PS, Ledbetter J (1993) The role of the CD28 receptor during T cell responses to antigen. *Annu Rev Immunol* 11: 191–212.
17. Lenschow DJ, Walunas TL, Bluestone JA (1996) CD28/B7 system of T cell co-stimulation. *Annu Rev Immunol* 14: 233–258.
18. Larsen CP, Ritchie SC, Hendrix R et al. (1994) Regulation of immuno-stimulatory function and co-stimulatory molecule (B7-1 and B7-2) expression on murine dendritic cells. *J Immunol* 152: 5208–5219.
19. Hart DN, Starling GC, Calder VL, Fernando NS (1993) B7/BB1 is a leucocyte differentiation antigen on human dendritic cells induced by activation. *Immunology* 79: 616–620.
20. June CH, Bluestone JH, Nadler JM, Thompson CB (1994) The B7 and CD28 receptor families. *Immunol Today* 15: 321–331.
21. Gross JA, Callas E, Allison JP (1992) Identification and distribution of the co-stimulatory receptor CD28 in the mouse. *J Immunol* 149: 380–388.
22. Freeman GJ, Lombard DB, Gimmi CD et al. (1992) CTLA-4 and CD28 mRNAa are co-expressed in most activated T cells after activation: expression of CTLA-4 and CD28 mRNA does not correlate with the pattern of lymphokine production. *J Immunol* 149: 3795–3801.
23. Harper K, Balzano C, Rouvier E, Mattei MG, Luciani MF, Goldstein P (1991) CTLA-4 and CD28 activated lymphocyte molecules are closely related in both mouse and human as to sequence, message, expression, gene structure and chromosomal location. *J Immunol* 147: 1037–1044.
24. Linsley PS, Greene JL, Tan P et al. (1992) Co-expression and functional co-operation of CTLA-4 and CD28 on activated T lymphocytes. *J Exp Med* 176: 1595–1604.
25. Krummel LF, Allison JP (1995) CD28 and CTLA-4 deliver opposing signals which regulate the response of T cells to stimulation. *J Exp Med* 182: 459–466.
26. Leach DR, Krummel MF, Allison JP (1996) Enhancement of anti-tumor immunity by CTLA-4 blockade. *Science* 271: 1734–1736.
27. Boussiotis VA, Freeman GJ, Gray G, Gribben J, Nadler LM (1993) B7 but not ICAM-1 co-stimulation prevents the induction of human alloantigen-specific tolerance. *J Exp Med* 178: 1753–1763.
28. Gimmi CD, Freeman GJ, Gribben JG, Gray G, Nadler LM (1993) Human T-cell clonal anergy is induced by antigen presentation in the absence of B7 co-stimulation. *Proc Natl Acad Sci USA* 90: 6586–6590.
29. Ding L, Linsley PS, Huang LY, Germain RM, Shevach EM (1993) IL-10 inhibits macrophage co-stimulatory activity by selectively inhibiting the upregulation of B7 expression. *J Immunol* 151: 1224–1234.
30. Lucas PJ, Negishi I, Nakayama K, Fields LE, Loh DY (1995) Naive CD-28 deficient T cells can initiate but not sustain an *in vitro* antigen-specific immune response. *J Immunol* 154: 5757–5768.
31. Green JM, Noel PJ, Sperling AI et al. (1994) absence of B7-dependent responses in CD28-deficient mice. *Immunity* 1: 501–508.
32. Boise LH, Minn AJ, Noel PJ et al. (1995) CD28 co-stimulation can promote T cell survival by enhancing the expression of Bcl-xL. *Immunity* 3: 87–98.
33. King CL, Stupi RJ, Craighead N, June CH, Thyphronitis G (1995) CD28 activation promotes Th2 subset differentiation by human CD4+ cells. *Eur J Immunol* 25: 587–595.

34. Seder RA, Germain RM, Linsley PS, Paul WE (1994) CD28 mediated co-stimulation of interleukin-2 (IL-2) production plays a critical role in T cell priming for IL-4 and interferon gamma production. *J Exp Med* 179: 299–304.
35. Chen L, McGowan P, Ashe S et al. (1994) Tumor immunogenicity determines the effect of B7 co-stimulation on t cell-mediated tumor immunity. *J Exp Med* 179: 523–532.
36. Chen L, Ashe S, Brady WA et al. (1992) Co-stimulation of anti-tumor immunity by the B7 counter receptor for the T lymphocyte molecules CD28 and CTLA-4. *Cell* 71: 1093–1102.
37. Townsend SE, Allison JP (1993) Tumour rejection after direct co-stimulation of the CD8+ T cells by B7 transfected melanoma cells. *Science* 259: 368–370.
38. Yang G, Hellstrom KE, Hellstrom I, Chen L (1995) Anti-tumor immunity elicited by tumor cells transfected with B7-2, a second ligand for CD28/CTLA-4 co-stimulatory molecules. *J Immunol* 154: 2794–2800.
39. Chong H, Hutchinson G, Hart IR, Vile RG (1996) Expression of co-stimulatory molecules by tumor cells decreases tumorigenicity but may also reduce systemic anti-tumor immunity. *Human Gene Ther* 7: 1771–1779.
40. Becker JC, Brablets T, Czerny C, Teermeer C, Brocker EB (1993) Tumour escape mechanisms from immunosurveillance in a specific MHC-restricted CD4+ human T-cell clone by the autologous MHC class II+ melanoma. *Int Immunol* 5: 1501–1508.
41. Dohring C, Angman L, Spagnoli G, Lanzavecchia A (1994) T helper and accessory cell independent cytotoxic responses to human tumour cells transferred with a B7 retroviral vector. *Int J Cancer* 57: 754–759.
42. Wu TC, Huang AY, Jaffee EM, Levitsky HI, Pardoll DM (1995) A reassessment of the role of B7-1 expression in tumor rejection. *J Exp Med* 182: 1415–1421.
43. Huang AYC, Bruce AT, Pardoll DM, Levitsky HI (1996) Does B7-1 expression confer antigen-presenting cell capacity to tumors *in vivo*? *J Exp Med* 183: 769–776.
44. Zitvogel L, Robbins PD, Storkus WJ et al. (1996) Interleukin-12 and B7-1 co-stimulation cooperate in the induction of effective anti-tumor immunity and therapy of established tumors. *Eur J Immunol* 26: 1335–1341.
45. Murphy EE, Terres G, Macatonia S et al. (1994) B7 and interleukin 12 cooperate for proliferation and interferon gamma production by mouse T helper clones that are unresponsive to B7 co-stimulation. *J Exp Med* 180: 223–231.
46. van der Bruggen P, Traversari C, Chomez P et al. (1991) A gene encoding an antigen recognised by cytolytic T lymphocytes on a human melanoma. *Science* 254: 1643–1647.
47. Ward PL, Koeppen HK, Hurteau T, Rowley DA, Schreiber H (1990) Major histocompatibility complex class I and unique antigen expression by tumors that escaped from CD8+ T cell dependent surveillance. *Cancer Res* 50: 3851–3858.
48. Ljunggren HG, Karre K (1990) In search of the "missing self": MHC molecules and NK recognition. *Immunol Today* 11: 237–244.
49. Levitsky HI, Lazenby A, Hayashi RJ, Pardoll DM (1994) *In vivo* priming of two distinct antitumour effector populations: role of MHC class I expression. *J Exp Med* 179: 1215–1224.
50. Colonna M, Samaridis J (1995) Cloning of immunoglobulin-superfamily members associated with HLA-C and HLA-B recognition by human natural killer cells *Science* 268: 405–408.
51. Phillips JH, Chang C, Mattson J, Gumperz JE, Parham P, Lanier LL (1996) CD94 and a novel associated protein (94AP) form a NK cell receptor in the recognition of HLA-A, HLA-B and HLA-C allotypes. *Immunity* 163–172.
52. Garrido F, Ruiz-Cabello F, Cabrera T et al. (1997) Implications for immunosurveillance of altered HLA class I phenotypes in human tumours. *Immunol Today* 18: 89–95.
53. Cromme FV, van Bommel P, Walboomers JMM et al. (1994) Differences in MHC and TAP-1 expression in cervical cancer lymph node metastases as compared with the primary tumours. *Brit J Cancer* 69: 1176–1181.
54. Ostrand-Rosenberg S, Roby C, Clements V (1991) Abrogation of tumorigenicity of MHC class II antigen expression requires the cytoplasmic domain of the class II molecule. *J Immunol* 147: 2419–2422.
55. Chen P, Anathaswamy H (1993) Rejection of K1735 murine melanoma in syngeneic hosts requires expression of MHC class I antigens and either class II antigens or IL-2. *J Immunol* 151: 155–162.
56. Baskar S, Ostrand-Rosenberg S, Habavi N, Nadler LM, Freeman GJ, Glimcher LH (1993) Constitutive expression of B7 restores immunology of tumor cells expressing truncated MHC class II molecules. *Proc Natl Acad Sci USA* 90: 5687–5690.
57. Clements V, Baskar S, Armstrong T, Ostrand-Rosenberg S (1992) Invariant chain alters the malignant phenotype of MHC class II + tumour cells. *J Immunol* 149: 2391–2396.
58. Subjeck JR, Thung-Tai S (1986) Stress protein systems of mammalian cells. *Am J Physiol* 250: C1–C17.
59. Multhoff G, Botzler C, Wiesnet M, Eissner G, Issels R (1995) CD-3 large granular lymphocytes recognize a heat-inducible immunogenic determinant associated with the 72-kD heat shock protein on human sarcoma cells. *Blood* 86: 1374–1382.
60. Udono H, Levey DL, Srivastava PK (1994) Cellular requirements for tumor-specific immunity elicited by heat shock proteins. *Proc Natl Acad Sci USA* 91: 3077–3081.
61. Srivastava PK, Udono H, Blachere NE, Li Z (1994) Heat shock protein transfer peptides during antigen antigen processing and CTL priming. *Immunogenetics* 39: 93–98.

62. Suto R, Srivastava PK (1995) A mechanism for the specific immunogenicity of heat shock protein-chaperoned peptides. *Science* 269: 1585–1588.
63. Davidoff AM, Iglehart JD, Marks JR (1992) Immune response to p53 is dependent upon p53/HSP70 complexes in breast cancers. *Proc Natl Acad Sci USA* 89: 3439–3442.
64. Winrow VR, Mojdehi GM, Ryder SD, Rhodes JM, Blake DR, Rampton DS (1993) Stress proteins in colorectal mucosa. *Dig Dis Sci* 38: 1994–2000.
65. Scott P, Kaufmann SHE (1991) The role of T-cell subsets and cytokines in the regulation of infection. *Immunol Today* 12: 346.
66. Bottomly K (1988) A functional dichotomy in CD4+ T lymphocytes. *Immunol Today* 9: 268–274.
67. Stevens TL, Bossie A, Sanders VM et al. (1988) Regulation of antibody isotype secretion by subsets of antigen-specific helper T cells. *Nature* 334: 255–258.
68. Finkelman FD, Holmes J, Katona IM et al. (1990) Lymphokine control of *in vivo* immunoglobulin isotype selection. *Annu Rev Immunol* 8: 303–329.
69. Mosmann TR, Cherwinski H, Bond MW, Giedlin MA, Coffman RL (1986) Two types of murine helper t cell clone. I. Definition according to profiles of lymphokine activities and secreted proteins. *J Immunol* 136: 2348.
70. Doherty TM, Kastelein R, Menon S, Andrade S, Coffman RL (1993) Modulation of murine macrophages function by IL-13. *J Immunol* 151: 7151–7160.
71. Seder RA, Paul WE (1994) Acquisition of lymphokine-producing phenotype by CD4+ T cells. *Annu Rev Immunol* 12: 635–673.
72. McIllmurray MB, Ambleton MJ, Reeves WG, Langsam M, Deane M (1977) Controlled trial of active immunotherapy in management of stage IIB malignant melanoma. *Brit J Med* 2: 540–542.
73. Mizoguchi H, O'Shea JJ, Longo DL, Loeffler CM, McVicar DW, Ochoa AC (1992) Alterations in signal transduction molecules in T lymphocytes from tumor-bearing mice. *Science* 258: 1795–1798.
74. Salvadori S, Gansbacher B, Pizzimenti A, Zier K (1994) Abnormal signal transduction by T cells of mice with parental tumors is not seen in mice bearing IL-2 secreting tumors. *J Immunol* 153: 5176–5182.
75. Finke JH, Zea AH, Stanley J et al. (1993) Loss of T-cell receptor zeta chain and p56lck in T cells infiltrating human renal cell carcinoma. *Cancer Res* 53: 5613–5616.
76. Farace F, Angevin E, Vanderplancke J, Escudier B, Triebel F (1994) The decreased expression of CD3 zeta chains in cancer patients is not reversed by IL-2 administration *Int J Cancer* 59: 752–755.
77. Ghosh P, Sica A, Young HA, Ye J, Franco JL, Wiltrout RH, Longo DL, Rice NR, Komschlies KL (1994) Alterations in NF kappa B/Rel family proteins in splenic T cells from tumor-bearing mice and reversal following therapy. *Cancer Res* 54: 2969–2972.
78. Herlyn D, Koprowski H (1982) IgG2a monoclonal antibodies inhibit human tumour growth through interaction with effector cells. *Proc Natl Acad Sci USA* 79: 4761–4765.
79. Uhr JW, Scheuerman RH, Street NE, Vitetta ES (1997) Cancer dormancy: opportunities for new therapeutic approaches. *Nature Med* 3: 505–509.
80. Racilla E et al. (1995) Tumor dormancy and cell signalling. II. Antibody as an agonist in inducing dormancy of a B cell lymphoma in SCID mice. *J Exp Med* 181: 1539–1550.
81. Yefenof E et al. (1993) Cancer dormancy: Isolation and characterization of dormant lymphoma cells. *Proc Natl Acad Sci USA* 90: 1829–1833.
82. Rughetti A, Turchi V, Ghetti CA et al. (1993) Human B-cell immune response to the polymorphic epithelial mucin. *Cancer Res* 53: 2457–2459.
83. Crawford LV, Pimm DC, Bulbrook RD (1982) Detection of antibodies against the cellular p53 in sera from patients with breast cancer. *Int J Cancer* 30: 403–408.
84. Livingstone PO, Calves MJ, Natoli EJ (1987) Approaches to augmenting the immunogenicity of the ganglioside GM2 is superior to whole cells. *J Immunol* 138: 1524–1531.
85. Portoukalian J, Carrel S, Dore JF, Rumke P (1991) Humoral immune response in disease-free advanced melanoma patients after vaccination with melanoma-associated gangliosides. *Int J Cancer* 49: 893–899.
86. Ravindranath MH, Morton DL, Irie RF (1989) An epitope common to gangliosides O-acetyl-GD3 and GD3 recognized by antibodies in melanoma patients after active specific immunotherapy. *Cancer Res* 49: 3891–3899.
87. Jones PC et al. (1981) Prolonged survival for melanoma patients with elevated IgM antibody to oncofetal antigen. *J Nat Cancer Inst* 66: 249–254.
88. Riethmuller G et al. (1994) Randomised trial of monoclonal antibody for adjuvant therapy of resected Dukes C colorectal carcinoma. *Lancet* 343: 1172–1174.
89. Lubin R, Zalcman G, Bouchet L, Tredanel J, Cazals D, Hirsch A, Soussi T (1995) Serum P53 antibodies as early markers of lung cancer. *Nature Med* 1: 701–702.
90. Labreque S, Naor N, Thompson D, Matlashewski G (1993) Analysis of the anti-P53 antibody response in cancer patients. *Cancer Res* 53: 3468–3471.
91. Herlyn M, Thurin J, Balaban G et al. (1985) Characteristics of human melanocytes isolated from different stages of tumour progression. *Cancer Res* 45: 5670.
92. Gupta RK, Golub SH, Morton DL (1979) Correlation between tumor burden and anti-complementary activity in sera from patients. *Cancer Immunol Immunother* 6: 63–69.

93. Sato T, McCue P, Masuoka K et al. (1996) Interleukin 10 production by human melanoma. *Clin Cancer Res* 2: 1383–1390.
94. Chang HL, Gillet N, Figari I, Lopez AR, Palladino MA, Derynck R (1993) Increasing transforming growth factor beta expression inhibits cell proliferation *in vitro*, yet increases tumorigenicity and tumour growth of Meth A sarcoma cells. *Cancer Res* 53: 4391–4398.
95. Gabrilovich DI, Chen HL, Girgis KR et al. (1996) Production of vascular endothelial growth factor by human tumors inhibits the functional maturation of dendritic cells. *Nature Med* 2: 1096–1103.
96. Nagata S, Golstein P (1995) The Fas death factor. *Science* 267: 1449–1456.
97. Watanabe-Fukunaga R et al. (1992) The cDNA structure, expression, and chromosomal assignment of the mouse Fas antigen. *J Immunol* 148: 1274–1279.
98. Hahne M, Rimoldi D, Schroter M et al. (1996) Melanoma cell expression of Fas (Apo-1/CD95) ligand: Implications for tumor immune escape. *Science* 274: 1363–1366.
99. O'Connell J, O'Sullivan G, Collins J, Shanahan F (1996) The Fas counterattack: Fas-mediated T cell killing by colon cancer cells expressing Fas ligand. *J Exp Med* 184: 1075–1082.
100. Alderson M, Tough T, Davis-Smith T et al. (1995) Fas ligand mediates activation-induced cell death in human T lymphocytes. *J Exp Med* 181: 71–77.
101. Golstein P, Ojcius D, Young J (1991) Cell death mechanisms and the immune system. *Immunol Rev* 121: 29–65.
102. Nagata S, Suda T (1995) Fas and Fas ligand: lpr and gld mutations. *Immunol Today* 16: 39–43.
103. Strand S, Hofmann WJ, Hug H et al. (1996) Lymphocyte apoptosis induced by CD95 (APO-1/Fas) ligand-expressing tumor cells: a mechanism of immune evasion? *Nature Med* 2: 1361–1366.
104. Tanaka M, Suda T, Haze K et al. (1996) Fas ligand in human serum. *Nature Med* 2: 317–322.
105. Pan G, O'Rourke K, Chinnaiyan AM, Gentz R, Ebner R, Ni J, Dixit VM (1997) The receptor for the cytotoxic ligand TRAIL. *Science* 276: 111–113.
106. Bodmer J-L, Burns K, Schneider P et al. (1997) TRAMP, a novel apoptosis-mediating receptor with sequence homology to tumor necrosis factor receptor 1 and Fas(Apo-1/CD95). *Immunity* 6: 79–88.

Molecular Aspects of Cancer and its Therapy
A. Mackiewicz and P.B. Sehgal (eds)
© 1998 Birkhäuser Verlag Basel/Switzerland

Cytokines in the host-tumor interaction[*]

P.B. Sehgal

Departments of Cell Biology & Anatomy and of Medicine, New York Medical College, Valhalla, NY 10595, USA

Introduction

Understanding the cellular, biochemical and immunological ramifications of the host-tumor interaction at both the local tumor level and the systemic level is key to the design of successful therapeutic modalities for human cancers. The participation of cytokines in both the local and systemic aspects of the host-tumor interaction has been extensively established. Indeed, there is now not only a vast literature on the involvement of cytokines in the biology of host-tumor interaction, but also on the therapeutic use in human cancer of cytokines such as the various interferons, interleukins, hematopoietic growth factors, and an ever-increasing list of new cytokines. These cytokines (or 'biological response modifiers') have been introduced into anti-cancer regimens, either for their direct anti-tumor effects on neoplastic cell elements, or for their indirect anti-tumor effects through enhancement of the host's immunological response to cancer or through enhancement of the recovery of the host after the use of other bone marrow suppressive anti-cancer agents. Effective therapeutic use of cytokines in human cancer (for example of interferon-α) is now definitely established.

In contemplating the present review, an approach could have been to present a compilation of the various cytokines in actual use, or under consideration for use, together with an evaluation of the underlying rationale in each instance. Today, the literature on cytokines and their use in human cancer is so extensive that it would be difficult to do justice to the subject within the scope of one review. Here we have used a different approach by focussing on one family of cytokines (the interleukin-6-type cytokines) whose members may prove clinically useful in cancer immunotherapy (see chapter by M. Wiznerowicz et al., this volume). The reader is referred to recent reviews devoted to discussions of the clinical use of cytokines and the scientific bases for it [1, 2].

Interleukin-6 (IL-6) is a frequent, if not invariant, participant in the host-tumor interaction and is often present in the local tumor environment [3, 4, reviewed in 5, 6]. Tumor-associated IL-6 can be derived from both the neoplastic cell elements and the stromal or tumor-infiltrating cells [3, 4, 7]. This IL-6 is thought to be responsible for the systemic 'paraneoplastic syndrome' which includes fever, weight loss, alterations in acute phase plasma protein levels, and altered immune responsiveness [8–11]. Aberrant paracrine or autocrine overexpression of IL-6 in the tumor environment clearly alters tumor cell biology (e.g., in multiple myeloma, in melanoma, in Castleman's and Hodgkin's diseases, etc) [6–11]. As their names indicate, leukemia inhibitory factor

---

[*]Dedicated to the memory of the late Mrs Indira Devi Sehgal

(LIF) and oncostatin M (OSM) were cytokines discovered by their ability to inhibit the proliferation of neoplastic cell lines (reviewed in [11]). Because LIF and OSM use the same gp130 signal transducing β chain as part of their cell surface receptors as IL-6, these cytokines are grouped together as the IL-6-type cytokines. This group also includes the cytokines IL-11, ciliary neurotrophic factor (CNTF) and cardiotrophin-1 (CT-1) [11]. In each of these instances, the high affinity cell surface receptor consists of the gp130 β chain together with one or more additional chains that bind the respective ligand and/or contribute additionally to signal transduction [11, 12]. It is currently believed that extracellular ligand-induced dimerization of the gp130 and/or additional signal transducing chains is responsible for mediating the signal to the intracellular environment, resulting in activation through Tyr-phosphorylation of respective Janus kinases (Jak1, Jak2, Tyk2) and the subseqeunt recruitment and activation through Tyr-phosphorylation of various members of the protein family termed Signal Transducer and Activators of Transcription (STATs) [12–15]. In this scheme, the role of the IL-6R or α chain, which can be cell-surface bound, or be soluble, is to bind the IL-6 ligand and deliver it to the gp130 chain, promoting ligand-induced dimerization of gp130 molecules [14]. Thus, from a functional standpoint, the manner of delivery of IL-6 to the cell surface can determine the local biological response. Tumor cell lines devoid of IL-6Rα can be rendered sensitive to IL-6 by delivery of IL-6 in the form of an IL-6/sIL-6R binary complex which can directly activate gp130-mediated cell signalling [14]. Thus tumor cells otherwise resistant to IL-6 can be made responsive (see chapter by M. Wiznerowicz et al., this volume, for a discussion of the clinical implications of this observation). It is now established that the Jak-STAT signal transduction pathway is activated by over 30 different cytokines and growth factors including the interferons, various interleukins and hematopoietic growth factors, many of which are well-established treatment modalities for human cancer (e.g., interferon-α/β, GM-CSF, G-CSF) [14–16].

This review is focussed on two aspects of ongoing research in the author's laboratory relevant to the involvement of IL-6-type cytokines in the host-tumor interaction: (i) the discovery of long-lasting high levels of circulating IL-6 in cancer patients subjected to different active specific anti-cancer immunization regimens, and (ii) the discovery of a novel indirect mechanism by which the p53 status of tumor cells can regulate IL-6-elicited signalling through the Jak-STAT signal transduction pathway.

Abnormalities of IL-6 transport in blood of cancer patients subjected to active specific immunotherapy: regulation of cytokine bioavailability

Active specific immunotherapy is increasingly in use as a treatment modality in human cancer. Cancer patients are repeatedly administered with various antigens (e.g., autologous tumor antigen preparations, anti-idiotypic (Id) monoclonal antibodies) coupled to immunopotentiating agents such as keyhole limpet hemocyanin (KLH) or tetanus toxoid, together with adjuvants such as Bacillus Calmette Guerin (BCG) [17]. The objective is to enhance the host's immune response to the tumor [17]. In using active immunization regimens, many investigators have attempted to identify predictive indicators of therapeutic success. As an example, in the case of immunotherapy of melanoma with the anti-Id mAb MK2-23, the appearance of an anti-anti-Id (Ab3) response and development of melanoma-specific cytotoxic T cells were positively correlated with an anti-tumor response [18, 19]. The administration of BCG as adjuvant and use of KLH as carrier together with the anti-Id mAb MK2-23 enhanced the Ab3 response [18, 19].

Recent data from this laboratory showed that melanoma patients administered active anti-cancer immunotherapy developed intravascular circulating reservoirs of IL-6 (a cytokine known to enhance cytotoxic T cell function and NK-cell activity), and raised the possibility that the development of such reservoirs may be a prerequisite for an anti-cancer therapeutic response [20, 21]. Patients subjected to active immunization with an anti-Id mAb MK2-23 ('mAb-KLH+BCG') [19] contained large amounts of 200-kDa IL-6 in their blood [20]. These complexes comprised ligand-occupied anti-IL-6 Ab and anti-IL-6R Ab, and were biologically inactive in the B9 and Hep3B assays [22]. In contrast, melanoma patients actively immunized with an autologous tumor cell membrane preparation 'AAAP' [23] contained large amounts of 30 and 450-kDa IL-6 in their blood [22]. These complexes were biologically active in the B9 and Hep3B assays. Despite this bioactivity, all patients were normothermic, suggesting limited tissue bioavailablity of the circulating IL-6 and/or tolerance to the pyrogenic effect of IL-6. Melanoma patients administered both mAb-KLH+BCG and AAAP displayed a composite profile of 30-, 200- and 450-kDa IL-6 each with its distinctive ELISA reactivity and bioactivity (Fig. 1) [22]. Thus, the nature of the particular active immunization regimen used regulated the generation of particular high molecular mass IL-6 complexes in blood. The new data suggest the provocative hypothesis that elicitation of high molecular mass IL-6 may be a prerequisite for the therapeutic efficacy of all active anti-cancer immunization. Indeed, the observation that high levels of IL-6 persisted in serum from melanoma patients who last received an mAb MK2-23+KLH booster over two years earlier, and who were alive and disease-free or disease-stable in the autumn of 1995 raises the possibility that circulating long-lived IL-6 may have contributed to the therapeutic response [22]. At a minimum, the new data show that aggressive active immunization in humans leads to characteristic and dramatic alterations in blood IL-6 transport and bioavailability.

The identification of several distinct abnormalities of IL-6 transport in blood emphasizes the complexity of the intravascular pool of this cytokine in cancer patients. That the particular active anti-cancer immunization protocol used determines which of these complexes predominates in blood points to the independent regulation of each transport modality. These observations in cancer patients find a parallel in the insulin-like growth factor-I (IGF-I) literature: the intravascular bioavailability of IGF-I is negatively or positively regulated by at least six different binding proteins (IGFBP1 to 6), each of which is independently expressed in different tissues [24–27]. Bioavailability of IGF-I from intravascular complexes with respective binding proteins is, in turn, regulated by specific proteases which cleave the binding proteins, reducing the latter's affinity for the ligand [24–27]. As an example, IGFBP-1 has an inhibitory effect on IGF-I function because it sequesters IGF-I in the vascular compartment; release of IGF-I from IGFBP-1 requires a specific IGFBP-1 protease. In contrast, binding of IGF-I to IGFBP-3 or 4 enhances IGF-1 function because these binding proteins enhance transit of IGF-I out of the vascular compartment increasing the delivery of IGF-I to target tissues. Proteases specific to each of these binding proteins are then involved in releasing IGF-I to the target tissues. Characteristic abnormalities in the levels of circulating IGFBP and of IGF-I transport occur in specific disease states such as an increase in circulating IGFBP-1 in diabetes, a decrease in circulating IGFBP-1 in hyperinsuline-

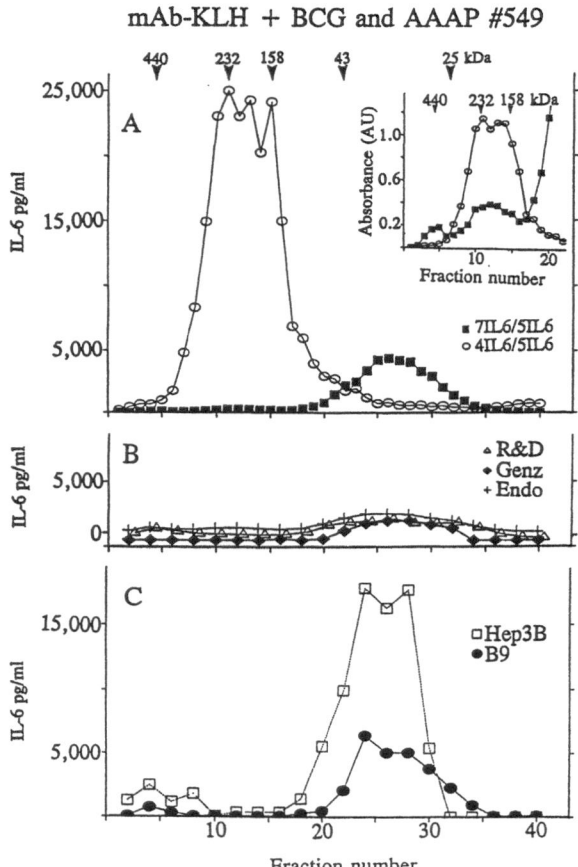

Figure 1. Abnormalities of IL-6 transport in blood from a melanoma patient (#549) who was first actively immunized using the mAb-KLH+BCG regimen and then using an autologous anti-cancer antigen preparation (AAAP) (as in [23]). 1 ml of serum was fractionated through a Sephadex-G-200 gel filtration column and the eluate fractions were assayed for IL-6 in five different ELISAs and two different bioassays.
Panel A. IL-6 concentrations as assayed in the 7IL6/5IL6 (■) and 4IL6/5IL6 (O) ELISAs. The inset illustrates the absorbance values recorded in each of these two ELISAs using the indicated elution fractions.
Panel B. IL-6 concentrations as assayed using three different commercial kits and expressed in terms of the kit standards: R & D (△); Genzyme (◆); Endogen (+).
Panel C. IL-6 concentrations as assayed using the B9 hybridoma proliferation (●) or the hepatocyte Hep3B stimulation bioassays (□). From [22].

mia of obese menopausal women, a decrease in IGFBP-2 in growth hormone deficiency, and an increase in IGFBP-3 in acromegaly (reviewed in [26, 28]).

In the case of IGF-I, the detection in serum of high molecular mass complexes of the ligand by Sephadex gel filtration chromatography, and the variable reactivity of the ligand in different ELISAs led to the discovery of circulating binding proteins which regulate IGF-I bioavailability *in vivo* [24, 25]. In the case of IL-6, the detection in serum of high molecular mass complexes of IL-6 by Sephadex gel filtration chromatography, and the variable reactivity of circulating IL-6 complexes in different ELISAs, led us to consider the role of various IL-6-binding proteins in regulating the bioavailability of this ligand *in vivo* [20, 29–31]. Potential IL-6-binding proteins include auto-antibodies, sIL-6R (without or with the additional association of sgp130), and other candidate proteins such as C-reactive protein, and fragments of complement C3 and C4 [20, 22, 30, 32, 33]. That the human circulation consistently contains high levels IL-6-binding proteins in the form of the soluble IL-6R (the soluble form of the α chain of the cell-surface receptor for IL-6; 'sIL-6R'; serum concentration 10–100 ng/ml) [32] and soluble gp130 (the soluble form of the β chain of the cell-surface receptor for IL-6; 'sgp130'; serum concentration 300–400 ng/ml) [33] suggests that free IL-6 may at best have only a transient existence in blood.

Anti-IL-6 IgG and anti-IL-6R IgG were detected in the IL-6/sIL-6R-containing 200 kDa complexes derived from cancer patients subjected to repeated polyclonal stimulation by BCG and KLH [22]. These autoantibodies appear to generate reservoirs of IL-6 from which functional IL-6 may be released over a long period of time [31]. Whether active release mechanisms such as specific proteases may be involved in this release process (as with IGF-I binding proteins [24–27]) remains to be examined. Why AAAP vaccination leads to the generation of the 30 and 450 kDa IL-6 complexes and not the 200 kDa complexes is unclear and remains a subject for future investigation. However, it is now clear that different active anti-cancer immunization regimens lead to different abnormalities of IL-6 transport in blood.

Considerable effort is being expended by various investigators in modelling complexes of recombinant IL-6, sIL-6R and sgp130 as monovalent trimeric and divalent hexameric complexes (the latter of molecular mass 440 kDa) and an evaluation of the structural interactions and biological properties of such complexes (reviewed in [34–36]). These studies, carried out with the underlying premise that dimerization of gp130 leads to intracellular signalling, seek to identify therapeutic derivatives that might have potent IL-6 antagonist, or even a superagonist activity, using free monomeric IL-6 as the basis for comparison [34]. The observation that IL-6 in blood exists in the form of differentially regulated high molecular mass complexes suggests caution in extrapolating the efficacy of a candidate IL-6 antagonist from cell culture to the *in vivo* situation.

Strategies to interfere with IL-6 function in human cancer include administration of anti-IL-6 or anti-sIL-6R mAb [37, 38] or chimeric bipartite 'ligand traps' consisting of an IgG Fc fragment dimer with one Fc portion covalently linked to the 'soluble' portion of IL-6R and the other to the 'soluble' portion of gp130 [39]. The dichotomy between the properties of IL-6 antagonists in cell culture experiments and properties observed in *in vivo* models point to a need to understand IL-6 transport in blood. As an example, in the case of anti-IL-6 mAb there is a paradoxical enhancement of IL-6 function *in vivo* despite the potent 'neutralizing' properties of these mAb in cell culture experiments [31, 37]. It appears that administration of anti-IL-6 mAb leads to the generation, *in vivo*, of a long-lived intravascular pool of IL-6 of endogenously-induced or exogenously-administered origin which circulates as a 200-kDa complex bound to the IgG, from within which active cytokine can be released to target tissues leading to an overall enhancement rather than an inhibition of cytokine function *in vivo* [31]. As for the chimeric bipartite IL-6 ligand trap [39], its *in vivo* properties remain to be elucidated.

Future investigations of abnormalities in IL-6 transport in blood in cancer patients adminstered active immunotherapy regimens should permit (i) elucidation of the biochemical and immunological effects of various circulating IL-6 complexes, (ii) studies of the regulation of IL-6 transport in blood and its biological consequences, and (iii) an evaluation of the relationship between circulating 'chaperoned' IL-6 and clinical outcome. That elicitation of high levels of 'chaperoned' circulating IL-6 in cancer patients during active anti-cancer immunization may be a predictor of therapeutic response is an exciting possibility awaiting investigation.

IL-6- and p53-dependent 'STAT-masking' in hepatoma cells

As has been mentioned earlier, a common feature of cytokines, such as the interferons, many interleukins, and hematopoietic growth factors, is that they engage cell-surface receptors which signal to the nucleus *via* the Janus kinases-STAT transcription factor (Jak-STAT) pathway [13–16]. Thus, alterations in the regulation of Jak-STAT signalling in cancer cells can determine the responsiveness of such cells to therapeutic cytokines. A focus of ongoing research in this laboratory is to investigate the regulation of the response of cancer cells to cytokines. Despite clear evidence of the influence of cytokines upon p53-induced cellular processes, for example the rescue of p53-induced apoptosis in myeloid cells by the cytokine IL-6 [40–42], there is little information concerning the influence, direct or indirect, of the transcription factor p53 upon cytokine-elicited cellular signalling through the Jak-STAT pathway. While mutations in p53 are among the commonest alterations observed in human cancer [43–49], many human cancer types are characterized by no or only rare mutations in p53 [50–56]. For example, B cell neoplasia such as myelomas rarely display mutations in p53, with the frequency of mutations rising only in advanced cases no longer responsive to therapy [51–56]. Thus, two categories of human cancers are treated with cytokines today: those in which the tumor cells carry a normal/wildtype *p53* gene and those in which the tumor cells carry mutations in *p53* or in which the *p53* gene is deleted. The biological functions of p53 and their alterations by mutations have been extensively studied in the context of the regulation of cell proliferation, of apoptosis and of repair of DNA damage [43–49]. With cytokines such as the various interferons and interleukins entering the mainstream of cancer therapy we have asked the following question: does *p53* status alter the ability of tumor cells to respond to cytokines?

In this section we shall summarize the discovery of a novel indirect mechanism by which p53 present in tumor cells can modulate Jak-STAT signalling elicited by cytokines. The available data are consistent with the mechanism that a wildtype p53-dependent gene product which accumulates in cancer cells is rapidly activated by IL-6 in a tyrosine-phosphorylation and proteasome-dependent step into a **'STAT-masking'** activity which, in turn, negatively regulates cytokine-induced Jak-STAT signalling and response in cancer cells (Fig. 2) [57].

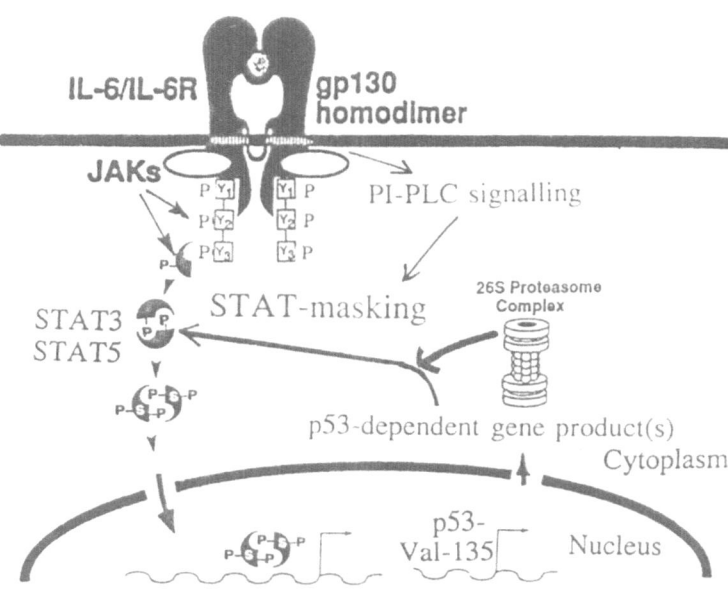

Figure 2. STAT-masking: a p53- and proteasome-dependent mechanism for negative regulation of Jak-STAT signalling.

The discovery of IL-6- and p53-dependent 'STAT-masking'

As part of a research program designed to evaluate the influence of wildtype *p53* and its mutant species on the production of cytokines by cancer cells, and on the response of cancer cells to cytokines [58–62], we used the IL-6-responsive human hepatoma Hep3B cells, which are deleted in their endogenous *p53* gene, to derive a panel of 11 cell lines ('Line 1' to 'Line 11') that can stably express p53-Val-135 which is a temperature-sensitive (ts) mutant such that it has wildtype p53 properties upon shift-down to 32.5 °C (Fig. 3). These Hep3B cell lines were obtained following cotransfection of Hep3B cells with a constitutive expression vector (off the HaSV LTR promoter) for the Val-135 temperature-sensitive mutant of murine *p53* together with pSVneo [62]. Following extensive selection in G418, eleven stable lines were derived. The use of the ts mutant of p53 allowed the derivation of these lines at 37 °C (*p53* in mutant conformation; no effect on cell proliferation) with the ability to investigate wt p53 effects by shifting the cells to 32.5 °C (Fig. 3). Compared to the parental hepatoma Hep3B cells and to pSVneo-alone Hep3B lines, p53-Val-135-containing Hep3B cells, at 32.5 °C, displayed reduced responsiveness to IL-6 as evaluated by (i) reduced secretion of β-fibrinogen and α1-antichymotrypsin in response to IL-6 [62], and (ii) reduced activation by IL-6 of a STAT3/5 responsive reporter construct containing two copies of the 36-bp β-fibrinogen IL-6RE [63]. In investigating the underlying mechanisms

Ts phenotype of p53
37°C   32.5°C

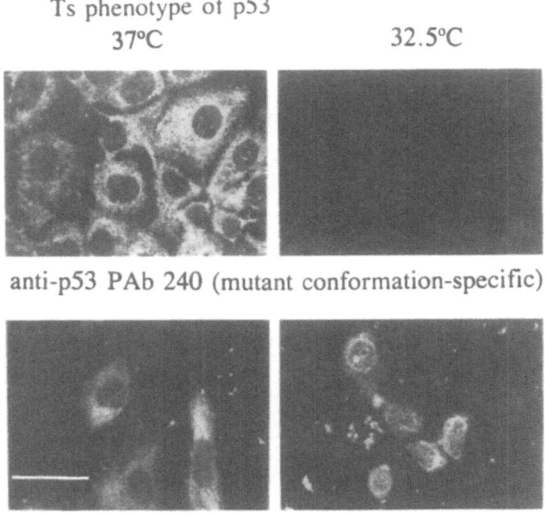

anti-p53 PAb 240 (mutant conformation-specific)

anti-p53 PAb 421 (panreactive)

Figure 3. Temperature-dependence of p53-Val-135 conformation in Line 5 Hep3B cells. Figure illustrates confocal immunofluorescence microscopy of cells first cultured at 37 °C for one day in eight-well chamber slides and then shifted to 32.5 °C for 18–20 h. The white bar in this and all subsequent immunofluorescence figures corresponds to 20 µM; all data within each experiment were collected at identical black level and gain settings. Immuno-staining for p53 was carried out using either the mutant p53 conformation-specific murine monoclonal antibody (mAb) PAb240 or the panreactive antibody PAb421. From [57].

for the reduced IL-6 responsiveness in these cells, we discovered a rapid and marked loss *selectively* of STAT3 and STAT5 immunostaining from both the cytoplasmic and nuclear com-partments within 30 minutes of addition of IL-6, as evaluated by confocal immunofluorescence microscopy (Fig. 4) [57]. All eleven p53-Val-135-containing Hep3B cell lines derived by us dis-played IL-6-induced STAT-masking [57] provided that the cells have been incubated at 32.5 °C for 18–20 h. Even though there was a dramatic reduction in STAT3 and STAT5 immunofluor-escence (Fig. 4), there was little degradation *per se* of STAT3 and STAT5 (Fig. 5). It is for this reason that we term this phenomenon 'STAT-masking' (Fig. 2).

The mechanistic basis for IL-6-induced STAT3 and STAT5-masking

The loss of STAT3 and STAT5 immunostaining as illustrated in Figure 3 was (i) IL-6 induced and rapid in that a reduction in immunostaining was observed within 10 min and there was almost complete loss by 20–30 min after IL-6 addition, (ii) transient in that STAT3 and STAT5 immun-ostaining returned 120–240 min after IL-6 addition, (iii) dependent upon cytokine concentration in that, when assayed 30 min after IL-6 addition, the loss of immunostaining was elicited by IL-6 at 0.3 ng/ml, was near maximal at 3–10 ng/ml, and was still evident at 100 ng/ml, (iv) selective in

All cultures IL-6 30 min

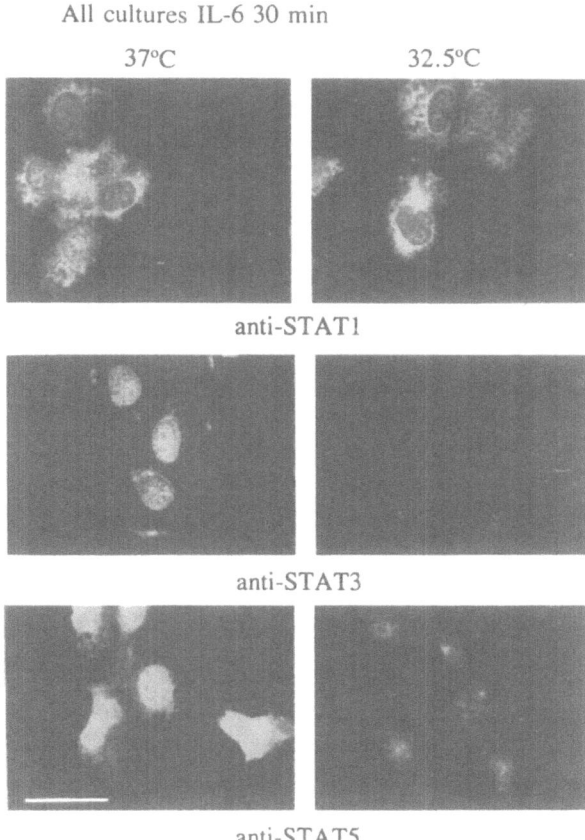

Figure 4. STAT3 and STAT5 masking in IL-6-treated Line 5 Hep3B cells incubated at 32.5 °C (wt p53 conformation) but not at 37 °C (mutant conformation). Cells were first cultured at 37 °C for one day and then shifted to 32.5 °C or continued at 37 °C for another 18 to 20 h. All cultures received IL-6 (30 ng/ml) for 30 min. Murine mAb to STAT1, STAT3 and STAT5 (which crossreacts with native STAT5b) were used in the immunostaining analyses illustrated. From [57].

that a loss of immunostaining was not observed for STAT1, STAT4, STAT6, NF-κB p65, C/EBPα, β, γ, and Sp1 transcription factors, (v) cytokine specific in that interferon-γ elicited a modest reduction in STAT3 immunostaining but no loss of STAT5 or STAT1 immunostaining, and epidermal growth factor elicited no changes in immunostaining of any transcription factor, (vi) required that the p53-Val-135-expressing Hep3B cells be incubated for at least 18–20 h at 32.5 °C, (vii) was observed using an anti-STAT3 monoclonal antibody or an anti-STAT3 polyclonal antibody each raised to different peptides from different regions of the STAT3 amino acid sequence, and (viii) was dependent upon proteins pre-existing at the commencement of IL-6 treatment, in that the protein synthesis inhibitor cycloheximide did not inhibit the IL-6-induced loss of STAT3 or STAT5 immunostaining. IL-6-induced and p53-dependent STAT-masking

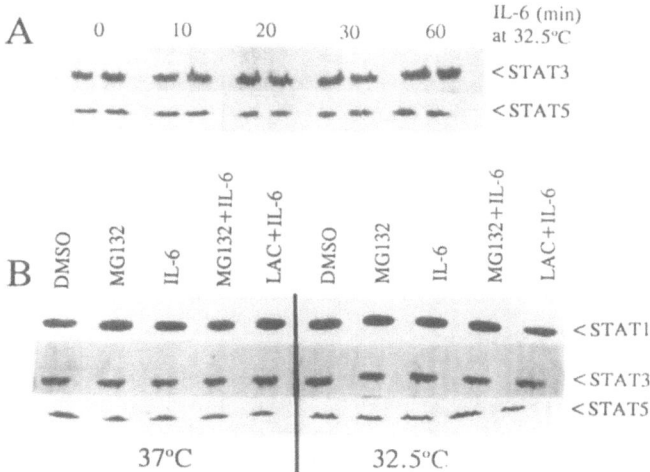

Figure 5. Western blot analyses of STAT3 and STAT5 content in IL-6-treated Line 5 cells exhibiting the IL-6-induced loss of STAT3 and STAT5-immunostaining. Experimental conditions were similar to those in Figure 4 except that cultures of Line 5 cells were prepared in 100 mm Petri dishes.
Panel A. STAT3 and STAT5b content of Line 5 cells at different times after IL-6 addition (30 ng/ml) at 32.5 °C.
Panel B. STAT1α, STAT3 and STAT5b content of Line 5 cells 30 min after IL-6 addition together with various proteasome inhibitors. From [57].

required tyrosine-kinase and proteasome activity in that genistein, staurosporine, MG132 and lactacystin, but not H7, added to cells 30 min before IL-6 blocked STAT-masking (Figs 6 and 7). The tyrosine-kinase- and proteasome-dependent events required for STAT-masking were completed by 30 min of IL-6 addition in that neither the protein kinase inhibitors genistein and staurosporine, nor the proteasome inhibitors MG132 and lactacystin, blocked STAT-masking when added 30 min after IL-6 [63]. Orthovanadate and pervanadate both blocked STAT-masking, indicating the additional involvement of a protein-tyrosine phosphatase in the mechanism of STAT-masking. Furthermore, U-73122, an inhibitor of agonist-receptor-coupled phosphatidyl-inositol-specific phospholipase C (PI-PLC) not only blocked STAT-masking when added 30 min prior to IL-6 but rapidly reversed the masked phenotype when added 30 min after IL-6 [63]. Additionally, PD98059, an inhibitor of mitogen-activated kinase kinase 1 (MAPKK1) which is activated by PI-PLC signalling, also blocked STAT masking when added 30 min prior to IL-6 [63]. Taken together, the data are consistent with a model in which the STAT-masking phenotype is the result of cross-engagement by IL-6 of a PI-PLC signalling pathway which, acting through a p53-dependent gene product(s) can inhibit IL-6-initiated signalling through the gp130-Jak-STAT pathway, an event microscopically visible in p53-Val-135-containing cells as IL-6-induced STAT-masking [57, 62, 63].

We infer that the IL-6-induced loss of STAT3/5 immunostaining is the result of the association of STAT3 and STAT5 with other proteins, rendering the former inaccesible to antibodies, or an alteration in the conformation of the STAT proteins, rendering these no longer reactive to antibodies. From our perspective, the phenomenon of STAT-masking captures a reaction-inter-

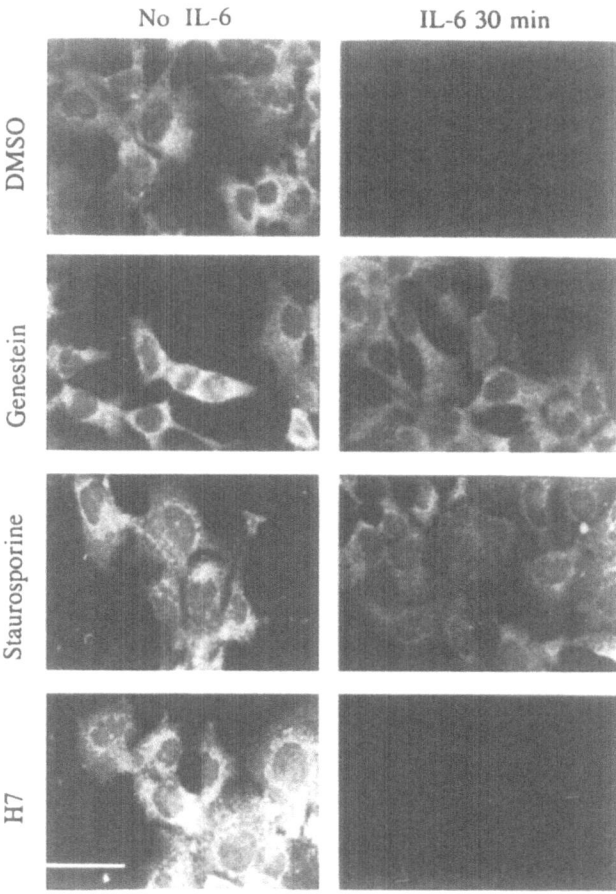

Figure 6. Loss of STAT3 immunostaining is IL-6-induced and requires Tyr-P kinase. Line 5 cultures were evaluated for the effect of genistein (100 μM), staurosporine (10 μM), and H7 (10 μM and 100 μM)(Sigma) upon the IL-6-induced loss of STAT3 and STAT5 immunostaining in cultures shifted down to 32.5 °C for 20 h. The various inhibitors were added 30 min prior to IL-6 treatment (30 ng/ml for 30 min). This figure illustrates data obtained using anti-STAT3 mAb for immunostaining; similar results were obtained using anti-STAT5 mAb for immunostaining (data not shown). From [57].

mediate during IL-6 signalling which can be observed in an inverse manner i.e., by loss of immunostaining. The open questions that remain are: what are the associated proteins that mask STAT3/5? How are they regulated? What is their physiological role in Jak-STAT signalling and in cytokine-stimulated gene expression?

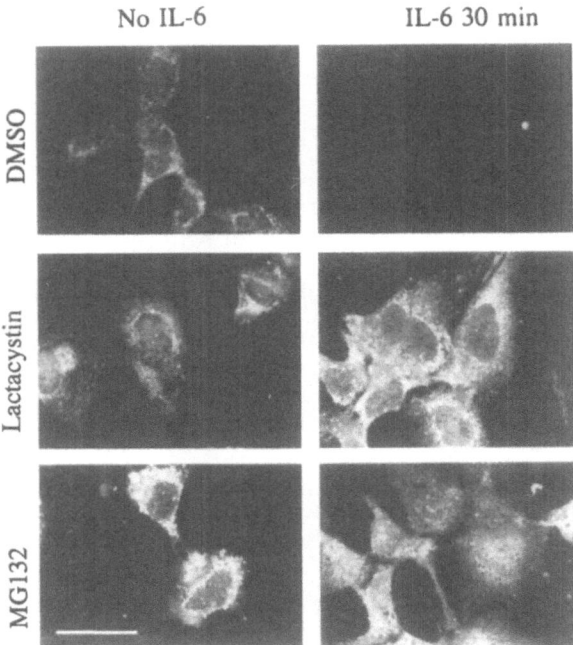

Figure 7. Proteasome dependance of IL-6-induced loss of STAT3 immunostaining. Line 5 cultures 20 h following shift-down to 32.5 °C as described in Figure 4 were treated with lactacystin (25 μM) or MG132 (40 μM) for 30 minutes prior to the addition of IL-6 (30 ng/ml) for 30 min. Following fixation immunostaining for STAT3 and STAT5 was evaluated using the respective anti-STAT mAb. This figure illustrates the anti-STAT3 immunostaining data; similar results were obtained using anti-STAT5 mAb (data not shown). From [57].

Functional implications of STAT-masking in Jak-STAT signalling: engagement of an inhibitory pathway

Cytokines and growth factors upon binding to their cell-surface receptors activate the Jak-STAT signalling pathway which consists of the activation of various Jak kinases, the subsequent tyrosine-phosphorylation of various STAT proteins, their dimerization, additional serine-phosphorylation, an increase in nuclear STAT-related DNA-binding activity and the consequent upregulation of target gene expression. Typically, STAT factor activation begins within 1–10 minutes, is maximal by 15–60 min and declines by 2–4 h [14–16, 64, 65]. In a number of experimental cell culture systems, biochemical and immunofluorescence studies have clearly revealed the rapid cytoplasm to nuclear transfer of STAT proteins upon cytokine addition [14, 16]. The decline in STAT-DNA binding activity by 2–4 h despite the continuous presence of the ligand is thought to be the combined result of (i) a cessation of continued STAT Tyr-phosphorylation at the cell membrane, and (ii) a loss of already activated DNA-binding competent STAT proteins (reviewed in [65]). The mechanism(s) suggested for the latter include tyrosine dephosphorylation by specific phosphatases [65] and/or ubiquitination selectively of Tyr-P-containing STAT proteins followed by proteasomal degradation [64]. The mechanisms by which continued STAT phosphorylation at the cell membrane is terminated are incompletely understood. Activation/recruitment of specific SH2 domain-containing protein-tyrosine phosphatases such as those designated SHP-1 or SHP-2 or an inositol-5'-phosphatase designated SHIP have been implicated in several experimental systems as components of receptor-mediated inhibitory signalling [66, 67], including involvement of SHP-1 in the termination of erythropoietin-EPO-R-Jak2 signalling [68] and in interferon-induced Jak-1-STAT1α signalling [69, 70]. The positive and negative involvement of SHP-1, SHP-2 and SHIP in regulating cell signalling have now been clearly documented, and the activation of SHP-1 and SHP-2 by receptor activation including *via* growth factors which activate the phospholipase C pathway have been reported [71–73]. However, despite one report showing the association of the IL-6-receptor β chain (gp130) with PLCγ and with SHP-2 upon IL-6 addition [74], the physiological significance of these associations remain completely unexplored. Very recently a family of at least fifteen proteins that bind SHP-2 and serve to inhibit receptor tyrosine-kinase signalling has been described [75]. These novel proteins bind SHP-2 through the latter's SH2 domains, and have been named signal-regulatory proteins or SIRPs [75]. The phenomenon of STAT-masking in wildtype p53-containing Hep3B cells provides us with a novel experimental system to investigate the inhibitory regulation of Jak-STAT signalling in cancer cells.

Proteasomal regulation of STAT-masking

A novel aspect of IL-6-induced STAT-masking is the proteasome dependence of the phenomenon. The only previous discussion of proteasomal involvement in Jak-STAT signalling is in two publications which report that the proteasomal inhibitor MG132 enhanced interferon-γ (IFN-γ) induced nuclear STAT1 DNA-binding activity [64, 65]. Haspel et al. [65] attribute their observations to the hypothesis that MG132 blocks proteasomal turnover of the IFN-γ receptor at the cell surface thus prolonging STAT signalling, and Kim and Maniatis [64] attribute their observations to the hypothesis that MG132 blocks proteasomal degradation of Tyr-phosphorylated and ubiquitinated DNA-binding competent STAT1. Haspel et al. [65] failed to detect degradation of STAT1 in IFN-γ-treated cells and point to nuclear dephosphorylation of STAT1 and the recycling of the dephosphorylated STAT1 back to the cytoplasm as the basis for the decline in nuclear STAT1 DNA-binding activity. They also [65] observed that vanadate, an inhibitor of protein-tyrosine phosphatase, prolonged STAT1 phosphorylation and DNA-binding activity.

We now recognize that the requirement for proteasomal activity in STAT-masking is neither in terms of the effect of proteasomes on degradation *per se* of STAT3/5, nor on the turnover of the relevant IL-6 cell surface receptors (IL-6Rα and gp130). Rather the proteasome activity appears to be required for a regulatory event which takes place in the first 10–20 min of IL-6 addition, and may reflect signal-induced proteasomal processing of masking proteins (roughly analogous to the processing NF-κB1 precursor to p50), or the signal-induced degradation of a negative regulator (analogous to the signal-induced degradation of I-κB)(reviewed in [57]). The molecular basis for the proteasomal regulation of STAT-masking is likely to be a new cellular process which regulates Jak-STAT signalling. STAT-masking may well reflect the proteasome-dependent association of regulatory proteins with STAT3/5, which control cytoplasm to nuclear trafficking of STAT3/5, and the recyling back to the cytoplasm of dephosphorylated STAT3/5. The observation that p53-Val-135-containing cultures need to be incubated at 32.5 °C for at least 18–20 h before the IL-6-induced loss of STAT3 and STAT5 immunostaining can be elicited suggests the hypothesis that a "wildtype" *p53*-dependent gene product which either increased or decreased in these cells in the 18–20 h period is involved in a tyrosine-kinase dependent step upon IL-6 addition into a STAT-masking activity (Fig. 2). The preferred hypothesis illustrated in Figure 2 is that a p53-induced gene product which increases in these cells is involved in STAT-masking. Once accumulated in p53-Val-135-containing Hep3B cell lines at 32.5 °C, this p53-dependent gene product(s) can subsequently function at 37 °C in mediating STAT-masking. When Line 1 cells were first incubated at 32.5 °C for 20 h, and then shifted up to 37 °C for 30 min, IL-6 was able to elicit STAT3 and STAT5 masking as assayed 30 min later, even with the cells having been kept continuously at 37 °C.

The functional consequences of the proteasomal activity-dependent STAT-factor masking and the effect of proteasomal inhibitors upon nuclear STAT-DNA binding activity was evaluated in experiments in which nuclear extracts prepared from IL-6-treated p53-Val-135 containing-cells incubated at either 37 °C or 32.5 °C were tested for their ability to bind a canonical STAT-binding DNA element (the 'short GAS' element from the *IRF-1* gene [57]. Consistent with the masking phenomenon illustrated in Figure 4, IL-6 in the concentration range 1–10 ng/ml [62] had a reduced ability to elicit STAT3 homodimer DNA-binding activity ('Complex A') in nuclear extracts prepared from Line 1 cells at 32.5 °C compared to cells at 37 °C (Fig. 8). At both temperatures, the inclusion of MG132 increased STAT-DNA binding corresponding to Complex C

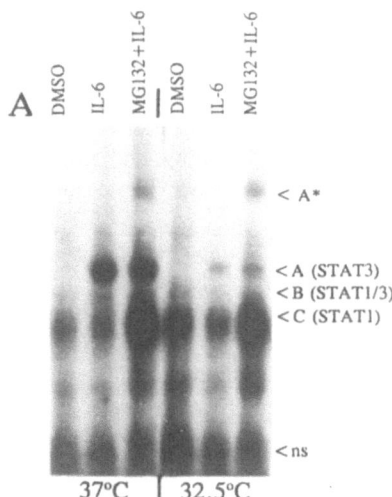

Figure 8. STAT-specific DNA binding activity in nuclear extracts of p53-Val-135 expressing Hep3B cells first cultured (in 100 mm Petri dishes) at 37 °C for one day, then shifted to the indicated temperature for 20 h, and then exposed to IL-6 or MG132 or both. Cell cultures were exposed to MG132 (40 µM) for 30 min prior to the addition of IL-6 (30 ng/ml) for another 30 min in the continued presence of MG132. ns, nonspecific DNA binding. From [57].

(STAT1 homodimer), Complex B (STAT1/3 heterodimer), and Complex A (STAT3 homodimer) as well as a slower mobility Complex A* previously shown to correspond to STAT5 homodimer (Fig. 8). Thus functionally (i) there was a reduction in the nuclear pool of DNA-binding competent STAT proteins during masking, and (ii) consistent with its ability to block masking, the proteasomal inhibitor MG132 enhanced STAT-DNA binding activity [20]. An additional functional consequence of STAT-masking was the reduced responsiveness of IL-6-(and STAT3/5)-responsive reporter constructs to this cytokine. We used the construct βFibCAT, which contains two copies of the IL-6 response element from the β-fibrinogen gene promoter linked to the basal adenovirus late promoter (2×IL-6RE/CAT is also abbreviated βFibCAT [62]. This construct is known to be responsive to STAT3 and STAT5. There was a reduction in the responsiveness of the βFibCAT reporter construct to IL-6 in p53-Val-135-containing cells that had been previously incubated at 32.5 °C, when compared to the p53-free parental Hep3B cells [63]. These data are consistent with the hypothesis that STAT-masking results in a functional alteration in the response of p53-containing cells to cytokines such as IL-6 (Fig. 2).

Conclusions

In this review we have briefly discussed two very recent insights into the involvement of IL-6 in cancer, derived from work in this laboratory. Research into the regulation of abnormalities in circulating chaperoned IL-6 in cancer patients is in its infancy. The potential implications of regulated bioavailability of cytokines from within the intravascular compartment are far-reaching, and include the possibility that the elicitation of chaperoned cytokines during active anti-cancer immunization regimens may be a prerequisite for clinical efficacy. At the cellular level, the discovery that Jak-STAT signalling elicited by IL-6 in hepatoma cells can be negatively regulated through p53- and proteasome-dependent STAT-masking points to new regulatory biochemical mechanisms that remain to be elucidated with respect to the responsiveness of cancer cells to cytokines. Uncovering the detailed molecular and cellular mechanisms involved in STAT-masking will be exciting.

Acknowledgements
The involvement of Dr. Ravi J. Rayanade, Dr. Abraham Mittelman, Dr. Lester T. May, Mr. Kirit Patel and Mr. MacKevin I. Ndubuisi in the experiments discussed is gratefully acknowledged. We thank Drs Joseph Etlinger, Sansar Sharma and Victor Fried for numerous discussions. Work in the author's laboratory would not have been possible without the help and encouragement of Elyse S. Goldweber, Josephine Lauriello, Suzanne Andrews, Benjamin Z. Holczer and Kimberly A. Sorrentino. Supported by research grants from the American Cancer Society (IM-701B and IM-735) and a contract from the National Foundation for Cancer Research.

References

1. Oppenheim J, Rossio JL, Gearing AJH (eds) (1993) *Clinical applications of cytokines: role in pathogenesis, diagnosis and therapy.* Oxford: Oxford University Press.
2. Kirkwood JM, Strawderman MH, Ernstoff MS, Smith TJ, Borden EC (1996) Interferon-alfa-2b adjuvant therapy of high-risk resected cutaneous melanoma: the Eastern Cooperative Oncology Group Trial EST 1684. *J Clin Invest* 14: 7–17.

3. Hirano T, Taga T, Yasukawa K, Nakajima K, Nakano N, Takatsuki F, Shimizu M, Murashima A, Tsunasawa S, Sakiyama F et al. (1987) Human B-cell differentiation factor defined by an anti-peptide antibody and its possible role in autoantibody production. *Proc Natl Acad Sci USA* 84: 228–231.
4. Tabibzadeh SS, Pouboridis D, May LT, Sehgal PB (1989) Interleukin-6 immunoreactivity in human tumors. *Am J Pathol* 135: 427–433.
5. Sehgal PB, Grieninger G, Tosato G (eds) (1989) Regulation of the acute phase and immune responses: interleukin 6. *Ann NY Acad Sci* 557: 1–583.
6. Sehgal PB (1990) Interleukin-6 in infection and cancer. *Proc Soc Exp Biol Med* 195: 183–191.
7. Kawano M, Hirano T, Matsuda T, Taga T, Horii Y, Iwato K, Assoku H, Tang B, Tanabe O, Tanaka H et al. (1988) Autocrine generation and requirement of BSF-2/IL-6 for human multiple myeloma. *Nature* 332: 83–85.
8. Yoshizaki K, Matsuda T, Nishimoto N, Kuritani T, Taeho L, Aozawa K, Nakahata T, Kawai H, Tagob H, Komori T et al. (1989) Pathogenic significance of interleukin-6 (Il-6/BSF-2) in Castleman's disease. *Blood* 74: 1360–1367.
9. Kishimoto T (1989) The biology of interleukin-6. *Blood* 74: 1–10.
10. Oldenberg HSA, Rogy MA, Lazarus DD, Van Zee K, Keeler BP, Chizzonite RA, Lowry SF, Moldawer LL (1993) Cachexia and the acute-phase protein response in inflammation are regulated by interleukin-6. *Eur J Immunol* 23: 1889–1894.
11. Mackiewicz A, Koj A, Sehgal PB (eds) (1995) Interleukin-6-type cytokines. *Ann NY Acad Sci* 762: 1–513.
12. Kishimoto T, Akira S, Taga T (1992) Interleukin-6 and its receptor: a paradigm for cytokines. *Science* 258: 593–597.
13. Kishimoto T, Akira S, Narazaki M, Taga T (1995) Interleukin-6 family of cytokines and gp130. *Blood* 86: 1243–1254.
14. Schindler C, Darnell JE Jr (1995) Transcriptional responses to polypeptide ligands: The Jak-STAT pathway. *Annu Rev Biochem* 64: 621–651.
15. Ihle JN (1996) STATs: Signal transducers and activators of transcription. *Cell* 84: 331–334.
16. Darnell JE Jr, Kerr IM, Stark GR (1994) Jak-STAT pathways and transcriptional activation in response to IFNs and other extracellular signaling proteins. *Science* 264: 1415–1421.
17. Bystryn JC, Ferrone S, Livingston P (eds) (1993) Specific immunotherapy of cancer with vaccines. *Ann NY Acad Sci* 690: 1–401.
18. Mittelman A, Chen ZJ, Kageshita T, Yand H, Yamada M, Baskind P, Goldberg N, Puccio C, Ahmed T, Arlin Z, Ferrone S (1990) Active specific immunotherapy in patients with melanoma. *J Clin Invest* 86: 2136–2144.
19. Mittelman A, Chen ZJ, Yang H, Wong GY et al. (1992) Human high molecular weight-melanoma associated antigen (HMW-MAA) mimicry by mouse anti-idiotypic monoclonal antibody MK2-23: induction of humoral anti-HMW-MAA immunity and prolongation of survival in patients with stage IV melanoma. *Proc Natl Acad Sci USA* 89: 466–470.
20. May LT, Patel K, Garcia D, Ndubuisi MI, Ferrone S, Mittelman A, Mackiewicz A, Sehgal PB (1994) Sustained high levels of circulating chaperoned interleukin 6 after active specific cancer immunotherapy. *Blood* 84: 1887–1895.
21. Sehgal PB (1996) Interleukin-6-type cytokines *in vivo*: regulated bioavailability. *Proc Soc Exp Biol Med* 213: 238–247.
22. Ndubuisi M, Patel K, Rayanade RJ, Mittelman A, May LT, Sehgal PB (1998) Distinct classes of chaperoned IL-6 in human blood: differential immunological and biological availability. *J Immunol* 160: 494–501.
23. Salantz CA Jr, McCollister DA, Kanor S (1982) Autologous anti-cancer preparation for specific immunotherapy in advanced cancer patients. *J Cancer Immunol Immunother* 13: 75–84.
24. Rechler MM (1993) Insulin-like growth factor binding proteins. *Vit and Horm* 47: 1–114.
25. Lee PDK, Conover CA, Powell DR (1993) Regulation and function of insulin-like growth factor-binding protein-1. *Proc Soc Exp Biol Med* 204: 4–29.
26. Katz LEL, Rosenfeld RG, Cohen SP (1995) Clinical significance of insulin-like growth factor binding proteins (IGFBPs). *Endocrinology* 5: 36–43.
27. Lowe WL Jr (1996) Insulin-like growth factors. *Sci Amer (Sci and Med)* 3: 62–71.
28. Mogul HR, Marshall M, Frey M, Burke HB, Wynn PES, Wilker S, Southern AL, Gambert SR (1996) Insulin like growth factor-binding protein-1 as a marker for hyperinsulinemia in obese menopausal women. *J Clin Endocrinol Met* 81: 4492–4495.
29. May LT, Santhanam U, Sehgal PB (1991) On the multimeric nature of human interleukin-6. *J Biol Chem* 266: 9950–9955.
30. May LT, Viguet H, Kenny JS, Ida N, Allison AC, Sehgal PB (1992) High levels of "complexed" interleukin 6 in human blood. *J Biol Chem* 267: 19698–19704.
31. May LT, Neta R, Moldawer LL, Kenny JS, Patel K, Sehgal PB (1993) Antibodies chaperone circulating IL-6. *J Immunol* 151: 3225–3236.
32. Honda M, Yamamoto S, Cheng M, Yasukawa K, Suzuki H, Saito T, Osigi T, Tokunaga T, Kishimoto T (1992) Human soluble IL-6 receptor: its detection and enhanced release by HIV infection. *J Immunol* 148: 2175–2180.

33. Narazaki M, Yasukawa K, Saito T, Ohsugi Y, Fukui H, Koishihar Y, Yancopoulos GD, Taga T, Kishimoto T (1993) Soluble forms of the interleukin-6 signal-transducing receptor component gp130 in human serum possessing a potential to inhibit signals through membrane-anchored gp130. *Blood* 82: 1120–1126.
34. Lahm A, Savino R, Salvati AL, Caribbo A, Ciapponi L, Demartis A, Toniatti C, Paonessa G, Altamura A, Cilberto G (1995) The molecular design of human IL-6 receptor antagonists. *Ann NY Acad Sci* 762: 136–151.
35. Ward LD, Howlett GJ, Discolo G, Yasukawa K, Hammacher A, Moritz RL, Simpson RJ (1994) High affinity interleukin-6 complex consisting of two molecules each of interleukin-6, interleukin-6 receptor and gp130. *J Biol Chem* 269: 23286–23289.
36. Ward LD, Hammacher A, Howlett GJ, Matthews JM, Fabri L, Moritz RL, Nice EC, Weinstock J, Simpson RJ (1996) Influence of interleukin-6 (IL-6) dimerization on formation of the high affinity hexameric IL-6 receptor complex. *J Biol Chem* 271: 20138–20144.
37. Lu ZY, Brochier J, Wijdenes J, Brailly H, Bataille R, Klein B (1992) High amounts of circulating interleukin (IL)-6 in the form of monomeric immune complexes during anti-IL-6 therapy. Towards a new methodology for measuring overall cytokine production in human *in vivo*. *Eur J Immunol* 22: 2819–2824.
38. Mihara M, Moriya Y, Kishimoto T, Ohsugi Y (1995) Interleukin-6 (IL-6) induces the proliferation of synovial fibroblastic cells in the presence of soluble IL-6 receptor. *Brit J Rheumatol* 34: 321–325.
39. Economides AN, Ravetch JV, Yancopoulos GD, Stahl N (1995) Designer cytokines: targeting actions to cells of choice. *Science* 270: 1351–1353.
40. Yonish-Rouach E, Resnitzky D, Lotem J, Sachs L, Kimchi A, Oren M (1991) Wildtype p53 induces apoptosis of myeloid leukemic cells that is inhibited by interleukin-6. *Nature* 352: 345–347.
41. Levy N, Yonish-Rouach E, Oren M, Kimchi A (1993) Complementation by wildtype p53 of interleukin-6 effects on M1 cells: Induction of cell cycle exit and co-operativity with c-myc suppression. *Mol Cell Biol* 13: 7942–7952.
42. Gottlieb E, Haffner R, von Ruden T, Wagner E, Oren M (1994) Down-regulation of wildtype p53 activity interferes with apoptosis of IL-3-dependent hematopoietic cells following IL-3 withdrawal. *EMBO J* 13: 1368–1374.
43. Levine AJ, Momand J, Finlay CA (1991) The p53 tumour suppressor gene. *Nature* 351: 453–456.
44. Hollstein M, Sidransky D, Vogelstein B, Harris CC (1991) p53 mutations in human cancers. *Science* 253: 49–54.
45. Michalovitz D, Halevy O and Oren M (1991) p53 mutations: Gains or losses? *J Cell Biochem* 45: 22–29.
46. Yin Y, Tainsky MA, Bishoff FZ, Strong LC, Wahl GM (1992) Wildtype p53 retores cell cycle control and inhibits gene amplification in cells with mutant p53 alleles. *Cell* 70: 937–948.
47. Vogelstein B, Kinzler KW (1992) p53 function and dysfunction. *Cell* 70: 523–526.
48. Koshland DE, Culotta E (1993) p53 sweeps through cancer research. *Science* 262: 1958–1961.
49. Oliner JD (1993) Discerning the function of p53 by examining its molecular interactions. *BioEssays* 15: 703–707.
50. Preudhomme C, Facon T, Zandecki M, Vanrumbeke M, Lai JL, Nataf E, Loucheux-Lefebvre MH, Kerckaert JP, Fenaux P (1992) Rare occurrence of p53 gene mutations in multiple myeloma. *Brit J Haematol* 81: 440–443.
51. Neri A, Baldini L, Trecca D, Cro L, Polli E, Maiolo AT (1993) p53 gene mutations in multiple myeloma are associated with advanced forms of malignancy. *Blood* 81: 128–135.
52. Willems PM, Kuypers AW, Meijerink JP, Holdrinet RS, Mensink EJ (1993) Sporadic mutations of p53 gene in mulitple myeloma and no evidence for germ line mutations in three familiar multiple myeloma pedigrees. *Leukemia* 7: 986–991.
53. Corradini P, Inghirami G, Astolfi M, Ladetto M, Voena C, Ballerini P, Gu W, Nilsson K, Knowles DM, Boccadoro M (1994) Inactivation of tumor suppressor genes, p53 and Rb, in plasma cell dyscrasias. *Leukemia* 8: 758–767.
54. Yasuga Y, Hirosawa S, Yamamoto K, Tomiyama J, Nagata K, Aokia N (1995) N-ras and p53 gene mutations are very rare events in multiple myeloma. *Int J Hematol* 62: 91–97.
55. Borsellino N, Belldegrun A, Bonavida B (1995) Endogenous interleukin-6 is a resistance factor for cis-diammincdichroplatinum and ectoposicle-mediated cytotoxicity of human prostate carcinoma cell lines. *Cancer Res* 55: 4633–4639.
56. Hangaishi A, Ogawa S, Imamura N, Miyawaki S, Muira Y, Uike N, Shimazaki C, Emi N, Takeyama K, Hirosawa S et al. (1996) Inactivation of multiple tumor-suppressor genes involved in negative regulation of the cell cycle, MTS1/p16INK4A/CDKN2, MTS2/p17INK4B, p53, and Rb genes in primary lymphoid malignancies. *Blood* 87: 4949–4958.
57. Rayanade RJ, Patel K, Ndubuisi M, Sharma S, Omura S, Etlinger JD, Pine R, Sehgal PB (1997) Proteasome- and p53-dependent masking of signal transducer and activator of transcription (STAT) factors. *J Biol Chem* 272: 4659–4662.
58. Santhanam U, Ray A, Sehgal PB (1991) Repression of the interleukin-6 gene promoter by p53 and the retinoblastoma susceptibility gene produce. *Proc Natl Acad Sci USA* 88: 7605–7609.
59. Margulies L, Sehgal PB (1993) Modulation of the human interleukin-6 (IL-6) promoter and transcription factor C/EBPβ (NF-IL6) activity by p53. *J Biol Chem* 268: 15096–15100.

60. Sehgal PB, Margulies L (1993) Cell type- and promoter-dependent ts phenotype of p53 Val^{135}. *Oncogene* 8: 3417–3419.
61. Sehgal PB, Wang L, Rayanade R, Pan H, Margulies L (1995) Interleukin-6-type cytokines. *Ann NY Acad Sci* 762: 1–13.
62. Wang L, Rayanade R, Garcia D, Patel K, Pan H, Sehgal PB (1995) Modulation of interleukin-6 induced plasma protein secretion in hepatoma cells by p53. *J Biol Chem* 270: 23159–23165.
63. Rayanade R, Ndubuisi MI, Etlinger JD, Sehgal PB (1998) Regulation of interleukin-6 signalling by p53: STAT3 and STAT5 "masking" in p53-Val-135-containing human hepatoma Hep3B cell lines. *J Immunol*; *submitted.*
64. Kim TK, Maniatis T (1996) Regulation of interferon-γ-activated STAT by the ubiquitin-proteasome pathway. *Science* 273: 1717–1719.
65. Haspel RL, Salditt-Georgieff M, Darnell JE Jr (1996) The rapid inactivation of nuclear tyrosine phosphorylated STAT1 depends upon a protein tyrosine phosphatase. *EMBO J* 15: 6262–6268.
66. Scharenberg AM, Kinet J-P (1996) The emerging field of receptor-mediated inhibitory signaling: SHP or SHIP? *Cell* 87: 961–964.
67. Tonks NK, Neel BG (1996) From form to function: Signaling by protein tyrosine phosphatases. *Cell* 87: 365–368.
68. Klingmüller U, Lorenz U, Cantley LC, Neel BG, Lodish HF (1995) Specific recruitment of SH-PTP1 to the erythropoietin receptor causes inactivation of JAK2 and termination of proliferative signals. *Cell* 80: 729–738.
69. David M, Chen HE, Goelz S, Larner AC, Neel BG (1995) Differential regulation of the alpha/beta interferon-stimulated Jak/STAT pathway by the SH2 domain-containing tyrosine phosphatase SHPTP1. *Mol Cell Biol* 15: 7050–7058.
70. David M, Zhou G, Pine R, Dixon JE, Larner AC (1996) The SH2 domain-containing tyrosine phsophatase PTP1D is required for interferon alpha/beta-induced gene expression. *J Biol Chem* 271: 15862–15865.
71. Lechleider RJ, Freeman RM Jr, Neel BG (1993) Tyrosyl phosphorylation and growth factor receptor association of the human corkscrew homologue, *SH-PTP2*. *J Biol Chem* 268: 13434–13438.
72. Tailor P, Jascur T, Williams S, von Willebrand M, Couture C, Mustelin T (1996) Involvement of Src-homology-2-domain-containing protein-tyrosine phosphatase 2 in T cell activation. *Eur J Biochem* 237: 736–742.
73. Bennett AM, Hausdorff SF, O'Reilly AM, Freeman RM, Neel BG (1996) Multiple requirements for *SHPTP2* in epidermal growth factor-mediated cell cycle progression. *Mol Cell Biol* 16: 1189–1202.
74. Boulton TG, Stahl N, Yancopoulos GD (1994) Ciliary neutrotrophic factor/ leukemia inhibitor factor/interleukin 6/oncostatin M family of cytokines induces tyrosine phosphorylation of a common set of proteins overlapping those induced by other cytokines and growth factors. *J Biol Chem* 269: 11648–11655.
75. Kharitonenkov A, Chen Z, Sures I, Wang H, Schilling J, Ullrich A (1997) A family of proteins that inhibit signalling through tyrosine kinases receptors. *Nature* 386: 181–186.

Molecular Aspects of Cancer and its Therapy
A. Mackiewicz and P.B. Sehgal (eds)
© 1998 Birkhäuser Verlag Basel/Switzerland

Gene therapy of cancer

M. Wiznerowicz, S. Rose-John[1] and A. Mackiewicz

Department of Cancer Immunology, University School of Medical Sciences at Great Poland Cancer Center, 15 Garbary St., PL-61-866 Poznan, Poland
[1]Abteilung Pathophysiologie. I Med. Klinik, Johannes Gutenberg-Universität, Obere Zahlbacher Str. 63, D-55101 Mainz, Germany

Introduction

Gene therapy may be defined as an alteration of the cell phenotype by insertion of the "correct" or removal of the "incorrect" genetic information into normal cells in order to control or treat a disease. Cells may be genetically modified *ex vivo* (cellular gene therapy) or *in vivo* (gene therapy) (Fig. 1).

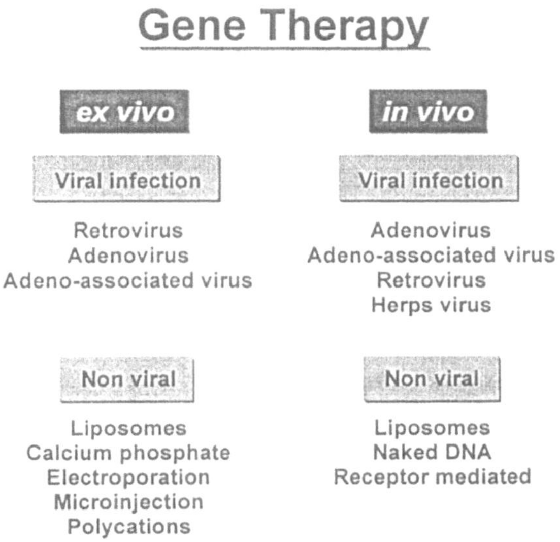

Figure 1. Two major approaches to gene therapy. Cells are genetically modified *in vitro* (*ex vivo*) and readministrated to the patient, or therapeutic gene is delivered directly to the patient and genetic modification occurs *in vivo*.

Gene therapy could be aimed either to cure hereditary diseases (the most common ones are due to enzymatic deficiencies) or to cure patients of acquired maladies such as cancer or AIDS. Since many hereditary diseases are caused by a single gene defect which induces the breakdown of some specific metabolic pathways, the therapeutic aproaches introduce a functional gene copy directly into the defective cell. These approaches are based on gene augmentation, improving the cellular phenotype and restoring proper metabolic function. Ideally, this need would be best achieved by replacement of the defective sequences with normal sequences through homologous recombination. Only this mechanism can ensure that the foreign genes will be regulated as faithfully and appropriately as the endogenous genes.

Gene therapy could be applied both to germ lines or somatic cells. However, for ethical and practical reasons, only somatic cell therapy is currently the focus of investigation.

Conventional treatment of cancer uses chemotherapy, radiotherapy or surgery to kill or remove transformed cells. These methods cause considerable damage to patients (especially radio- and chemotherapy) and/or give very unreliable results in cases of metastatic cancer.

So far about 120 clinical protocols of human cancer gene therapy have been designed, involving about 300 patients.

Gene delivery systems

The technological basis of gene therapy are the gene delivery systems. An ideal system should have the following characteristics: (1) protect and deliver DNA into cells efficiently, preferably to a specific cell type; (2) be nontoxic and nonimmunogenic; and (3) be easily produced in large quantities. No existing system meets all of the requirements. However, each of the gene vehicles so far developed possesses at least one of those properties.

Gene delivery systems currently employed can be divided into two major groups: nonviral and viral. In nonviral systems the therapeutic gene is placed into a common DNA plasmid. DNA in this form ("naked"), or in a complex with cationic lipids, or conjugated with ligands, is delivered to the cells of interest. Usually, naked or complexed DNA is able to transfect both dividing and nondividing cells. Plasmid DNA does not integrate into the genome of the target cell, resulting in transient gene expression. The most important advantages of the system are: no limits to the size of therapeutic DNA, safety, and low cost production which allows large scale preparations.

Viral-based systems use prepared *in vitro* recombinant viruses (retroviruses, adenoviruses or adeno-associated viruses) which contain the therapeutic gene within their chimeric genome, and utilizes their natural ability to infect eukaryotic cells.

In all viral systems used thus far, packaging cells for production of the recombinant viruses are needed. Limitations of the system are the constrained insert size (usually 5–10 kb, depending on the vector used) and preparation (time consuming and expensive). Moreover, adenoviral vectors were shown to be immunogenic when administrated *in vivo*. However, efficiency of gene transfer by means of viral systems is much higher than non-viral methods. In addition, retroviral and adeno-associated viral vectors permit stable integration of therapeutic genes with the cellular genome, allowing stable and continuous production of therapeutic protein.

Nonviral delivery systems

The concerns over safety, and the difficulty in obtaining large quantities of recombinant viral vectors, have directed research into the efficient, nonimmunogenic and low-cost nonviral vector systems. Approaches using naked DNA, polylysine conjugates and cationic liposomes are the most promising.

Naked DNA immunization

The idea of *in vivo* DNA delivery, referred to as DNA or polynucleotide vaccination, came from the plant biology gene gun techinque, which was developed to overcome the problems of introducing plasmids into plants. Originally, small gold particles were coated with plasmids containing target genes and such complexes were delivered by bombardment into plant cells with rigid cellulose walls. This technology was subsequently applied to animal cells *in vitro* [1], and *in vivo* by delivering plasmids deep into murine tissues using a gunpowder discharge that accelerates DNA-coated microprojectiles [2]. More simply, plasmids may be inoculated into a mouse skeletal muscle using a normal hypodermic needle and syringe [3]. It was found that skeletal muscle cells have a unique ability to take up naked DNA and express it more efficiently than cells of other tissues. Host muscle cells take up foreign DNA by pinocytosis, express the therapeutic gene, and produce the corresponding protein in the cytoplasm. An important issue is that the produced proteins enter the cell's major histocompatibility complex (MHC) class I pathway. The protein is processed, complexed with MHC-I and presented on the cell surface, where, by stimulating CD8+ cytotoxic T cells, it evokes a cell-mediated reaction. In muscle cells effective presentation of expressed antigens to cytotoxic T lymphocytes (CTLs) is speculative because myocytes express only low levels of MHC-I molecules and probably do not express enough accessory costimulatory molecules required for T cell activation. In such a case one would expect promotion of anergy and tolerance rather than priming of a CTL response. The mechanism of immune system activation probably involves antigen presenting cells. Most likely it is mediated by macrophages which infiltrate and phagocytose injured muscle tissue expressing target proteins. Following presentation *via* MHC-II molecules, CD4+ cells are activated and provide necessary helper functions to CD8+ lymphocytes.

Direct *in vivo* DNA delivery has found several applications in cancer gene therapy.

A number of studies reported the posibilities of immunizing animals against tumour antigens such as carcinoembryonic antigen (CEA) [4] or melanoma associated antigens (MART) or oncogene products e.g., Her-neu [5] or large T antigen of SV40 [6].

Not only muscle cells are capable of taking up injected DNA particles. It has been shown that direct injection of malignant melanomas with a plasmid carrying the herpes simplex thymidine kinase gene under the control of a melanoma-specific tyrosinase promotor caused significant tumour reduction after ganciclovir treatment [7].

This technology can also be applied to deliver cytokine genes directly into the tumour tissue. High local levels of given cytokine would be an effective stimulator of primed CTLs. Recently, it was reported that a plasmid containing the cDNA for human GM-CSF was transfected using a gene gun into human melanoma and sarcoma cells *in vitro* in order to prepare an autologous antimelanoma vaccine for a phase I/IB clinical trial [8]. Another study demonstrated the feasibility of transferring cDNAs coding LacZ, IL-2, IL-6 and GM-CSF by gene gun into canine oral mucosa and epidermis, resulting in protein expression [9]. Naked DNA can also be targeted to a tumour site by coupling a plasmid carrying a therapeutic cDNA molecule to a substance for which membrane receptors are present on a target cell, or a monoclonal antibody specific for a particular cell type, using polylysine (protamine or histones have also been proposed) (Fig. 2). In this system, following specific binding the DNA-ligand conjugate reaches the cytoplasm using the receptor-mediated endocytosis pathway and forms endosomes. After endosome disruption DNA is released into the cytoplasm where expression of the target gene takes place. Escape from the cell vesicle system is achieved by some viral agents incorporated into the DNA-polylysine-ligand/antibody conjugate, which disrupts the endosome.

This gene transfer system has been used in several *in vitro* tumour systems. It has been shown that DNA conjugated with HPV capsid protein was efficiently taken up by cervical carcinoma cells [10]. In another study an EGF receptor, overexpressed in many tumours, was used to target DNA to lung cancer [11]. The same principle has also been used in the case of folate, receptors for which are overexpressed in ovarian cancer cells [12]. Insertion into mice of syngeneic melanoma cells genetically modified to secrete IL-2, *via* the receptor-mediated endocytosis system, resulted in long-term protection of these animals against challenge with wildtype parental cells and induced elimination of pre-existing cancer cell deposits. These data have served as a basis for a clinical protocol for the treatment of melanoma [13].

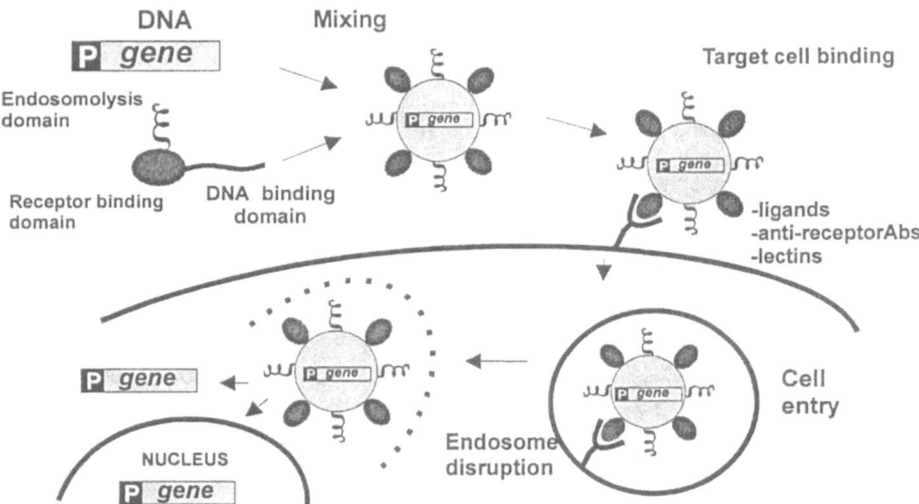

Figure 2. Plasmid DNA carrying therapeutic gene might be complexed with the ligand and in such form targetted to a specific cell type. Endosomolysis domain, often incorporated into the complex, allows endosome disruption within the transfected cell. In most cases the therapeutic gene does not stably integrate into the cell genome.

Liposomes

Liposomes may be used to encapsulate pharmacological agents, as well as plasmid DNA, and serve as delivery vehicles for the genetic modification of mammalian cells [14]. DNA forms a complex with lipids through charge interactions. Cationic liposomes normally contain a positively charged lipid and a neutral helper lipid, dioleoylphosphatidylethanolamine (DOPE). DOPE helps nonbilayer-forming cationic lipids to form stable liposomes. The group of cationic lipids includes: cationic cholesterol derivatives [15], lipopolylysine [16], and some surfactants [17]. Most double-chain cationic lipids form liposomes by themselves, or as a mixture with DOPE. DNA in liposome complexes is protected from degradation by endonucleases or ionizing radiation.

A cationic complex binds to a negatively charged cellular membrane due to the excess of positively charged residues on the liposome (Fig. 3). After binding plasmid DNA enters the cell. For most cell lines liposomes can be taken up *via* coated and noncoated pathways. Larger complexes reach the cytoplasm using noncoated vesicles. The size of liposome particles varies, depending on the charge ratio between liposome and DNA, and the final concentration of the complex. Various cell types may differ in their ability to take up particles of different size, which may partially explain why some cells are more difficult to transfect than others.

Following internalisation the DNA usually stays in the cytoplasm and in most cases does not integrate into the cellular genome. Following transcription and translation of the target gene,

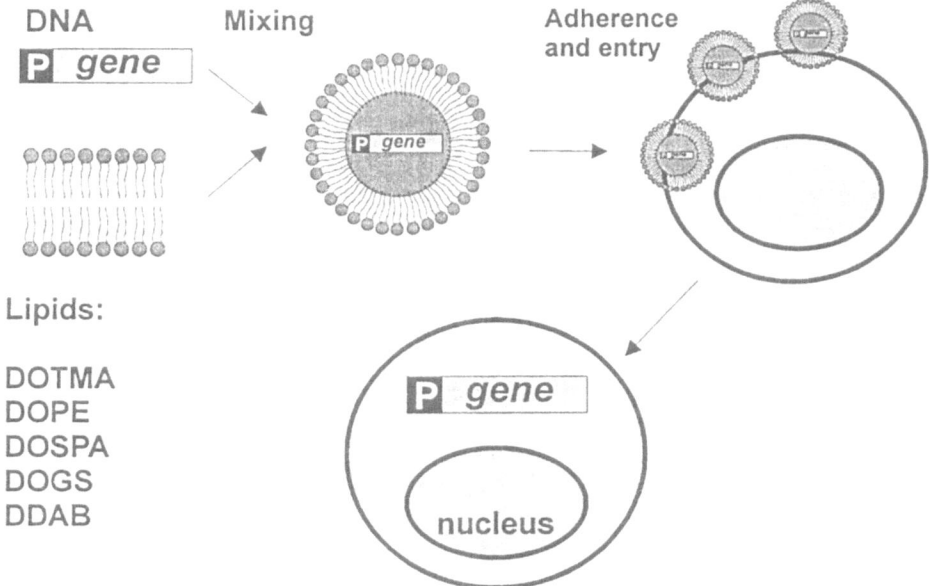

Figure 3. Plasmid DNA containing therapeutic gene can be complexed with lipids which increase adherence and entry to the target cell. Sometimes liposomes are modified by incorporation of ligands or monoclonal antibodies specific for a given cell type for cell-specific targetting. In most cases the therapeutic gene does not stably integrate into the cell genome.

therapeutic protein is produced. Due to its episomal character, the plasmid DNA is almost totally lost after cell division (usually within less than one week). Only a few copies incorporate into the cellular genome, giving rise to stable transfectants. Due to its relative simplicity, efficiency and reproducibility, cationic liposome-mediated transfection has been widely used to introduce foreign genes into a variety of primary and established cell lines.

In vivo DNA-liposome complexes were delivered to lung [18, 19] and nasal epithelium [20] by aerosol [21–23], to arterial epithelium by catheters [24], or by direct injection into brain [25] and tumours [26, 27] or by systemic administration [18, 28].

In cancer gene therapy the last approach, using *in situ* therapeutic gene delivery directly into the tumour mass, has been extensively studied in murine models. Cationic liposomes have been chosen for this purpose for several reasons. First, transient gene expression is sufficient to prime an efficient CTL response. Second, direct injection into the tumour mass is simple, convenient, and reproducible. Finally, cationic liposomes are nonimmunogenic and are therefore safe for multiple injections, an advantage compared to adenoviral vectors used in a similar approach.

Antisense

In order to eliminate expression of unwanted genes, antisense and ribozyme strategies were developed. The antisense approach to gene therapy utilizes synthetic oligonucleotides (oligos) or cDNA of the target gene expressed in the antisense orientation in the target cell to interfere with the natural processing of genetic information, in order to block protein expression [29]. Antisense oligos are short fragments (7–30 nucleotides in length) of DNA or modified DNA that are complementary to a target RNA (Fig. 4). Antisense cDNAs are delivered to the target cells by means of viral or nonviral vectors and antisense mRNA is transcribed. The oligos are normally added to the culture medium and are thought to enter the cell *via* endocytosis [30]. Both oligos and antisense mRNA selectively hybridize with the target mRNA sequence by hydrogen base-pair bonds. Ideally, this hybridization should interfere with the RNA transport, splicing and translation resulting in inhibition of pathological protein production. In some cases such antisense-RNA duplexes are more prone to degradation by a cellular RNAase H. Antisense oligos are also designed to inhibit transcription *via* triplex formation by binding to the major groove of DNA and forming triple-strand helix. The specificity of this binding is not Watson-Crick pairing, since the base pair is already formed, but is due to Hoogsten hydrogen-bonded interactions of a third base with the pair [31]. Some antisense molecules display their activity through direct interaction with the target proteins.

However, several obstacles have been encountered during the development of antisense technology. Nonmodified oligos are susceptible to degradation by cellular and extracellular nucleases [32]. Chemical modification of phosphodiester linkages of oligos by a variety of methods confers resistance to degradation in culture [33]. Another problem is the efficient delivery of synthesized oligos to the target cells in culture. Direct microinjection, electroporation or application of cationic liposomes as vehicles was shown to enhance antisense activity greatly.

For almost twenty years extensive studies have been carried out to apply antisense oligos in cancer therapy. A number of *in vitro* experiments demonstrated their role as antiproliferative agents. However, in some instances their activity was mediated through sequence-dependent rather than antisense mechanisms. For example, oligos containing four guanosine residues exerted

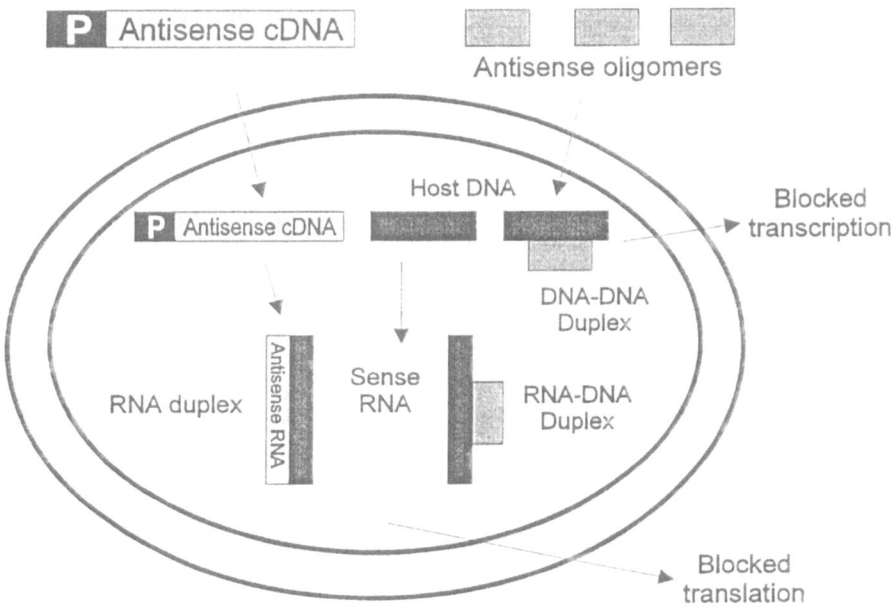

Figure 4. Antisense technology. Antisense cDNA may be expressed in the target cell following delivery by a vector (viral or non-viral). Short antisense oligos may be taken up by the target cells. Antisense oligos bind to DNA and inhibit mRNA synthesis, or hybridize with mRNA and block translation.

antiproliferative activity in a number of cell types tested. Anticancer therapies using antisense oligos are mainly focused on inhibiting the activity of intracellular proteins that control or have some influence on the cell cycle, such as oncogenes or mutated tumour suppressor genes.

Using animal tumour models the potential therapeutic effect of inhibiting different oncogenes has been demonstrated including *bcl-2* [34], c-*fos* [35], *IGF-I* [36], *E6/E7* of HPV [37], *mdr-1* [38], *AKT-2* [39], *TGF-β* [40], *cyclin-D* [41], *VEGF* [42], and *BCR-ABL* [43]. However, complete suppression of tumour formation has not been achieved in many instances. One possible explanation is the presence of multiple factors playing a role in tumorigenesis.

Clinical gene therapy trials using antisense oligos against two types of cancers are currently underway. One of them is treating acute lymphoblastic leukaemia (AML) using antisense oligonucleotides against p53. Levels of the tumour suppressor gene product p53 is markedly elevated in AML patients. This formed the basis for studies in which antisense oligos targeting p53 caused the death of abnormal cells. However, a phase I clinical trial failed to demonstrate therapeutic effects in patients. A phase I/II clinical trial is currently underway, applying a combined approach in which patients are treated with anti-p53 antisense oligomer along with mitoxantrone and cytosine arabinoside. In an independent clinical trial, bone marrow cells have been exposed *ex vivo* to p53 antisense oligomer for 36 h before reinfusion. The treatment was combined with conventional chemotherapy using agents such as VP-16 or BCNU.

Recently, the results of a clinical trial employing *BCL-2* antisense therapy in patients with non-Hodgkin lymphoma have been reported [34]. Antisense oligonucleotides targeted to the open reading frame of the BCL-2 mRNA caused a specific down-regulation of BCL-2 expression which led to increased apoptosis. Subcutaneous infusion of an 18-base, fully phosphorothioated antisense oligonucleotide administered daily for 2 weeks to nine patients who had BCL-2-positive relapsed non-Hodgkin lymphoma demonstrated no treatment-related toxic effects beside local inflammation at the infusion site. In two patients, the number of circulating lymphoma cells decreased during treatment. In some patients improvement of clinical status, objective biochemical and radiological evidence of tumour response, and down-regulation of the BCL-2, were observed.

Ribozymes
Ribozymes are naturally existing molecules which have been adapted to degrade specific mRNA molecules and inhibit expression of target protein [44]. Ribozymes are essentially antisense oligos in which the complementary fragments flank an active site, which cleaves a bound mRNA molecule (Fig. 5). The cleavage renders mRNA unstable and prevents protein production. Because of the flexibility of design and the extraordinary sequence specificity, trans-cleaving catalytic RNA, such as the "hammerhead" or "hairpin" ribozymes, might be useful as therapeutic

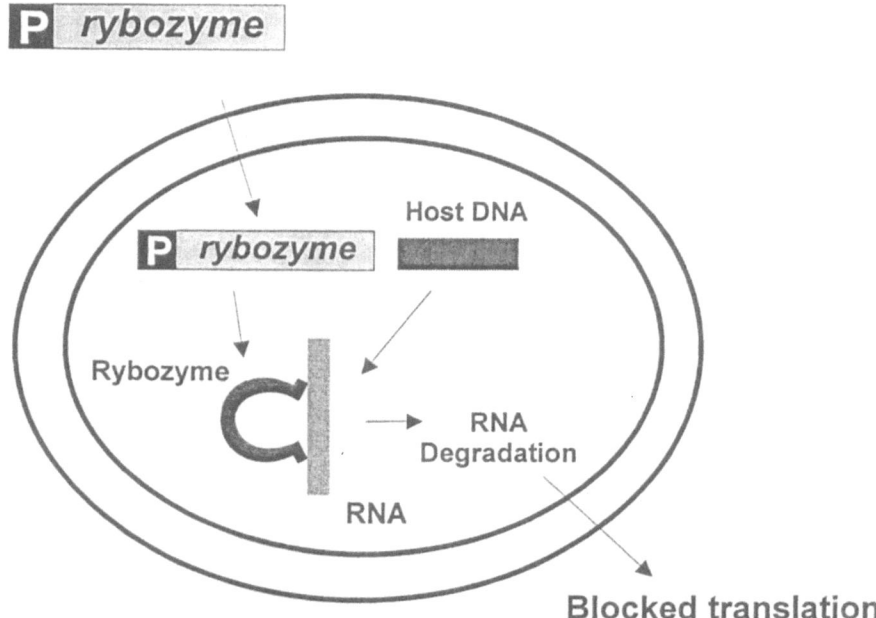

Figure 5. Ribozyme cDNAs are delivered to the target cells in a vector. After transcription this catalytic molecule specifically hybridizes with target gene mRNA, leading to its degradation.

agents [45]. Distinct advantages of ribozymes include low immunogenicity and small size, which facilitates insertion of multiple copies into a gene therapy vector in place of a gene encoding a single protein. Since ribozymes are functional as RNA molecules and do not depend on the activity of polymerase II, polymerase III-based promoters (e.g., tRNA or U6 snRNA promoter) are often used to drive their expression [46, 47]. A ribozyme under control of a given promoter is placed into a plasmid-liposome complex, retroviral or adenoviral vector and delivered to the target tumour cells. Ribozymes targetting oncogenes, transport proteins or growth factors have been designed for the specific inhibition of tumour cell proliferation, drug resistance and angiogenesis. The efficacy of expression of a ribozyme construct in tumour cells has been demonstrated for ribozymes targeting mRNA for H-RAS (bladder cancer) [48], c-FOS [49], p53 (lung cancer) [50], BCR/ABL [51], CD44 (glioma) [52], CAPL (osteosarcoma) [53], matrix metalloproteinase-9 (H-ras and myc-transformed cells) [54], telomerase (HepG2, Huh-7) [55], VLA-6 integrin (fibrosarcoma) [56] the multidrug resistance gene product P-glycoprotein (lung cancer, mesothelioma, pancreatic cancer, acute leukemia) [57, 58] and pleiotrophin (melanoma) [59]. Several laboratories are exploring a novel application of this technology which employs the splicing ability of ribozymes to introduce new functions or correct pre-existing defects, rather than inhibit gene expression. One group engineered a ribozyme to correct a mutated *lacZ* gene in *Escherichia coli*. This innovative approach would find an application in cancer gene therapy for correction of mutated forms of different tumour suppressor genes occurring commonly in a variety of tumours.

Viral delivery systems

Viral vectors are the most frequently used vehicles for therapeutic gene delivery in gene therapy trials. Their advantages over nonviral system are (1) high effectiveness in transduction of dividing (retroviral, adenoviral, adeno-associated vectors) and nondividing (adenoviral, adeno-associated vectors) cells, and (2) stability of integrated therapeutic genes.

However, the high cost of production and possibilitiy of contamination with helper virus (which is however very low) produce some limitations.

Retroviral vectors
Retroviral vectors are the most powerful tools of gene transfer into mammalian cells [60–62]. The advantages of using these genetically modified RNA viruses as carriers of foreign genetic material are significant. They include relatively simple design, the well-understood biology of retroviruses, their nonpathogenic nature, facility of integration into the host cell genome, and high gene expression and stability of viral particles. However, the relatively low viral titre (compared to adenoviral vectors), limited capacity for foreign DNA (7–8 kb), inability to infect non-dividing cells, possible insertional mutagenesis, and complement inactivation *in vivo*, create some important disadvantages.

Retroviral genetic material consists of two molecules of homologous RNA. After internalization following binding to the surface receptors, viral RNA is transcribed through the action of reverse transcriptase to form a proviral DNA. The provirus is translocated into the nucleus and integrated into the genome of the target cell.

The proviral DNA consists of functional sequences, the so-called "long terminal repeats" (LTR), containing promotor sequences and sites for mRNA polyadenylation, and sequences encoding the viral core (*gag*), envelope proteins (*env*), reverse transcriptase and integrase (*pol*).

The system for production of recombinant viral particles has two components: the retroviral vector, and packaging cells (Fig. 6). In the retroviral vector, genes encoding viral proteins are replaced by the genes of interest. Usually, beside the therapeutic gene, a positively selectable marker gene (for antibiotic resistance) is used. Viral proteins are provided *in trans* by the so-called packaging cells, which are mouse fibroblasts transfected with plasmids containing the viral genome depleted of packaging sequence, thus enabling replication of the wildtype virus. After transfection of retroviral vector into packaging cells, RNA translated from the vector containing the gene of interest and the packaging sequence combines with *gag*, *env* and *pol* proteins produced in the packaging cells. The recombinant virus is used to infect (transduce) target cells.

In classical constructs the 5' LTR drives expression of the therapeutic gene. In most gene transfer protocols, vectors containing genes to be expressed also carry a positively selectable marker (e.g., neomycin, hygromycin, or puromycin resistance). Transfected or transduced target cells are usually selected in the presence of antibiotic and then analysed for the expression of foreign gene. Classically, the selectable gene in recombinant vectors is placed under the control of separate, internal promoter. Due to the interference of the promoters, leading to downregulation of internal promoter activity, such constructs yield a population of resistant cells within which only small proportion (5–10%) express the therapeutic gene [63]. Accordingly, cells expressing thera-

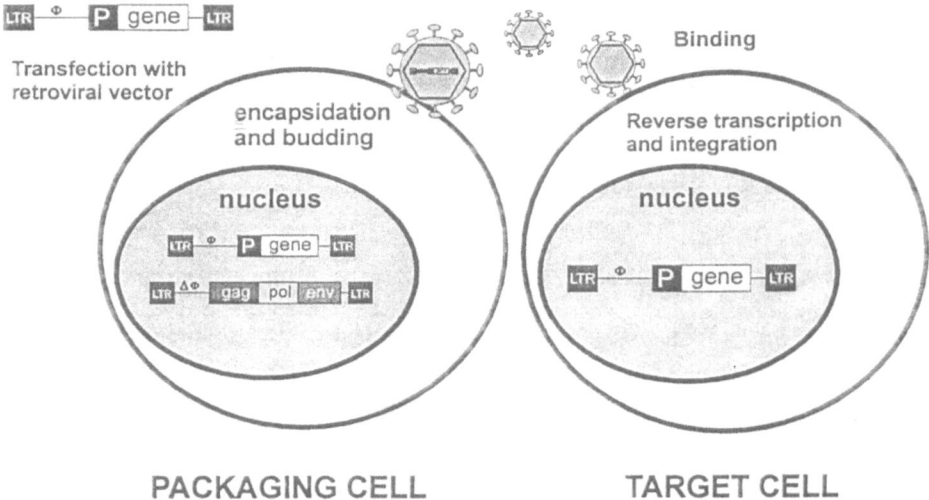

Figure 6. Retroviral vector carrying therapeutic gene is transfected *in vitro* into packaging cells. mRNA transcribed from the vector combines with viral proteins provided by packaging cells *in trans*. Packaging sequence in the wildtype mRNA was mutated thus enabling packaging into viral particles. Recombinant viral particles are continously released without cell disruption and are able to integrate therapeutic genes stably into target cell genome during division.

peutic gene have to be cloned, which is time-consuming and costly. One way to overcome this problem is to create a bifunctional chimaeric protein by fusing the therapeutic gene in-frame with the selectable marker gene [64]. However, this is not practical when the product of the therapeutic gene is a secreted protein.

Another approach which avoids transcriptional interference involves the use of internal ribosome entry site (IRES) sequences from the 5'-untranslated regions of picornaviruses such as polio virus or encephalomyocarditis virus (EMCV), to create polycistronic transcripts encoding multiple gene products [65]. The unique three-dimensional structure of IRES enables binding of ribosomes in the middle of the mRNA molecule and 5' cap-independent translation. IRES are used in retroviral vectors to join therapeutic and selectable marker cDNAs in order to create a dicistronic gene. In our studies we used the bacterial betagalactosidase gene (*lacZ*) as a marker and *neo* as a resistance gene. A lacZ-IRES-neo cassette was inserted into various retroviral vectors, replacing the lacZ-pgk-neo cassette in which pgk was used as an internal promoter (Fig. 7A). Due to simultaneous translation of both genes, such constructs ensured almost 100% expression of the marker gene in the pooled resistant cell population [66].

Another way to avoid promoter interference is to insert the target gene outside the transcriptional unit of the vector [67–69]. In such constructs the cassette containing the gene of interest under control of the exogenous promoter is inserted into the U3 region of the 3'LTR. mRNA transcription is terminated by the action of the pA site within the R region. Thus the expression of target gene is not influenced by the viral LTR and should depend on the promoter used. Moreover, due to the unique activity of reverse transcriptase which copies 3'LTR sequences to 5'LTR, the therapeutic gene in target cells is duplicated, which produces its high level of expression. Usually in such constructs the resistance gene remains under the control of the exogenous promoter. Vectors designed as described above are referred to as double-copy.

In our studies, we created an original version of a double-copy vector, inserting a cassette containing a dicistronic gene under the control of a strong HCMV-IE promoter, into the U3 region of the 3'LTR. These vectors provided high levels of human interleukin-6 (hIL-6) and soluble IL-6 receptor (sIL-6R) mRNA expression, and production of corresponding proteins [66] (Fig. 7B, C, D).

Adenoviral vectors;
Adenoviral (Ad) vectors are also widely used in gene therapy protocols due to their ability to transduce nondividing cells. These vectors can be produced at higher viral titres ($>10^{11}$) than retroviral vectors [70]. However, the therapeutic gene is not integrated into the genome of the target cell, which leads to transient expression of the therapeutic protein.

Adenoviruses have a relatively large DNA genome (around 36 kb). Most genes are essential for the viral life cycle and so there is not much space for insertion of additional genes. However, using a similar approach to the retroviral packaging system, a packaging cell line based on human embryonic kidney cells and referred to as 293 has been established [71]. This cell line carries and expresses adenoviral *E1* gene whose product complements *in trans* the adenoviral genome lacking this sequence.

To obtain recombinant adenoviral vectors, 293 cells have to be cotransfected with plasmid carrying a cassette containing the therapeutic gene inserted into a fragment of the Ad genome (0–

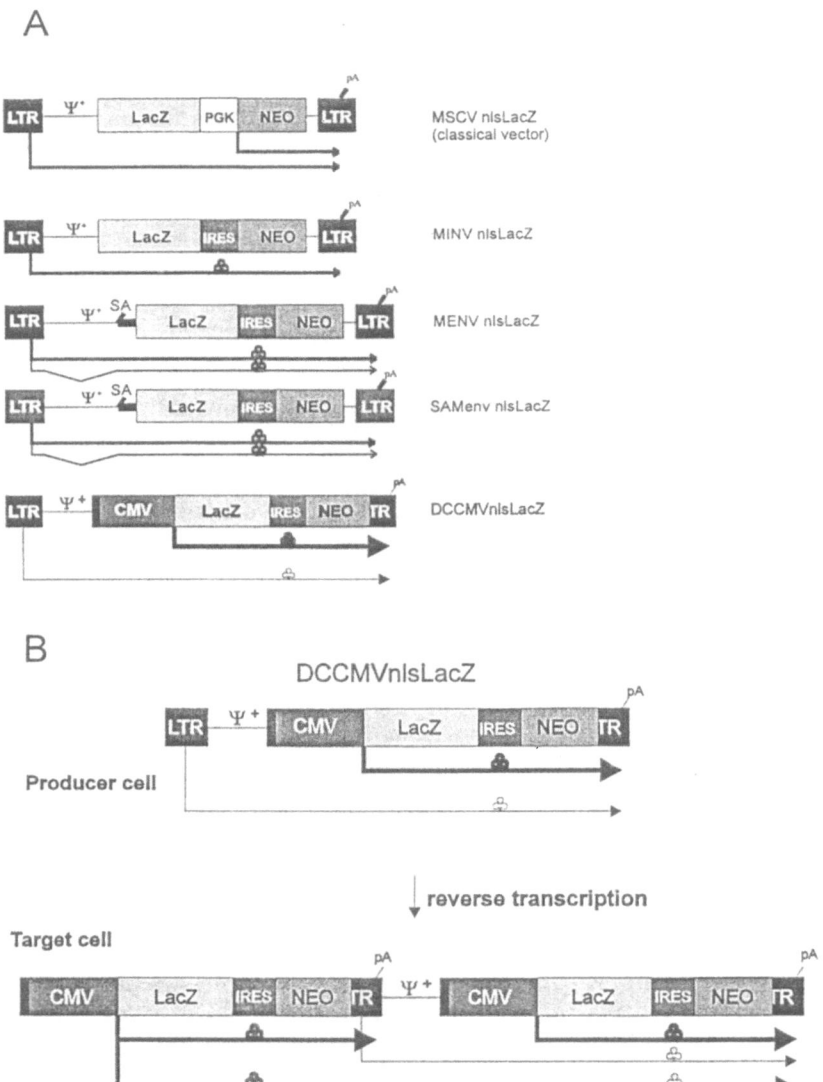

Figure 7. (A) Structure of MSCV-based bicistronic retroviral vectors. All vectors contain the *nlsLacZ* gene which is translated from LTR-directed transcripts from hCMV-IE-directed transcripts in DCCMVnlsLacZ. Abbreviations and symbols: CMV, hCMV-IE promoter; LacZ, *nuclear localizing sequence (nls) LacZ* gene; SA, *env* splice acceptor; ψ^+, extended packaging signal; arrows represent transcripts; ♣, IRES stem-loop structure; pA, polyadenylation site. (B) Reverse transcription of DCCMVnlsLacZ vector RNA in target cells results in the duplication of hCMV-IE-*nlsLacZ*-IRES-*neo* transcriptional unit in the U3 region of 3' LTR to the 5' LTR. (C, D) Characterization of human melanoma cell lines transduced with double-copy bicistronic retroviral vectors expressing hIL-6 and hsIL-6R. (C) Northern blot analysis of hIL-6 and shIL-6R transcripts in four melanoma cell lines transduced

C

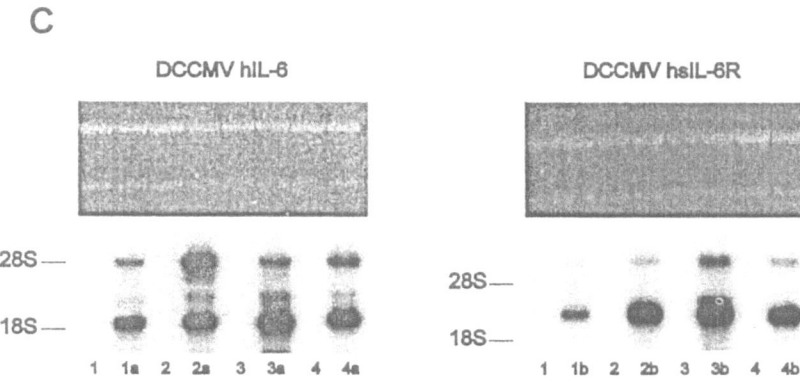

DCCMV hIL-6   DCCMV hsIL-6R

28S —   28S —

18S —   18S —

1 1a 2 2a 3 3a 4 4a   1 1b 2 2b 3 3b 4 4b

D

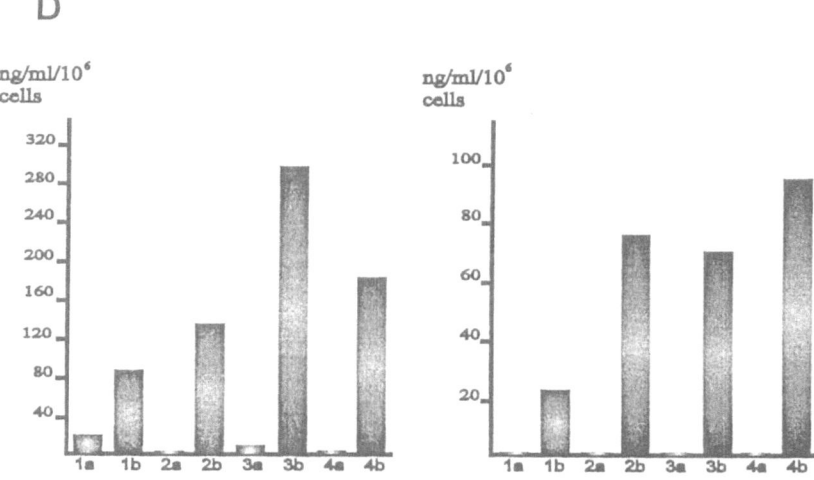

ng/ml/10^6 ng/ml/10^6
cells   cells

320   100

280

240   80

200

160   60

120
                                                    40
80

40   20

1a 1b 2a 2b 3a 4a 4b   1a 1b 2a 2b 3a 3b 4a 4b

with the DCCMVhIL-6 and DCCMVhsIL-6R vectors, which carry either the hIL-6 or hsIL-6R cDNA, respectively, in place of the *nlsLacZ* gene in DCCMVnlsLacZ. In each case, the smallest transcripts correspond to mRNAs initiated from the hCMV-IE promoter. Additional transcripts represent RNA species initiated from the retroviral LTR and the 5' situated hCMV-IE promoter. The upper panels show ethidium bromide staining of equal amounts of the RNA samples. (D) Production of hIL-6 (left panel) and hsIL-6R (right panel) by four melanoma cell lines transduced with the DCCMVhIL-6 and DCCMVhsIL-6R vectors, respectively, as determined by specific enzyme-linked immunosorbent assays 1, 1a (WM35); 2, 2a (WM902b); 3, 3a (WM9); 4, 4a (WM239): nontransduced cell lines and transduced cell populations, respectively.

17 map units) in place of the *E1* gene and *E3*-deleted linear adenoviral genome (Fig. 8). The *E3* gene product, which is involved in modulating the host immune response to adenovirus [72], is not essential for the viral life cycle and its removal would increase the space for therapeutic gene insertion up to 7.5 kb [70]. However, removing the immunosuppressive activity of the *E3* gene product would lead to an enhanced immune response against the virus.

After homologous recombination between common sequences in plasmid and Ad genome, full-length (0–100 map units; *E1⁻, E3⁻*) adenoviral DNA containing therapeutic gene is generated and can be efficiently packaged into viral particles. The recombinant virus obtained is able to transduce target cells without further replication since it lacks an *E1* gene. In accordance with the adenoviral life-cycle, genetic information is maintained as unintegrated, efficiently transcribed DNA.

The most frequent application of Ad vectors in gene therapy is in the treatment of cystic fibrosis [73]. In cancer gene therapy, adenoviral vectors are currently being used in gene therapy clinical protocols dealing with brain and liver tumours. In these trials recombinant viruses carrying suicide genes (e.g., *herpes simplex* thymidine kinase – HSV-tk) are delivered stereotactically directly into the tumour. Other examples include application of Ad to deliver tumour suppressor p53 gene into lung, head and neck, or liver cancer cells by direct tumour injection.

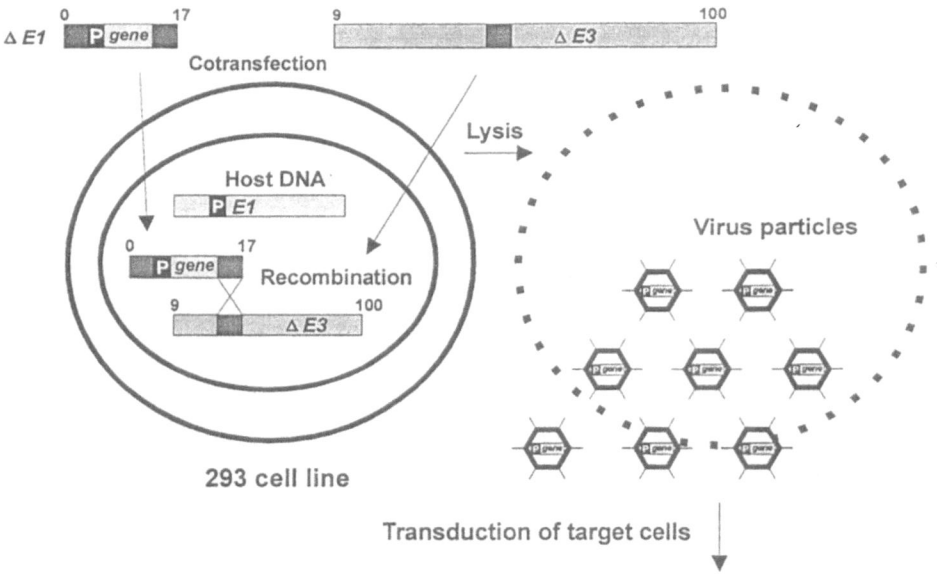

Figure 8. Adenoviral vector is cotransfected with adenovirus type 5 genomic DNA deleted in *E3* region into 293 cells. Due to the homologous recombination between corresponding sequences in Ad vector and Ad5 genome, and activity of *E1* gene product provided by 293 cells, viral particles containing therapeutic genes are released after cell lysis. Such recombinant adenoviruses are able to transduce dividing and non-dividing target cells, however the therapeutic gene does not enter the nucleus and integrate into the cell genome but exists episomally in the cell cytoplasm and usually is lost after a few divisions.

The transient fashion of gene expression requires multiple administration of the vector. Such aprocedure may induce an immune response to the vector. On the other hand the adenoviral vector can also be highly immunogenic to the patient who already posseses either antibodies to the virus or immunocompetent cells [74]. The efforts to improve adenoviral vectors focus on the removal of genes encoding adenoviral proteins from the vector. Such manipulation is expected to reduce immunogenicity and enable insertion of larger therapeutic gene cassettes. These constructs, named "coatless vectors", are so far very difficult to obtain because of instability of the viral particles. However, recently isolation of an adenoviral vector with 25% deletion of its genome was reported [75].

Adeno-associated vectors

Adeno-associated vectors (AAV), naturally defective, single-stranded DNA parvoviruses, were discovered as a satellite viruses which were present in preparations of adenoviruses. They were found not to be pathogenic. The unique feature of AAV is inability to infect cells in culture in the absence of co-infection by a helper virus (adenovirus, herpesvirus or vaccinia virus) [76, 77]. In the absence of helper virus, the infecting AAV genome undergoes integration at a specific site on the *q* arm of chromosome 19, and remains latent for a prolonged period of time [78]. This is actually the only known example of site-specific integration of a virus, providing an opportunity to construct a vector for insertion of therapeutic genes into a known site within the cellular genome. After infection of latently infected cells, AAV may be rescued from the integrated site *via* excision and replication.

All developed vectors contain foreign sequences inserted between inverted terminal repeats (ITR) of the AAV genome (Fig. 9). The ITR is required for packaging and along with one of the two major viral proteins (Rep) mediates site-specific integration.Vectors lacking the *rep* gene integrate into the genome but the specificity of this integration is unknown. Thus the *rep* gene has been deleted from vectors to leave more room for exogenous genetic information. Moreover, the product of this gene is toxic to many types of cells, making creation of stable packaging lines very difficult.

AAV vectors are currently produced by transient cotransfection of plasmids containing a therapeutic gene between ITRs along with the second plasmid providing *rep* and *cap*, products which are responsible for encapsidation. Following infection of the transfected cells by helper adenovirus, the recombinant AAV genome carrying therapeutic gene is packed into AAV particles. AAV and adenovirus are released after cell lysis, heat inactivated (to inactivate adenovirus since the AAV particle is more stable) and separated by centrifugation (AAV and Ad have different densities). After the treatment the recombinant AAV particles are used to transduce target cells.

The high titre of the viral vector after concentration (up to 10^{12} CFU/ml), the extreme stability of the virus particles and the ability to transduce non-dividing cell stably, are considerable advantages over retroviral and Ad vectors. However, the useful site-specific integration is abrogated in the absence of *rep* gene function sacrificed to increase cloning capacity (4.5 kb). Moreover, the inability to obtain stable packaging cells shows that the currently used vector constructs need to be modified.

There is an increasing number of attempts to apply AAV vectors to cancer gene therapy. One group stereotactically delivered AAV vector particles carrying a dicistronic gene containing HSV-

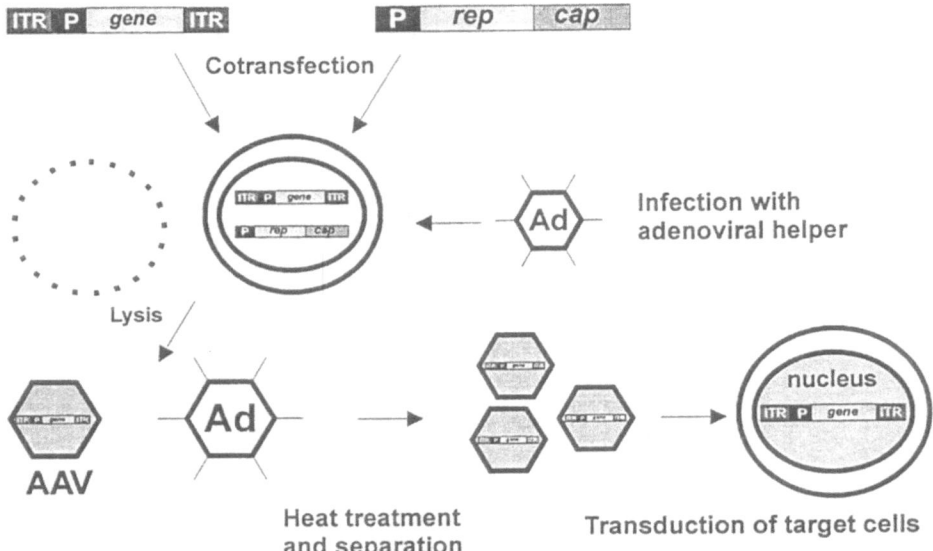

Figure 9. Adeno-associated vector (AAV) carrying therapeutic gene is cotransfected with plasmid containing viral *rep* and *cap* genes. After infection with helper adenovirus transfected cells are lysed and recombinant AAV particles are released together with helper Ad. AAVs can be purified from the mixture by heat treatment and centrifugal separation and used to transduce the target cells. Therapeutic gene delivered to the cells by the AAVs stably integrates into the cellular genome of dividing and non-dividing cells. (ITR – inverted terminal repeat – AAV promoter and sequences mediating integration)

tk and IL-2 cDNAs into human glioma in a nude mouse experimental tumour model. After ganciclovir administration they observed a dramatic decrease in the tumour size, indicating that high titre AAV vector treatment may be safe and effective in *in vivo* gene therapy of human brain tumours [79].

Another group used the same strategy, using an of AAV vector specifically to express HSV-tk gene in human hepatocellular carcinoma cell lines displaying different levels of α-fetoprotein (AFP) and albumin production, as well as in nonhepatocyte tumour cell lines. Ganciclovir treatment caused death only of AFP and albumin-positive hepatoma cells, but not of tumour cells of other than hepatocyte origin, or AFP and albumin-negative hepatoma cells. Moreover, the dose required to kill the cancer cells was inversely proportional to the level of AFP expression in these cells (see below).

Since AAV vectors transduce nondividing S-phase cells, they can transfer genes into noncycling tumour cells. This is very important for *in vivo* gene therapy because only a small portion of cells within the tumour mass are dividing.

However, up to now there are no published data available from gene therapy clinical trials using AAV vectors.

Targetting of gene therapy vectors

Targetting of vectors in gene therapy may be divided into two major approaches. The first, referred to as targetting of entry, is to direct the vectors to a particular cell type. The second approach involves cell specific or regulatable promoters for expression of therapeutic genes. Targetting of therapeutic genes is a very important issue for *in vivo* applications, where genetic modification of specific cell types, and cell specific or suitable levels of expression, is highly desirable.

Targetting of entry

Viral entry to the target cell is mediated through the interaction of viral envelope proteins with receptors on the cell surface. Recombinant retroviral and adenoviral viruses, which are most extensively manipulated to direct therapeutic genes to a specific cell type, are able to enter virtually any cell type. This is an advantage in *ex vivo* approches but in *in vivo* gene therapy transduction of other cells than those specified may have fatal consequences. The manipulations of viral tropism may be divided into two approaches: immunological and molecular. The immunological approach involves the coupling of ligand or monoclonal antibody specific for a cell receptor with viral surface proteins using an artificial bridge (avidin-streptavidin complex is commonly used). The molecular approach involves the creation of fusion proteins with viral surface proteins and ligands or antigen-binding fragments of monoclonal antibodies which recognise specific receptors on the target cell surface. However, there is little evidence for effective targetting of recombinant viruses to cancer cells *in vivo* (for a recent review see [80]).

Transcriptional targetting of therapeutic gene expression

The ability to direct therapeutic gene expression to a particular cell type is a very important issue in gene therapy [81]. First, controlling therapeutic genes by using regulatable or tissue-specific promoters accomplishes restricted expression even after nonspecific delivery. Moreover, cell-specific promoters usually give more stable and predictable patterns of expression than exogenous promoters. Depending on the cell type and gene used this affects safety and effectiveness, especially when the therapeutic gene product might be toxic when produced by other cell types than those which should have been modified, for example in the case of *in situ* or *in vivo* delivery of suicide genes. After expression of a suicide enzyme and prodrug activation, a metabolite would be potentially toxic to normally dividing cells.

Most of the promoters used drive expression of genes whose protein products are restricted to cancer cells. They include tissue associated antigens, tumour-specific antigens, and oncogene products. For example, a high level of melanin synthesis in melanoma cells depends on activity of the tyrosinase promoter and promoters of the tyrosinase-related protein genes *(TRP-1, -2)*. These promoters have been used to achieve specific expression of HSV-tk in human melanoma cells [82, 83]. Carcinoembryonic antigen (CEA) is a tumour antigen mainly expressed in colorectal, gastric, breast and lung cancers. Fragments of the CEA promoter have been used to obtain specific activation of HSV-TK or cytosine deaminase (CD) prodrugs in the above mentioned types of tumours [84, 85]. However, *in vivo* results have been disappointing; no regression of tumour transfected with the CD gene under the control of the CEA promoter was observed [85]. The promoter of another tumour antigen (AFP) has been applied for effective expression of HSV-TK in hepatoma cells using retroviral [86], adenoviral [87], and AAV vectors [88]. The latter studies evaluated the ability of the AFP promoter to restrict suicide gene expression *in vivo* using AFP-producing and nonproducing xenografts in mice. Transduction of AFP-positive xenografts with adenoviral vector carrying HSV-TK gene resulted in complete tumour regression after ganciclovir treatment [89]. Another study used AAV vector with a chimaeric promoter containing the liver-specific albumin promoter and the AFP enhancer, and demonstrated that albumin and AFP-producing hepatoma cells were sensitive to ganciclovir treatment in proportion to the level of AFP expression [88].

Another tissue-selective system utilizes the *MUC1* gene promoter. MUC-1 is a heavily glycosylated protein and is aberrantly expressed in pancreatic, breast and ovarian cancers. Linking of the *MUC-1* gene promoter to the HSV-TK gene revealed cytotoxity specific to breast cancer cells *in vitro* and *in vivo* [90].

It has been found that many oncogenes are overexpressed in tumour cells, and this is due to abnormal activity of specific promoters. The best studied is the promoter of *ERB-B-2* growth factor receptor, whose overexpression leads to tumourogenesis of epithelial cells lining the ducts of the breast and pancreas. Accordingly, the *ERB-B-2* promoter has been used to direct the expression of suicide genes, including cytosine deaminase in breast and pancreatic cancers [91]. *Myc/Max* response elements were used to control transcription of HSV-TK in small cell lung cancer cells overexpressing those oncogenes. *c-myc*-overexpressing cancer cells were found to be more sensitive to ganciclovir treatment than normal cells [92]. Transcriptional control elements of prostate-specific antigen (PSA) have been reported to limit the expression of heterologous constructs to prostate cancer cell lines *in vitro* [93], which would be useful for suicide gene therapy for prostate cancer.

Targetted gene expression is a very promising approach, and with increasing understanding of mechanisms controlling overexpression of tumour-specific proteins, and information derived from the Human Genome Project, more specific vectors will be developed for therapeutic purposes.

Strategies of cancer gene therapy

Gene therapy clinical protocols approved for trials are based on four major approaches:
(1) Immuno-gene therapy.
(2) Administration of so-called suicide genes (e.g., HSV-TK or CD) and activation of a suicide mechanism for direct killing of cancer cells.
(3) Inactivation of oncogenes or activation of tumour suppressor genes which regulate the cell-cycle (e.g., p53, Rb, ras, raf).
(4) Introduction of multidrug resistance genes (MDR) into patient bone marrow cells as a protection against massive chemotherapy.

Genes might be delivered into target cells both *in vivo* or *ex vivo*. When applied *in vivo*, by means of viral or nonviral molecular vehicles, the therapetic gene is delivered directly into the patient target tissue. In contrast, in the *ex vivo* approach cells are isolated from the patient, modified to express the therapeutic gene *in vitro* and readministered to the patient.

According to the strategic needs different approaches are employed. In the case of clinical protocols exploiting genetically modified tumour vaccine (GMTV) or introduction of *MDR* genes into bone marrow, cells are modified *ex vivo*. However, in the case of a suicide gene-based strategy or manipulation of oncogene or tumour suppressor gene expression, the genetic vectors need to be delivered directly *in situ* into the tumour or administered systemically *in vivo*.

Immuno-gene therapy

The concept of immunization against cancer emerged from the observation that cancer cells are able to escape immune system surveillance and may then form a tumour. Paul Ehrlich in early 1900 suggested that cancer cells randomly arise in the body but are quickly eliminated by the immune system. Many years later the immune surveillance theory was developed based on the finding that T cell-mediated immune response is able to eliminate some tumour cells. The hypothesis was confirmed by observation of increased incidence of tumours among immunosuppressed patients e.g., those undergoing transplantation. However, those patients were more susceptible to cancer of the immune system than to other types of malignances (e.g., brain, breast, lung) whose incidence was the same as in the healthy population. Similarly, HIV patients with impaired CD4+ T lymphocyte function frequently develop only certain types of tumours, such as Kaposi's sarcoma, while the incidence of other more common cancers is not increased.

However, another observation in opposition to the immune surveillance theory comes from the nude mouse model. These mice lack a thymus and do not possess functional T cells. Despite that fact these animals are no more susceptible to cancer than other animals.

Nevertheless, it is now quite obvious that an effective immune response may be generated against at least some tumours and therapeutic approaches may be aimed to boost the response against malignant cells. Although the immune system often recognizes tumour epitopes on cancer cells, in most cases it is not able to generate an effective response. This might be due to inhibitory mechanisms developed by tumour cells to escape cytotoxic effector reactions. They include:
(1) Modulation of tumour antigen expression and presentation
(2) Reduction in class I MHC molecules (lack of proper β2-microglobulin expression)
(3) Lack of costimulatory signal (B-7 family)
(4) Expression of apoptotic molecules (Fas)
Most gene therapy approaches based on activation of the immune response use transfer of genes encoding proteins displaying immunomodulatory activity (e.g., cytokines or membrane-bound costimulatory molecules) and can mediate direct or indirect antitumour effect. There are two major strategies of using these factors. The first, referred to as adoptive immuno-gene therapy, is based on the concept of *ex vivo* delivering of immunomodulatory factors to the immune cells including T lymphocytes or antigen presenting cells (APC), to develop more effective responses against cancer. The second approach includes transfer of genes encoding potent immunomodulators into the cancer cell. The autologous or allogeneic cancer cells may be modified *ex vivo* and given as a genetically modified tumour vaccine (GMTV), which would provide the necessary costimulatory signals and induce an effective immune response against remaining metastatic tumour cells. In one protocol cytokine-secreting autologous fibroblasts are used for this purpose. On the

other hand, tumour cells may be engineered to produce immunomodulatory proteins *in situ*, at the site of tumour growth.

Historically, IL-2 was the first cytokine believed to display antitumour biological activities. In animal models IL-2 was shown to be effective in decreasing tumour size when injected intravenously to tumour-bearing animals [94]. In human studies IL-2 was used to activate lymphocytes isolated from cancer patients. Such lymphocytes (lymphokine activated killers, or LAK) [95], were subsequently reinfused to the patient in the hope that they would kill cancer cells [96]. The results obtained led to the design of the one of the first gene therapy protocols which involved transduction of lymphocytes obtained from melanoma patients with retrovirus carrying IL-2 cDNA.

In order to obtain lymphocytes of a high specificity for cancer cells, the patient's T cells were isolated directly from the metastatic lesion. This tumour-specific population, referred to as tumour infiltrating lymphocytes (TIL), was shown to be 100-fold more potent *in vitro* than LAKs in killing autologous melanoma cells [97]. TILs modified to secrete IL-2 were reinfused to melanoma patients and were expected to eliminate existing melanoma cells specifically [98]. However, this promising approach did not fulfill expectations since IL-2-secreting TILs were found to accumulate in the liver and spleen of treated patients rather than in the tumour mass [99]. Currently, IL-7 modified TILs are being used in trials against melanoma and kidney cancers (Tab. 1A, see Appendix at the end of this chapter).

Dendritic cells (DCs) are potent APCs that can activate quiescent T lymphocytes. In one study human DCs were retrovirally transduced with a melanoma TAA gene – *MART-1*. *In vitro* stimulation using MART-1-transduced DCs raised specific antitumour CTLs from autologous quiescent cells [100].

The strategy of GMTV is based on the concept of *ex vivo* genetic modification of autologous or allogeneic tumour cells in order to provide costimulatory signals for the immune system to be activated in order to eliminate cancer cells specifically (Fig. 10A–D) [101]. On the other hand soluble costimulatory molecules might be locally provided by other cell types such as fibroblasts which were genetically modified, admixed with autologous tumour cells and administered to the patient.

The rationale of this strategy is that tumour cells secreting high doses of costimulatory molecules, such as cytokines, would more effectively present tumour antigens or more effectively prime MHC-I-mediated CTL response, since cancer cells in most cases lack expression of MHC molecules and/or their peptide-processing machinery is defective. Moreover, cytokines may activate antigen presenting cells (APC) [94]. However, the mechanisms governing cytokine costimulation need further study. It is likely that following administration of GMTV, an MHC-II-based mechanism is involved. APCs take up tumour antigens released from disrupted cancer cells and present them to CD4+ cells utilizing the MHC-II dependent pathway. Delayed type hypersensitivity (DTH) reaction in patients receiving GMTV at the site of injection, which is commonly observed after 48–72 h, supports the above concerns. CD4+ helpers, activated at the injection site, sectrete a variety of cytokines which attract many other immune system cells including CTLs or macrophges.

In another version of GMTV, tumour cells are modified by insertion of genes encoding membrane-bound costimulatory molecules. It was shown that effective costimulation of CD4+ and

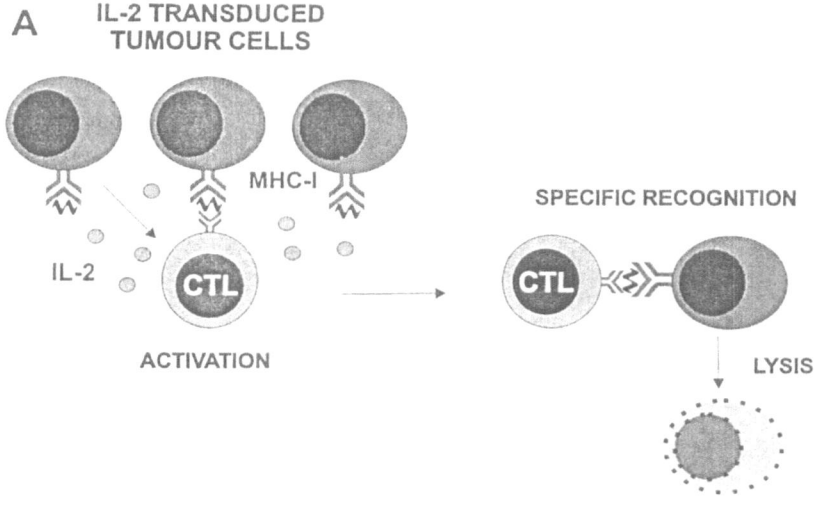

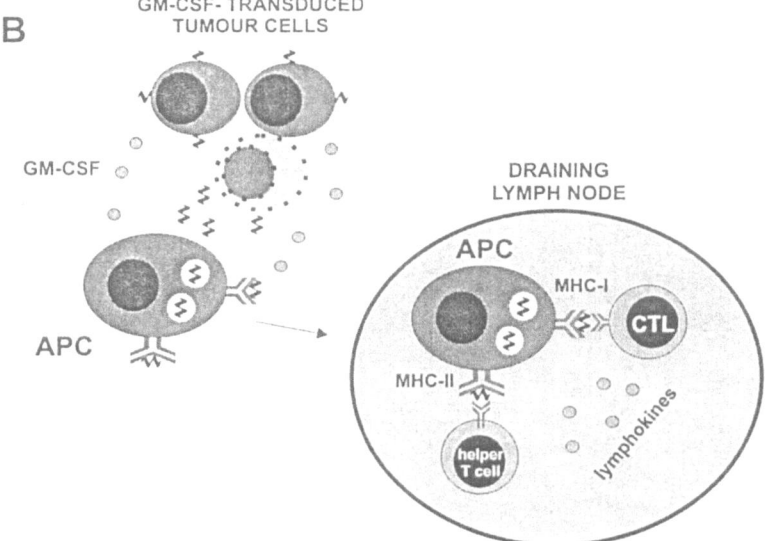

Figure 10. Activation of immune system by different variants of GMTV (A) IL-2 secreted by genetically modified tumour cells bypasses helper T lymphocytes and directly activates specific CTLs which recognize tumour antigens. The activation leads to specific recognition and lysis of patient wildtype cells. (B) GM-CSF secreted by genetically modified tumour cells activates antigen presenting cells (APCs). Activated APCs take up more efficiently the tumour antigens released by disrupted tumour cells, move to draining lymph nodes and present the antigens to helper and cytotoxic T lymphocytes either *via* MHC-I or MHC-II-restricted pathways.
(continued on next page)

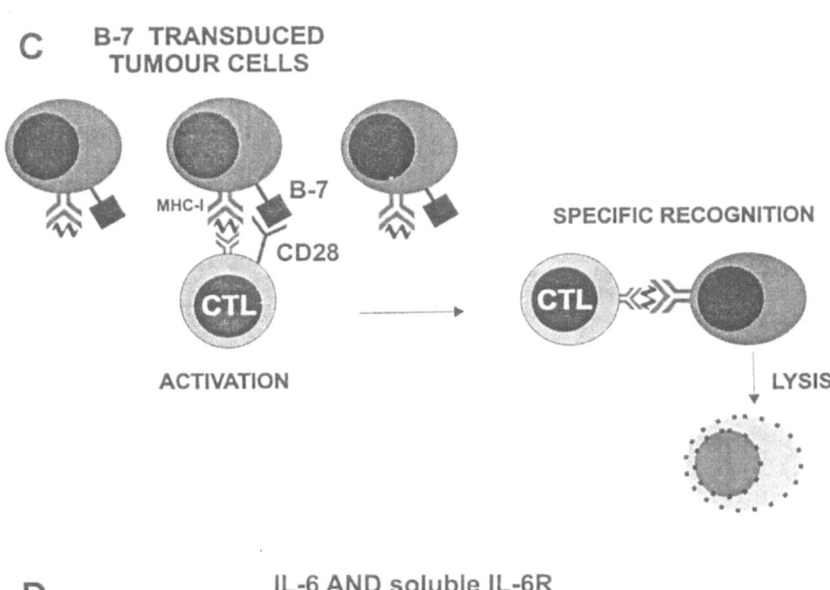

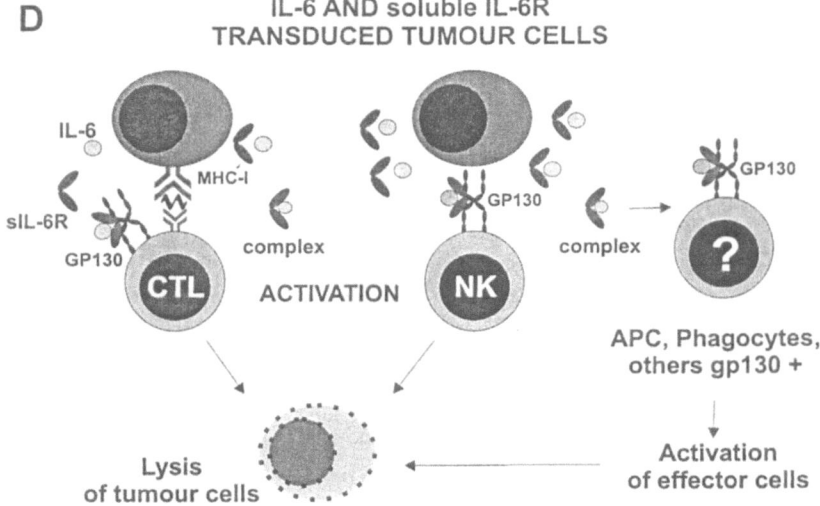

Figure 10. (continued) (C) B7 expressed on the surface of genetically modified tumour cells, activates CTL which recognize MHC-I-restricted tumour antigens. Activation leads to the specific recognition and lysis of patient wildtype cells. (D) IL-6 and soluble IL-6R secreted by genetically modified tumour cells form an active complex and activate gp130 present on almost all cells of the immune system. Activation of CTLs and NK cells leads to specific recognition and lysis of patient wildtype cells.

CD8+ T cells might be achieved only in the context of antigen presentation *via* MHC-TCR complex. This type of costimulation is triggered by the interaction of a B-7 molecule expressed on the target cells with CD28 protein present on the surface of lymphocytes. When lymphocytes recognize antigen presented in the context of MHC molecules without stimulation *via* B-7 they do not respond and may develop anergy to the antigen. Many tumour cells lack B-7 and escape from destruction by the immune system [102]. Accordingly, restoration of B-7 gene expression might enhance tumour cell immunogeneticy. When melanoma cell lines transfected with B-7 cDNA were injected into syngeneic animals, complete tumour regression was observed [103].

Another immunological approach involves GMTV modified to express tumour rejection antigens. Most studies use melanoma antigens, whose epitopes have been found to be recognized by T cells. They include MAGE and MART whose presentation is associated with melanoma regression [104]. However, there are very similar problems as encountered in other vaccination approaches. First, the cancer cell population was found to be very heterogeneous in terms of expression of these antigens. Thus, immunization using one or even two antigens will not prime the CTL response against all existing cancer cells. Another limitation is that tumour rejection antigens were only found on few tumours, including melanoma, renal carcinoma or prostate cancer. Identification of such antigens on other tumours would be of importance for future studies.

Other cells used as vehicles to deliver cytokines into the tumour microenvironment were autologous fibroblasts [105–107]. Fibroblasts were isolated from the patient, grown in culture and genetically modified to secrete cytokines. Subsequently, they were injected in the vicinity of the metastatic melanoma lessions. However, there were certain limitations to the system. It appeared that autologous fibroblasts were rather difficult to obtain in culture in high quantities in a relatively short time. Currently, there is one ongoing trial using the above strategy and IL-12 modified fibroblasts (Tab. 1A, see Appendix at the end of this chapter).

Another potential approach to immunomodulation uses the introduction of strong immuno-stimulators, like HLA-B7 gene, into tumour cells *in situ*.Transfection of $H-2K^s$ antigen cDNA into experimental mouse tumour *in situ* was shown to increase the antitumour activity of murine TIL against both the modified and unmodified cells. This was probably due to the stimulation of the immune system within the tumour mass, which increased local production of cytokines like interferons, in turn augmenting MHC class I and II expression and tumour antigen presentation. After injection of tumours with foreign MHC gene, both allogeneic and tumour-specific CTLs were detected in the spleen of treated animals. Significant extension of survival time was also observed [27]. These encouraging results have led to the approval of a clinical protocol for the treatment of five HLA-B7 negative patients with advanced melanoma using the HLA-B7 gene complexed with DC-chol/DOPE liposomes. Plasmid DNA vector carrying HLA-B7 complexed with liposome was directly injected into metastatic tumours of these melanoma patients. Gene transfer, recombinant gene expression, and safety and potential toxicity of this therapy was demonstrated. Six courses of treatment were completed without complications in five HLA-B7-negative patients with stage IV melanoma. Plasmid DNA was detected within biopsies of treated tumour nodules 3–7 days after injection but was not found in the serum at any time, assayed by the polymerase chain reaction. Recombinant HLA-B7 protein was demonstrated in tumour biopsy tissue in all five patients by immunochemistry, and immune responses to HLA-B7 and autologous tumours could be detected. No antibodies to DNA were detected in any patient. One patient demonstrated regression of injected nodules on two independent treatments, which was accompanied by regression at distant sites. These studies demonstrate the feasibility, safety, and therapeutic potential of direct gene transfer in humans [26]. Further analysis of immune response revealed T cell migration into treated lesions. However, the frequency of cytotoxic T lymphocytes against autologous tumours in circulating peripheral blood lymphocytes was not altered significantly. Local inhibition of tumour growth was detected after gene transfer in two patients, one showing partial regression [108].

Administration of so-called suicide genes and activation of a suicide mechanism for direct killing of cancer cells

Suicide gene therapy (SGT) uses transduction of tumour cells with bacterial enzyme genes which display a unique ability to convert a non-toxic prodrug into intracellular toxin [109]. The prodrug is applied shortly after suicide gene transfer, and after conversion blocks cell division and induces apoptosis. Disruption of tumour cells induces host inflammatory reaction which augments a therapeutic effect [110].

However, to exert their activity suicide genes (SGs) have to be delivered *in vivo* or *in situ* into the tumour site. Fortunately, as shown by *in vitro* experiments, only 1–5% of tumour cells need to express SG to kill the remaining nontransfected cells [111].

This is due to the phenomenon referred to as the "bystander effect", based on toxin diffusion through gap junctional intercellular communication (GJIC) to the other cancer cells [112]. Another study suggested a strong cell-mediated immune component to the bystander effect. In murine melanoma (B16) tumours killed *in vivo* with GC treatment, a pronounced intratumoural infiltrate of macrophages, CD4+ and CD8+ T cells was observed. In addition expression of interleukin IL-2, IL-12, IFN-gamma, tumour necrosis factor-alpha (TNF-alpha) and granulocyte/macrophage colony-stimulating factor (GM-CSF) but not IL-4, IL-6 or IL-10, was observed, a profile of cytokine expression which resembles that of a Th1 immune response. The data show that B16 cells died predominantly by necrosis, rather than apoptosis, on exposure to GC, a process which may be associated with the generation of antitumour inflammatory responses [113].

Usually the vector carrying SG is delivered directly into the tumour site. However, in the case of retroviral vectors, tumour cell transduction can be achieved by injection of virus-producing packaging cells. The first SGT clinical protocol approved for human trials involved stereotactic injection into human brain glioma of retroviral packaging cells producing recombinant virus carrying HSV-TK gene, and a subsequent GC administration mechanism [114].

Targetted expression of suicide genes within tumour cells might be the most promising cancer gene therapy strategy. Several studies have reported application of tumour-specific promoters including *ERB-B-2* promoter, von Willebrand factor promoter, CEA promoter, and AFP promoter (see above).

Modulation of oncogenes and tumour suppressor gene expression

Extensive studies which led to the identification of a number of possible mechanisms of tumorigenesis created new opportunities to modulate these mechanisms in order to treat or prevent cancer. It is believed that most cancers arise due to overexpression or amplification of oncogenes or mutation of tumour suppression genes. Protooncogene products are normally homologues of oncogenes and play an important role as growth factor receptors, signal transducers or transcription factors. Cancer-causing mutations of oncogenes involve point mutations, amplifications, translocations, and rearrangments, leading to disregulation of the cell cycle and promoting tumour growth. Tumour suppressor genes, on the other hand, control cell proliferation. Thus deletion of oncogenes or expression of tumour suppressor genes could mediate reversion of tumour phenotype, tumour cell death or immune reaction against cancer cells.

The *ras* family of oncogenes is the most commonly activated in tumours. The *ras* (including H-*ras*, K-*ras*, N-*ras*) genes encode a membrane-bound protein with guanosine triphosphatase (GTPase) activity, and participate in signal transduction and promotion of cell cycling. Antisense approaches involve delivery of a vector carrying antisense cDNA for ras into tumour cells *in vivo* [115]. Antother oncogene, c-*myb*, was found to be abnormally expressed in leukaemic cells. Clinical trials evaluating the therapeutic efect of antisense c-*myb* oligos are currently in progress for treatment of acute and chronic forms of myelogenous leukemia (Tab. 1C, see Appendix at the end of this chapter).

It has been found that the mutated form of the p53 tumour suppressor is a potent oncogene promoting the cell cycle. Adenovirus-mediated delivery of p53 antisense cDNA to tumour cells has been used in treatment of head and neck squamous cell carcinoma (Tab. 1C, see Appendix).

Restoration of function of wildtype tumour suppressor genes in tumour cells inhibits tumour formation and growth. In 1996 the results from a trial involving retrovirus-mediated transfer of *p53* gene to tumours in patients with lung cancer were reported. Retroviral supernatant was directly injected into tumours with documented p53 mutation using a fibreoptic bronchoscope or percutaneous needle. Three of the seven treated patients showed evidence of tumour regression in the treated lesion. Safety and lack of toxicity suggest a potential clinical application of this technology, especially for patients with unresectable local tumours [116].

However, manipulation of oncogenes and tumour suppressor gene expression has considerable limitations. The administration of viral vectors to patients is limited to local and regional tumours. Moreover, immune reaction to Ad vectors and low transduction efficiency of retroviral vectors create another obstacles. Improvements in vector construction, including manipulation, targetted delivery and tumour-specific expression, are necessary for progress in this field.

Multi-drug resistance genes (MDR)

The rationale of this strategy is to transfer genes conferring resistance to existing chemotherapeutic agents to isolated patient bone marrow or blood-derived bone marrow cells. The *MDR1* gene product, P-glycoprotein, functions as an efflux pump and is responsible for the drug resistance of many tumours. This gene was found to be amplified in tumour cells, which led to ineffectiveness of hydrophobic cytotoxic drugs in the treatment of various types of cancer. Patient bone marrow cells transfected with the vector carrying the MDR gene are selected in the presence of a cytostatic to obtain a population that will be resistant to that drug when administrated systemically [117, 118].

Such a procedure would allow high-dose chemotherapy, with reinfusion of drug-resistant patient blood cells prior to treatment. Mouse haematopietic cells expressing methotrexate-resistance dihydrofolate reductase were protected against systemically administrated methotrexate when reinjected into syngeneic recipients [119].

Clinical protocols involving *ex vivo* transfer of MDR cDNA into a patient's bone marrow cells were approved for the high dose chemotherapeutic treatment of breast and ovarian cancers. To date eight clinical protocols have been approved for clinical trials.

However there are some problems with this type of treatment: high doses of chemotherapy do not seem to induce a better response. Moreover, the nonhaematological side effects may be limiting. There is also a possible risk of transduction of metastatic cancer cells which may be present in patient bone marrow. So far there is insufficient information to evaluate the potential therapeutic efficacy of this approach.

Clinical trials

About 113 cancer gene therapy clinical protocols have so far been approved by the FDA or equivalent agencies in various countries [120]. About half of these clinical protocols have entered phase I or I/II trials. There are a few journals or institutions which list and update gene marker/therapy protocols as well as patents granted in the field of gene therapy. However, not all accepted protocols are included in a single list, which can be confusing. Table 1 (see Appendix) presents a current list prepared from various sources. Numbers of protocols listed below are given on the basis of a list published in August 1997 [121]. The majority of protocols (72), are based on an immuno-gene therapy strategy (Tab. 1A, see Appendix), 21 protocols deal with a suicide gene strategy (Tab. 1B, see Appendix), 12 with modulation of oncogenes and tumour suppressor gene expression (Tab. 1C, see Appendix), and 8 with MDR-1 gene modification of bone marrow cells (Tab. 1D, see Appendix). Most of the immuno-gene therapy protocols were designed to treat malignant melanoma (26 protocols), 19 to treat various types of advanced cancer, 6 to treat prostate cancer, 5 to treat glioma, glioblastoma or neuroblastoma, 4 to treat renal cancer, 4 colon carcinoma, 3 breast cancer, and one or two protocols to treat ovarian, lung, cervical, or squamous cell carcinoma, or lymphoma and leukaemia. Beyond a relatively large number of approved protocols only a few papers have published the results of clinical trials.

A clinical trial of 12 patients with grade IV melanoma vaccinated with allogenic cells transduced with the IL-2 gene showed a mixed clinical response in three patients (stabilization of the disease with regression of some subcutaneous nodules or decreased progression with regression of one subcutaneous nodule) [122]. Phase I trial of immunotherapy with IFN-gamma gene-modified autologous melanoma cells demonstrated that 13 of 20 patients completed the immunization protocol [123]. Eight of these 13 patients developed a humoral response (IgG) against autologous and allogenic melanoma cells. Other patients showed no or weak IgG response. Two patients who developed significant increases in serum IgG demonstrated tumour regression, and two patients with low serum IgG response had transient shrinkage of metastatic nodules during therapy. The antibodies recognized different antigens, indicating that individual patients may develop different responses to the same immunization protocol. Finally, one report of IL-2 gene transfer into TILs which were reinfused to advanced lung cancer patients with pleural effusions demonstrated that in six of ten patients pleural effusions did not re-accumulate for at least 6 weeks. In one patient, in addition to resolution of pleural effusions the size of the original tumour decreased [124]. During the 3rd European Conference on Gene Therapy of Cancer held in Berlin in September 1997, S. Osanto (Leiden, The Netherlands) reported results of immunization of 27 patients with an HLA class I-matched allogenic melanoma cell line modified to secrete IL-2. Five patients showed regression of one or more metastases, including one patient with complete regression of small intradermal metastases. Others (E.M. Rankin et al. Amsterdam, The Netherlands and Somatix Therapy Co., USA) reported vaccination of 24 patients with autologous melanoma cells modified to secrete GM-CSF. Six of 24 patients with long enough follow-up showed protracted (> 6 months) stabilization of previously progressive disease.

Three papers describing direct gene transfer of an allogenic class I MHC (HLA-B7) into patients with metastatic melanoma have been published [26, 108, 125]. The original report by Nabel et al. [26] has already been discussed. Subsequent studies carried out by the same group [108] involving 10 patients demonstrated T cell migration into treated lesions and enhanced reactivity of TILs. Interestingly, the frequency of CTL against autologous tumour in circulating peripheral blood lymphocytes (PBL) was not altered, suggesting that PBL reactivity is not indicative of local tumour responsiveness. In two patients local inhibition of tumour growth was observed. One of these patients subsequently received TIL treatment derived from a gene-modified tumour, which resulted in a complete regression of residual disease. In another study [125] involving 17 patients, seven had tumour responses to the injected nodule, while one patient with a single site of disease achieved a complete remission.

Promising results were reported for direct p53 gene transfer into non-small lung cancer [116]. Nine patients were enrolled. Tumour regression was noted in three patients, and tumour growth stabilized in three other patients. A clinical trial of BCL-2 antisense therapy involved 9 patients with non-Hodgkin's lymphoma [34]. In two patients a reduction in tumour size (one minor, one complete response) was observed. In another two patients a reduction in the number of circulating lymphoma cells was seen. In a further two patients, symptoms of the disease had improved.

Results of MDR-1 vector modification of bone marrow cells demonstrated that only a very small subset of the granulocyte/macrophage colony forming unit cell fraction of myeloid cells, contributes to the repopulation of the haematopoietic tissues following mega-chemotherapy and transplantation of autologous haematopoietic cells [126].

GMTV – admixture of autologous tumour cells and an HLA-A1/A2-positive allogenic melanoma cell line modified to secrete IL-6 and sIL-6R

Interleukin-6 (IL-6) is a multifunctional cytokine that exerts its activity *via* a receptor complex (IL-6R) composed of two subunits, an IL-6-binding α chain (gp80) and a signal transducing β

chain (gp130) [127]. The soluble form of the α subunit (sIL-6R) acts agonistically with IL-6 to enhance its activity both *in vitro* and *in vivo* [128, 129]. Moreover, the IL-6/sIL-6R complex displays a broader range of biological activities than IL-6 alone, since it is capable of activating cells which possess gp130 but lack gp80 [128]. In preclinical studies, introduction of the IL-6 and sIL-6R genes into a weakly immunogenic murine melanoma cell line (B-78-H1) inhibited tumour growth potential and ability to metastasize concomitant with the stimulation of a potent, specific and long-lasting anti-melanoma immune response [129, 130]. The IL-6/sIL-6R complex was significantly better at inducing anti-melanoma activity than IL-6 alone. Analysis of tumour infiltrates demonstrated that IL-6/sIL-6R-secreting melanoma cells attracted CD8+ T cells and NK cells but not CD4+ T cells or dendritic cells (A. Mackiewicz et al., unpublished results).

These results formed the basis for the design of a phase I/II human melanoma gene therapy clinical protocol [131] which was approved by the Committee for Ethics of Scientific Research of USMS in Poznan on November 26, 1993, and the trial was started on January 6, 1995. The aim of the study was to immunize melanoma patients of the HLA-A1 and/or HLA-A2 haplotype with an IL-6/sIL-6R GMTV, in an attempt to elicit specific as well as non-specific anti-melanoma immune responses of potential therapeutic benefit (Fig. 11).

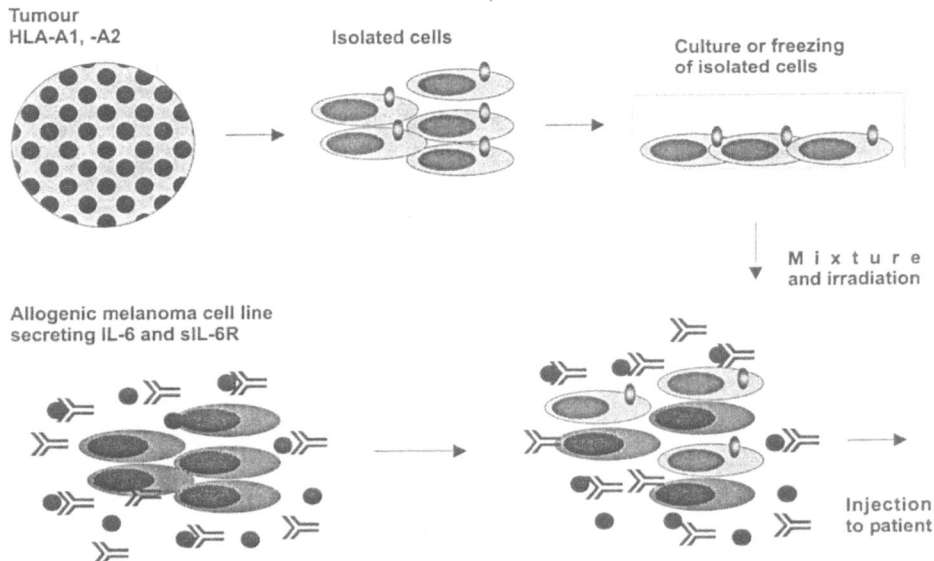

Figure 11. Strategy of IL-6/sIL-6R gene therapy immunogene therapy protocol. Autologous cells from HLA-A1 or/and HLA-A2 positive patients are isolated from metastatic tumour tissue, frozen in liquid nitrogen, thawed when required, and mixed with an allogeneic human melanoma cell line transduced with retroviral vector containing cDNAs encoding hIL-6 and hsIL-6R. The mixture is irradiated and subsequently administered to the patients.

Clinical design

Twenty two patients with advanced stage malignant melanoma (MM), all of whom signed an informed consent form, were enrolled into the study. Patients were evaluated as described [131]. Immunological tests (immunophenotyping of peripheral blood lymphocytes (PBL); natural killer (NK) cell activity) were performed before each vaccine administration. NK cell activity was analyzed using K652 erythroleukaemia cells as targets. In patient No. 9, a biopsy from the site of vaccination was taken two weeks following the fifth injection. In patient No. 1, biopsies from skin metastases were taken before treatment and after the third and fourth vaccinations. Biopsy specimens were analyzed for immune cell infiltration.

The HLA-A1/A2-positive melanoma cell line Mich-1, which expresses MART1, MAGE 1 and 3, was transduced with human IL-6 and sIL-6R cDNAs using a MSCV-based double-copy bicistronic retroviral vector. Following expansion, cultured cells were trypsinized, aliquoted (2.5×10^7 viable cells) and frozen in liquid nitrogen. Metastatic melanoma lesions were surgically excised, the tissue minced into 2–3 mm pieces, and single cells released by enzymatic digestion with collagenase and separated by density gradient centrifugation. Tumour cell preparations were aliquoted (2.5×10^7) and frozen. Prior to injection, the two types of cells were mixed 1:1 (5×10^7 cells total) and irradiated with 100 Gy. They were then injected into the patient at 3–4 sites (usually in the arm); in the vicinity of draining nonaffected lymph nodes on days 0, 14, 28, 32, further injections were given once a month for three consecutive months and subsequently at two-month intervals for a year.

Cellular responses

In biopsies obtained from the sites of vaccine inoculation, only a few melanoma cells were found which were, however, heavily infiltrated by activated T cells (CD3+, DR+) of both CD8+ and CD4+ subsets, with a prevalence of CD8+ cells. Analysis of the PBL phenotype (CD3, CD8, CD4, HLA-DR, CD25, CD16, CD56, CD19) demonstrated a considerable increase in activated T cells (CD3+DR+, CD3+CD25+) after the third and fourth injections. In most patients, the peripheral NK cell activity before treatment was markedly lower than that determined for the corresponding controls. Upon additional injections, all patients exhibited a considerable increase in NK cell activity which exceeded initial levels and was similar to that of controls.

Following the second vaccination, the sites of distant subcutaneous metastases in some patients became discoloured (a dark blue) and warm. In patient No. 1 some of the affected metastases regressed; however, new ones appeared later on. In patient No. 7, a significant reduction in the number and size of skin metastases was observed, with no evidence of new lesions. A biopsy of a subcutaneous metastatic nodule taken from patient No. 1 before treatment revealed the presence of T cells at the margin of the neoplastic infiltration which did not penetrate the tumour proper. Inspection of a biopsy specimen taken from a subcutaneous metastatic lesion from the same patient two weeks after the third vaccination indicated substantial migration of CD3+ T cells into the malignant tissue. In the dispersed infiltrate, CD8+DR+ T cells predominated; however CD4+ cells were also present. In a subsequent biopsy taken from another subcutaneous metastatic nodule 2 weeks after the fourth vaccination, a heavy T cell infiltrate was observed in the melanoma mass which consisted mainly of CD8+DR+ cells. In neither biopsy specimens were NK cells detected.

Selected clinical courses

Patient No. 4 developed MM (left cheek, Clark III, ulceration) at the age of 15. Three years later, multiple metastases were detected in the neck lymph nodes and were treated by surgery followed by high-dose combination chemotherapy and radiotherapy. In the following year, metastases in mediastinal lymph nodes were diagnosed and remained unchanged over the next 3 years. After that time they began to grow progressively. During this period, a metastatic tumour (18×12 cm) was found in the left ovary. The tumour was surgically excised and used for vaccine preparation. Vaccination was initiated three months following surgery. At that time, multiple mediastinal metastases were pressing the trachea and oesophagus, causing problems with breathing and swallowing. After two months of treatment, a substantial reduction in mediastinal tumour burden was observed, with the metastatic nodules continuing to regress until they were no longer detectable at 8 months.

Patient No. 11 developed MM (left thigh, Clark III, ulceration) at the age of 42. Five months after initial treatment, metastases were detected in inguinal lymph nodes. These tumours were surgically excised and used for vaccine preparation. Vaccination was started 3 months after surgery. After 8 months of treatment, this patient remains free of detectable disease.

Clinical response
Out of 22 patients, one complete response (CR), two partial responses (PR), 6 cases of stable disease (SD), 5 SD followed by progression of the disease (PD), and 2 mixed responses were observed. In 6 patients PD was seen.

Conclusions
(i) The procedure has a good safety profile with no toxicity; (ii) the vaccine induced cellular (anti-tumour) immune responses associated with significant T cell infiltration of distant metastatic nodules; and (iii) although clinical efficacy requires further testing, the feasibility of this approach as a potential treatment of metastatic melanoma was demonstrated.

Concluding remarks

Although very promising, cancer gene therapy is still in its infancy. The incompletely understood pathogenesis of cancer and the still primitive technology of gene delivery are both factors which limit successful treatment. Improvement to the existing gene transfer technology and the design of new ones are the major directions for further development. In addition new information gained from the molecular studies of cancer biology and provided by the Human Genome Project will identify targets for further gene therapy strategies.

Acknowledgements
This work was supported by the State Committee for Scientific Research (Warsaw) and the Deutsche Forschungs-gemeinschaft (Bonn, Germany). Figures 7A, B, C, D are reproduced with the permission of Stockton Press.

References

1. Yang NS, Burkholder J, Roberts B, Martinell B, Mc Cabe D (1990) *In vitro* gene transfer to mammalian somatic cells by particle bombardment. *Proc Natl Acad Sci USA* 87: 9568–9572.
2. Wiliams RS (1991) Introduction of foreign genes into tissues of living mice by DNA-coated microprojectiles. *Proc Natl Acad Sci USA* 88: 2726–2730.
3. Wolff JA (1990) Direct gene transfer into muose muscles *in vivo*. *Science* 247: 1465–1468.
4. Conry RM, LoBuglio AF, Loechel F, Moore SE, Sumerel LA, Barlow DL, Pike J, Curiel DT (1995) A carcinoembryonic antigen polynucleotide vaccine for human clinical use. *Cancer Gene Ther* 2: 33–38.
5. Concetti A, Amici A, Petrelli C, Tibaldi A, Provinciali M, Venanzi FM (1996) Autoantibody to p185erbB2/neu oncoprotein by vaccination with xenogenic DNA. *Cancer Immunol Immunother* 43: 307–315.
6. Bright RK, Shearer MH, Kennedy RC (1995) Nucleic acid vaccination against virally induced tumours. *Ann NY Acad Sci* 772: 241–251.
7. Vile RG, Hart IR (1993) Use of tissue-specific expression of herpes simplex virus thymidine kinase gene to inhibit growth of established murine melanomas following direct intratumour injection of DNA. *Cancer Res* 53: 3860–3864.
8. Mahvi DM, Sondel PM, Yang NS, Albertini MR, Schiller JH, Hank J, Heiner J, Gan J, Swain W, Logrono R (1997) Phase I/IB study of immunization with autologous tumour cells transfected with the GM-CSF gene by particle-mediated transfer in patients with melanoma or sarcoma. *Hum Gene Ther* 8: 875–891.
9. Keller ET, Burkholder JK, Shi F, Pugh TD, McCabe D, Malter JS, MacEwen EG, Yang NS, Ershler WB (1996) *In vivo* particle-mediated cytokine gene transfer into canine oral mucosa and epidermis. *Cancer Gene Ther* 3: 186–191.
10. Muller M, Grissmann L, Cristiano RJ et al. (1995) Papillomavirus capsid binding and uptake by cells from different tissues and species. *J Virol* 69: 948–954.
11. Chen J, Gamou S, Takayanagi A, Shimizu N (1994) A novel gene delivery system using EGF receptor-mediated endocytosis. *FEBS Lett* 338: 167–169.
12. Gottschalk S, Cristiano R, Smith L, Woo S (1994) Folate-mediated gene delivery and expression *in vitro*. *Gene Ther* 1: 185–191.
13. Zatloukal K, Schneeberger A, Berger M et al. (1995) Elicitation of a systemic and protective anti-melanoma immune response by an IL-2-based vaccine. *J Immunol* 154: 3406–3419.
14. Felgner PL, Gadek TR, Holm M, Roman R, Chan HW, Wenz M, Northrop JP, Ringold GM, Danielsen M et al. (1987) Lipofection a highly efficient, lipid-mediated DNA transfection procedure. *Proc Natl Acad Sci USA* 84: 7413–7417.
15. Farhood H, Bottega R, Epand RM, Huang L (1992) Effect of cationic cholesterol derivatives on gene transfer and protein kinase C activity. *Biochim Biophys Acta* 1111: 239–246.
16. Zhou X, Klibanov AL, Huang L (1991) Lipophylic polylysinesmediate efficient DNA transfection in mammalian cells. *Biochim Biophys Acta* 1065: 8–14.
17. Rose JK, Buonocore L, Whitt MA (1991) A new cationic liposome reagent mediating nearly quantitative transfection of animal cells. *Biotechniques* 10: 520–525.
18. Brigham KL, Meyrick B, Christman, Magnuson M, King G, Berry LC Jr (1989) *In vivo* transfection of expression of murine lungs with a functioning procaryotic gene using a liposome vehicle. *Am J Med Sci* 298: 278–281.
19. Hazinski TA, Ladd PA, De Matteo CA (1991) Localization and induced expression of fusion genes in the rat lung. *Am J Respir Cell Mol Biol* 4: 206–210.
20. Caplen NJ, Alton EW, Middleton PG, Dorin JR, Stevenson BJ, Gao X, Durham SR et al. (1995) Liposome-mediated CFTR gene transfer to the nasal epithelium of patients with cystic fibrosis. *Nature Med* 1: 39–46.
21. Alton EW, Middleton PG, Caplen NJ, Smith SN, Steel DM, Munkonge FM, Jeffrey PK, Geddes DM, Hart SL, Williamson R et al. (1994) Non-invasive liposome mediated gene delivery can correct the ion transport defective chloride channel regulation in cystic fibrosis mutant mice. *Nat Genet* 5: 135–142.
22. Stribling R, Brunette E, Liggitt D, Gaensler K, Debs R (1989) Aerosol gene delivery *in vivo*. *Proc Natl Acad Sci USA* 86: 3474–3478.
23. Hyde SC, Gill DR, Higgins CF, Trezise AE, MacVinish LJ, Cuthbert AW, Ratcliff R, Evans MJ, Colledge WH (1993) Correction of the ion transport defect in cystic fibrosis transgenic mice by gene therapy. *Nature* 362: 250–255.
24. Nabel EG, Plautz G, Boyce FM, Stanley JC, Nabel GJ (1989) Recombinant gene expression *in vivo* within endothelial cells of the arterial wall. *Science* 244: 1342–1343.
25. Ono T, Fujino Y, Tsuhiya T, Tsuda M (1990) Plasmid DNAs directly injected into mouse brain with lipofectin can be incorporated and expressed by brain cells. *Neurosci Lett* 117: 259–263.

26. Nabel GL, Nabel EG, Yang ZY, Fox BA, Plautz GE, Gao X, Huang L, Shu S, Gordon D, Chang AE (1993) Direct gene transfer with DNA liposome complexes in melanoma: expression, biological activity, lack of toxicity in humans. *Proc Natl Acad Sci USA* 90: 11307–11311.
27. Plautz GE, Yang ZY, Wu BY, Gao X, Huang L, Nabel GJ (1993) Immunotherapy of malignancy by *in vivo* gene transfer into tumours. *Proc Natl Acad Sci USA* 90: 4645–4649.
28. Zhu N, Liggit D, Liu Y, Debs R (1993) Systemic gene expression after intravenous DNA delivery into adult mice. *Science* 261: 209–211.
29. Stein CA, Cheng Y-C (1993) Antisense oligonucleotides as therapeutic agents – is the bullet really magical? *Science* 261: 1004–1012.
30. Thierry AR, Dritschilo A (1992) Intracellular activity of unmodified, phosphorothioated and liposomally encapsulated oligodeoxynucleotides for antisense activity. *Nucl Acids Res* 20: 5691–5698.
31. Helen C, Thoung NT, Haqrel-Bellen A (1992) Control of gene expression by triple helix-forming oligonucleotides. The antigene strategy. *Ann NY Acad Sci* 660: 27–34.
32. Akhtar S, Kole R, Juliano RL (1992) Stability of antisense oligodeoxynucleotide analogs in cellular extracts and sera. *Life Sci* 49: 1793–1801.
33. Cohen JS (1993) Gene mimetic substances. *Adv Pharmacol* 25: 319–339.
34. Webb A, Cunningham D, Cotter F, Clarke PA, di Stefano F, Ross P, Corbo M, Dziewanowska Z (1997) BCL-2 antisense therapy in patients with non-Hodgkin lymphoma. *Lancet* 9059: 1137–1141.
35. Arteaga CL, Holt JT (1996) Tissue-targeted antisense c-fos retroviral vector inhibits established breast cancer xenografts in nude mice. *Cancer Res* 56: 1098–1103.
36. Lee CT, Wu S, Gabrilovich D, Chen H, Nadaf-Rahrov S, Ciernik IF, Carbone DP (1996) Antitumour effects of an adenovirus expressing antisense insulin-like growth factor I receptor on human lung cancer cell lines. *Cancer Res* 56: 3038–3041.
37. Steele C, Sacks PG, Adler-Storthz K, Shillitoe EJ (1992) Effect on cancer cells of plasmids that express antisense RNA of human papillomavirus type 18. *Cancer Res* 52: 4706–4711.
38. Liu C, Qureshi IA, Ding X, Shan Y, Huang Y, Xie Y, Ji M (1996) Modulation of multidrug resistance gene (mdr-1) with antisense oligodeoxynucleotides. *Clin Sci (Colch)* 91: 93–98.
39. Cheng JQ, Ruggeri B, Klein WM, Sonoda G, Altomare DA, Watson DK, Testa JR (1996) Amplification of AKT2 in human pancreatic cells and inhibition of AKT2 expression and tumourigenicity by antisense RNA. *Proc Natl Acad Sci USA* 93: 3636–3641.
40. Fakhrai H, Dorigo O, Shawler DL, Lin H, Mercola D, Black KL, Royston I, Sobol RE (1996) Eradication of established intracranial rat gliomas by transforming growth factor beta antisense gene therapy. *Proc Natl Acad Sci USA* 93: 2909–2914.
41. Schrump DS, Chen A, Consoli U (1996) Inhibition of lung cancer proliferation by antisense cyclin D. *Cancer Gene Ther* 3: 131–135.
42. Martiny-Baron G, Marme D (1995) VEGF-mediated tumour angiogenesis: a new target for cancer therapy. *Curr Opin Biotechnol* 6: 675–680.
43. Garcia-Hernandez B, Sanchez-Garcia I (1996) Retroviral vector design for gene therapy of cancer: specific inhibition and tagging of BCR-ABLp190 cells. *Mol Med* 2: 124–133.
44. Cech TR, Bass BL (1986) Biological catalysis by RNA. *Annu Rev Biochem* 55: 599–629.
45. Kashani-Sabet M, Scanlon KJ (1995) Application of ribozymes to cancer gene therapy. *Cancer Gene Ther* 2: 213–223.
46. Ojwang JO, Hampel A, Looney DJ et al. (1992) Inhibition of human immunodefficiency virus type I expression by a haipin ribozyme. *Proc Natl Acad Sci USA* 89: 10802–10806.
47. Noonberg SB, Scott GK, Garovoy MR, Benz CC, Hunt CA (1994) *Nucl Acids Res* 22: 293–300.
48. Eastham JA, Ahlering TE (1996) Use of an anti-ras ribozyme to alter the malignant phenotype of a human bladder cancer cell line. *J Urol* 56: 1186–1188.
49. Scanlon KJ, Jiao L, Funato T, Wang W, Tone T, Rossi JJ, Kashani-Sabet M (1991) Ribozyme-mediated cleavage of c-fos mRNA reduces gene expression of DNA synthesis enzymes and metallothionein. *Proc Natl Acad Sci USA* 88: 10591–10595.
50. Cai DW, Mukhopadhyay T, Roth JA (1995) Suppression of lung cancer cell growth by ribozyme-mediated modification of p53 pre-mRNA. *Cancer Gene Ther* 2: 199–205.
51. Shore SK, Nabissa PM, Reddy EP (1993) *Oncogene* 8: 3183–3188.
52. Ge L, Resnick NM, Ernst LK, Salvucci LA, Asman DC, Cooper DL (1995) Gene therapeutic approaches to primary and metastatic brain tumours: II. ribozyme-mediated suppression of CD44 expression. *J Neurooncol* 26: 251–257.
53. Maelandsmo GM, Hovig E, Skrede M, Engebraaten O, Florenes VA, Myklebost O, Grigorian M, Lukanidin E, Scanlon KJ, Fodstad O (1996) Reversal of the *in vivo* metastatic phenotype of human tumour cells by an anti-CAPL (mts1) ribozyme. *Cancer Res* 56: 5490–5498.
54. Hua J, Muschel RJ (1996) Inhibition of matrix metalloproteinase 9 expression by a ribozyme blocks metastasis in a rat sarcoma model system. *Cancer Res* 56: 5279–5284.
55. Kanazawa Y, Ohkawa K, Ueda K, Mita E, Takehara T, Sasaki Y, Kasahara A, Hayashi N (1996) Hammerhead ribozyme-mediated inhibition of telomerase activity in extracts of human hepatocellular carcinoma cells. *Biochem Biophys Res Commun* 225: 570–576.

56. Yamamoto H, Irie A, Fukushima Y, Ohnishi T, Arita N, Hayakawa T, Sekiguchi K (1996) Abrogation of lung metastasis of human fibrosarcoma cells by ribozyme-mediated suppression of integrin alpha6 subunit expression. *Int J Cancer* 65: 519–524.
57. Kiehntopf M, Brach MA, Licht T, Petschauer S, Karawajew L, Kirschning C, Herrmann F (1994) Ribozyme-mediated cleavage of the MDR-1 transcript restores chemosensitivity in previously resistant cancer cells. *EMBO J* 13: 4645–4652.
58. Holm PS, Scanlon KJ, Dietel M (1994) Reversion of multidrug resistance in the P-glycoprotein-positive human pancreatic cell line (EPP85-181RDB) by introduction of a hammerhead ribozyme. *Brit J Cancer* 70: 239–243.
59. Czubayko F, Schulte AM, Berchem GJ, Wellstein A (1996) Melanoma angiogenesis and metastasis modulated by ribozyme targeting of the secreted growth factor pleiotrophin. *Proc Natl Acad Sci USA* 93: 14753–14758.
60. Miller AD, Miller DG, Garcia JV, Lynch CM (1993) Use of retroviral vectors for gene transfer and expression. *Methods Enzymol* 217: 581–599.
61. Mulligan RC (1993) The basic science of gene therapy. *Science* 260: 926–932.
62. Hawley RG (1996) Therapeutic potential of retroviral vectors. *Transfus Sci* 17: 7–14.
63. Emerman M, Temin HM (1984) Genes with promoters in retrovirus vectors can be independently suppressed by an epigenetic mechanism. *Cell* 39: 459–467.
64. Lupton SD, Brunton LL, Kalberg VA, Overell RW (1991) Dominant positive and negative selection using a hygromycin phosphotransferase-thymidine kinase fusion gene. *Mol Cell Biol* 11: 3374–3378.
65. Ghattas IR, Sanes JR, Majors JE (1991) The encephalomyocarditis virus internal ribosome entry site allows efficient coexpression of two genes from a recombinant provirus in cultured cells and in embryos. *Mol Cell Biol* 11: 5848–5859.
66. Wiznerowicz M, Fong AZC, Mackiewicz A, Hawley RG. Double-copy bicistronic retroviral vector platform for gene therapy and tissue engineering: application to melanoma vaccine development. *Gene Ther* 10: 1061–1068.
67. Hantzopoulos PA, Sullenger BA, Ungers G, Gilboa E (1989) Improved gene expression upon transfer of the adenosine deaminase minigene outside the transcriptional unit of a retroviral vector. *Proc Natl Acad Sci USA* 86: 3519–3523.
68. Rittner K, Stoppler H, Pawlita M, Sczakiel G (1991) Versatile eucaryotic vectors for strong and constitutive transient and stable gene expression. *Meth Mol Cell Biol* 2: 176–181.
69. Hawley RG et al. (1996) Retroviral vectors for production of interleukin-12 in the bone marrow to induce a graft-*versus*-leukemia effect. *Ann N. Y. Acad Sci*; 795: 341–345.
70. Graham FL, Prevec L (1991) *Manipulation of adenoviral vectors.* Humana press.
71. Graham FL, Smiley J, Russel WC, Nairu R (1977) Characteristics of a human cell line transformed by DNA from human adenovirus type 5. *J Gen Virol* 36: 59–72.
72. Wold WSM, Gooding LR (1991) Region E3 of adenovirus: a cassette of genes involved in host immuno-surveillance and virus-cell interaction. *Virology* 184: 1–9.
73. Engelhardt JF, Simon RH, Yang Y, Zepeda M, Weber-Pendleton S, Doranz B et al. (1993) Adenovirus-mediated transfer of the CFTR gene to lung of nonhuman primates: biological efficiacy study. *Hum Gene Ther* 4: 759–769.
74. Knowles MR et al. (1995) A controlled study of adenoviral-vector-mediated gene transfer in the nasal epithelium of patients with cystic fibrosis. *N Eng J Med* 333: 823–831.
75. Mitani K, Graham FL, Caskey CT, Kochanek S (1995) Rescue, propagation, and partial purification of a helper virus-dependent adenovirus vector. *Proc Natl Acad Sci USA* 92: 3854–3858.
76. Carter BJ (1990) The growth cycle of adeno-associated virus. *In*: Tjissen P (ed.): *Handbook of Parvoviruses.* CRC Press, Boca Raton, 155–168.
77. Carter BJ, Mendelson E, Trempe JP. AAV DNA replication, integration, and genetics. *In*: Tjissen P (ed.):. *Handbook of Parvoviruses.* CRC Press, Boca Raton, 169–226.
78. Samulski RJ, Zhu X, Xiao X, Brook JD, Housman DE, Epstein N, HUnter LA (1991) Targeted integration of adeno-associated virus (AAV) into human chromosome 19. *EMBO J* 10: 3941–3950.
79. Okada H, Miyamura K, Itoh T, Hagiwara M, Wakabayashi T, Mizuno M, Colosi P, Kurtzman G, Yoshida J (1996) Gene therapy against an experimental glioma using adeno-associated virus vectors. *Gene Ther* 3: 957–964.
80. Cosset F-L, Russel SJ (1996) Targetting retroviral entry. *Gene Ther* 3: 946–956.
81. Miller N, Whelan J (1997) Progress in transcriptionally targeted and regulatable vectors for genetic therapy. *Hum Gene Ther* 8: 803–815.
82. Vile RG, Hart IR (1993) *In vitro* and *in vivo* targeting of gene expression to melanoma cells. *Cancer Res* 53: 962–967.
83. Vile RG, Hart IR (1993) Use of tissue-specific expression of the herpes simplex virus thymidine kinase gene to inhibit growth of established murine melanomas following direct intratumoural injection of DNA. *Cancer Res* 53: 3860–3864.

84. Osaki T, Tanio Y, Tachibana I, Hosoe S, Kumagai T, Kawase I, Oikawa S, Kishimoto T (1994) Gene therapy for carcinoembryonic antigen-producing human lung cancer cells by cell-type specific expression of herpes simplex thymidine kinase gene. *Cancer Res* 54: 5258–5261.
85. Richards CA, Austin EA, Huber BE (1995) Transcriptional regulatory sequences of carcinoembryonic antigen: Identification and use with cytosine deaminase for tumour specific gene therapy. *Hum Gene Ther* 6: 881–893.
86. Ido A, Nakata K, Kato Y, Nakao K, Murata K, Fujita M, Ishii N, Tamao (1995) Gene therapy for hepatoma cells using a retrovirus vector carrying herpes simplex virus thymidine kinase gene under the control of human alpha-fetoprotein gene promoter. *Cancer Res* 55: 3105–3109.
87. Arbuthnot PB, Bralet MP, Le Jossic C, Dedieu JF, Perricaudet M, Brechot C, Ferry N (1996) *In vitro* and *in vivo* hepatoma cell-specific expression of a gene transferred with an adenoviral vector. *Hum Gene Ther* 7: 1503–1514.
88. Su H, Chang JC, Xu SM, Kan YW (1996) Selective killing of AFP-positive hepatocellular carcinoma cells by adeno-associated virus transfer of the herpes simplex virus thymidine kinase gene. *Hum Gene Ther* 7: 463–470.
89. Kaneko S, Hallenbeck P, Kotani T, Nakabayashi H, McGarrity G, Tamaoki T, Anderson WF, Chiang YL (1995) Adenovirus-mediated gene therapy of hepatocellular carcinoma using cancer-specific gene expression. *Cancer Res* 55: 5283–5287.
90. Chen L, Chen D, Manome Y, Dong Y, Fine HA, Kufe DW (1995) Breast cancer selective gene expression and therapy mediated by recombinant adenoviruses containing the DF3/MUC1 promoter. *J Clin Invest* 96: 2775–2782.
91. Harris JD, Gutierrez AA, Hurst HC, Sikora K, Lemoine NR (1994) Gene therapy for cancer using tumour-specific prodrug activation. *Gene Ther* 1: 170–175.
92. Kumagai T, Tanio Y, Osaki T, Hosoe S, Tachibana I, Ueno K, Kijima T, Horai T, Kishimoto T (1996) Eradication of Myc-overexpressing small cell lung cancer cells transfected with herpes simplex virus thymidine kinase gene containing Myc-Max response elements. *Cancer Res* 56: 354–358.
93. Lee CH, Liu M, Sie KL, Lee MS (1996) Prostate-specific antigen promoter driven gene therapy targeting DNA polymerase-alpha and topoisomerase II alpha in prostate cancer. *Anticancer Res* 16: 1805–1811.
94. Gansbacher B, Zier K, Daniels B, Cronin K, Bannerji R, Gilboa E (1990) Interleukin 2 gene transfer into tumour cells abrogates tumourigenicity and induces protective immunity. *J Exp Med* 172: 1217–1224.
95. Kawakami Y, Custer MC, Rosenberg SA, Lotze MT (1989) IL-4 regulates IL-2 induction of lymphokine-activated killer activity from human lymphocytes. *J Immunol* 142: 3452–3461.
96. Rosenberg SA, Lotze MT, Yang JC, Topalian SL, Chang AE, Schwartzentruber DJ, Aebersold P, Leitman S, Linehan WM, Seipp CA et al. (1993) Prospective randomized trial of high-dose interleukin-2 alone or in conjunction with lymphokine-activated killer cells for the treatment of patients with advanced cancer. *J Nat Cancer Inst* 85: 622–632.
97. Aebersold P, Hyatt C, Johnson S, Hines K, Korcak L, Sanders M, Lotze M, Topalian S, Yang J, Rosenberg SA (1991) Lysis of autologous melanoma cells by tumour-infiltrating lymphocytes: association with clinical response. *J Nat Cancer Inst* 83: 932–937.
98. Rosenberg SA, Aebersold P, Cornetta K, Kasid A, Morgan RA, Moen R, Karson EM, Lotze MT, Yang JC, Topalian SL et al. (1990) Gene transfer into humans – immunotherapy of patients with advanced melanoma, using tumour-infiltrating lymphocytes modified by retroviral gene transduction. *N Engl J Med* 323: 570–578.
99. Nerrouche Y, Negrier S, Bain C, Combaret V, Mercatello A, Coronel B et al. (1995) Clinical application of retroviral gene transfer in oncology: results of a French study with tumour-infiltrating lymphocytes transduced with the gene of resistance to neomycin. *J Nat Cancer Inst* 87: 280–285.
100. Reeves ME, Royal RE, Lam JS, Rosenberg SA, Hwu P (1996) Retroviral transduction of human dendritic cells with a tumour-associated antigen gene. *Cancer Res* 56: 5672–5677.
101. Tepper R, Mule J (1994) Experimental and clinical studies of cutokine gene-modified tumour cells. *Hum Gene Ther* 5: 153–164.
102. Chen L, Ashe S, Brady WA, Hellstrom I, Hellstrom KE, Ledbetter JA, McGowan P, Linsley PS (1992) Costimulation of antitumour immunity by the B7 counterreceptor for the T lymphocyte molecules CD28 and CTLA-4. *Cell* 71: 1093–1102.
103. Townsend SE, Allison JP (1993) Tumor rejection after direct costimulation of CD8+ T cells by B7-transfected melanoma cells. *Science* 259: 368–370.
104. Rosenberg SA (1997) Cancer vaccines based on the identification of genes encoding cancer regression antigens. *Immunol Today* 4: 175–182.
105. Zitvogel L, Tahara H, Robbins PD, Storkus WJ, Clarke MR, Nalesnik MA, Lotze MT (1995) Cancer immunotherapy of established tumours with IL-12. Effective delivery by genetically engineered fibroblasts. *J Immunol* 155: 1393–1403.
106. Tahara H, Lotze MT, Robbins PD, Storkus WJ, Zitvogel L (1995) IL-12 gene therapy using direct injection of tumours with genetically engineered autologous fibroblasts. *Hum Gene Ther* 6: 1607–1624.

107. Lotze MT, Rubin JT, Carty S, Edington H, Ferson P, Landreneau R, Pippin B, Posner M, Rosenfelder D, Watson C et al. (1994) Gene therapy of cancer: a pilot study of IL-4-gene-modified fibroblasts admixed with autologous tumour to elicit an immune response. *Hum Gene Ther* 5: 41–55.
108. Nabel GJ, Gordon D, Bishop DK, Nickoloff BJ, Yang ZY, Aruga A, Cameron MJ, Nabel EG, Chang AE (1996) Immune response in human melanoma after transfer of an allogeneic class I major histocompatibility complex gene with DNA-liposome complexes. *Proc Natl Acad Sci USA* 93: 15388–15393.
109. Deonaraian MP, Spooner RA, Epenetos AA (1995) Genetic delivery of enzymes for cancer therapy. *Gene Ther* 2: 235–244.
110. Barba D, Hardin J, Sadelain M, Gage FH (1994) Development of anti-tumour immunity following thymidine kinase-mediated killing of experimental brain tumours. *Proc Natl Acad Sci USA* 91: 4348–4352.
111. Freeman SM, Abboud CN, Whartenby KA, Packman CH, Koeplin DS, Moolten FL, Abraham GN (1993) The "bystander effect": tumour regression when a fraction of the tumour mass is genetically modified. *Cancer Res* 53: 5274–5283.
112. Mesnil M, Piccoli C, Tiraby G, Willecke K, Yamasaki H (1996) Bystander killing of cancer cells by herpes simplex virus thymidine kinase gene is mediated by connexins. *Proc Natl Acad Sci USA* 93: 1831–1835.
113. Vile RG, Castleden S, Marshall J, Camplejohn R, Upton C, Chong H (1997) Generation of an antitumour immune response in a non-immunogenic tumour: HSVtk killing *in vivo* stimulates a mononuclear cell infiltrate and a Th1-like profile of intratumoural cytokine expression. *Int J Cancer* 71: 267–274.
114. Culver KW, Van Gilder J, Link CJ, Carlstrom T, Buroker T, Yuh W, Koch K, Schabold K, Doornbas S, Wetjen B et al. (1994) Gene therapy for the treatment of malignant brain tumours with *in vivo* tumour transduction with the herpes simplex thymidine kinase gene/ganciclovir system. *Hum Gene Ther* 5: 343–379.
115. Alemany R, Ruan S, Kataoka M, Koch PE, Mukhopadhyay T, Cristiano RJ, Roth JA, Zhang WW (1996) Growth inhibitory effect of anti-K-ras adenovirus on lung cancer cells. *Cancer Gene Ther* 5: 296–301.
116. Roth JA, Nguyen D, Lawrence DD, Kemp BL, Carrasco CH, Ferson DZ, Hong WK, Komaki R, Lee JJ, Nesbitt JC et al. (1996) Retrovirus-mediated wildtype p53 gene transfer to tumours of patients with lung cancer. *Nature Med* 2: 985–991.
117. Mickisch GH, Aksèntijevich I, Schoenlein PV, Goldstein LJ, Galski H, Stahle C et al. (1992) Transplantation of bone marrow cells from transgenic mice expressing the human MDR-1 results in long term protection against the myelosuppressive effect of chemotherapy in mice. *Blood* 79: 1087–1093.
118. Sorentino BP, Brandt SJ, Bodine D, Gottesman M, Pastan I, Cline A et al. (1992) Selection of drug-resistance bone marrow cells *in vivo* after retroviral transfer of the human MDR1. *Science* 257: 99–103.
119. May C, Gunther R, McIvor RS (1996) Protection of mice from lethal doses of methotrexate by transplantation with transgenic marrow expressing drug resistance dihydrofolate-reductase activity. *Blood* 87: 2579–2587.
120. Roth JA, Cristiano RJ (1997) Gene therapy for cancer: what we done and where are we going? *J Nat Cancer Inst* 89: 21–39.
121. Human Gene Marker Protocols/Therapy Clinical Protocols (1997) *Hum Gene Ther* 8: 1499–1530.
122. Arienti F, Sule-Suso J, Belli F, Mascheroni L, Rivoltini L, Melani C, Maio M, Cascinelli N, Colombo MP, Parmiani G (1996) Limited antitumour T cell response in melanoma patients vaccinated with interleukin-2 gene-transduced allogeneic melanoma cells. *Hum Gene Ther* 16: 1955–1963.
123. Abdel-Wahab Z, Weltz C, Hester D, Pickett N, Vervaert C, Barber JR, Jolly D, Seigler HF (1997) A Phase I clinical trial of immunotherapy with interferon-gamma gene-modified autologous melanoma cells: monitoring the humoral immune response. *Cancer* 80: 401–412.
124. Tan Y, Xu M, Wang W, Zhang F, Li D, Xu X, Gu J, Hoffman RM (1996) IL-2 gene therapy of advanced lung cancer patients. *Anticancer Res* 16: 1993–1998.
125. Stopeck AT, Hersh EM, Akporiaye ET, Harris DT, Grogan T, Unger E, Warneke J, Schluter SF, Stahl S (1997) Phase I study of direct gene transfer of an allogeneic histocompatibility antigen, HLA-B7, in patients with metastatic melanoma. *J Clin Oncol* 15: 341–349.
126. Hanania EG, Giles RE, Kavanagh J, Fu SQ, Ellerson D, Zu Z, Wang T, Su Y, Kudelka A, Rahman Z et al. (1996) Results of MDR-1 vector modification trial indicate that granulocyte/macrophage colony-forming unit cells do not contribute to posttransplant hematopoietic recovery following intensive systemic therapy. *Proc Natl Acad Sci USA* 93: 15346–15351.
127. Mackiewicz A, Koj A, Sehgal P (eds) (1995) Interleukin 6-type Cytokines. *Ann N Y Acad Sci* 762: 1–510.
128. Mackiewicz A, Schooltink H, Heinrich PC, Rose-John S (1992) Complex of soluble human IL-6-receptor/IL-6 up-regulates expression of acute-phase proteins. *J Immunol* 149: 2021–2027.
129. Mackiewicz A, Wiznerowicz M, Roeb E, Karczewska A, Nowak J, Heinrich PC, Rose-John S (1995) Soluble interleukin 6 receptor is biologically active *in vivo*. *Cytokine* 7: 142–149.
130. Mackiewicz A, Wiznerowicz M, Roeb E, Pawlowski T, Baumann H, Heinrich P, Rose-John S (1995) Interleukin-6-type cytokines and their receptors for gene therapy of melanoma. *Ann NY Acad Sci* 762: 361–374.
131. Mackiewicz A, Górny A, Laciak M, Malicki J, Murawa P, Nowak J, Wiznerowicz M, Hawley RG, Heinrich PC, Rose-John S (1995) Gene therapy of human melanoma. Immunization of patients with autologous tumour cells admixed with allogeneic melanoma cells secreting interleukin 6 and soluble interleukin 6 receptor. *Hum Gene Ther* 6: 805–811.

Appendix

Table 1. Cancer gene therapy protocols approved for clinical trials

A. Immunogene therapy protocols.

Principal Investigator	Protocol Title	Gene Transduction	Target	Vector Name	Delivery
Berchuck A. Duke University, Durham, USA	IL-2 gene modified tumour cells in patients with metastatic ovarian cancer	*Ex vivo*	Metastatic ovarian cancer cells	IL-2	Lipid
Black KL. UCLA, School of Medicine, Los Angeles, USA	Injection of glioblastoma patients with TGF-β_2 gene-modified autologous tumour cells	*Ex vivo*	Autologous glioblastoma cells	IL-2/ TGF-β_2	Retrovirus
Bozik ME. Univ. of Pittsburg Cancer Institute, USA	Gene therapy of malignant gliomas: IL-4 gene modified autologous tumour cells	*Ex vivo*	Malignant glial cells	IL-4	Retrovirus
Brenner M. St. Jude Children's Research Hospital, Memphis, USA	Cytokine gene-modified autologous neuroblastoma cells for treatment of relapse/refractory neuroblastoma	*Ex vivo*	Neuroblasts	IL-2	Retrovirus, Adenovirus
Cascinelli N. Sylvester Cancer Center/Univ. of Miami Hospital, USA	Immunization of metastatic melanoma patients with IL-4-transduced, allogeneic melanoma cells	*Ex vivo*	Human melanoma cell line	IL-4	Retrovirus
Cascinelli N. Sylvester Cancer Center/Univ. of Miami Hospital, USA	Immunization of metastatic melanoma patients with IL-2 gene-transduced, allogeneic melanoma cells	*Ex vivo*	Human melanoma cell line	IL-2	Retrovirus
Chang AE. Univ. of Michigan Medical Center, Ann Arbor, USA	Immunotherapy for cancer by direct gene transfer into tumours	*In vivo*	Melanoma cells	HLA-B7	Lipid β2-micro-globulin
Chang AE. Univ. of Michigan Medical Center, Ann Arbor, USA	Phase II study of immunotherapy of metastatic cancer by direct gene transfer	*In vivo*	Cancer cells	HLA-B7	Lipid β2-micro-globulin
Chang AE.Univ. of Michigan Medical Center, Ann Arbor, USA	Activated lymph node cells primed with autologous tumour cells transduced with GM-CSF gene	*Ex vivo*	Tumour cells	GM-CSF	Retrovirus
Chen AP. NCI, National Naval Medical Center, Bethesda, USA	Recombinant vaccinia virus expressing PSA vaccine in patient with adenocarcinoma of the prostate	*In vivo*	Prostate cancer cells	PSA	Vaccinia
Cole DJ. Medical Univ. of South Carolina, Charleston, USA	CEA vaccinia virus vaccine	*In vivo*	Fibroblasts	CEA	Vaccinia
Conry RM. Univ. of Alabama, Birmingham, USA	Polynucleotide immunization to human CEA in patients with metastatic colorectal cancer	*In vivo*	Myocytes	CEA	Plasmid

Table 1A. (continued)

Principal Investigator	Protocol Title	Gene Transduction	Target	Vector Name	Delivery
Das Gupa T. Univ. of Illinois at Chicago, USA	Allogeneic melanoma cells transduced with retroviral vector expressing IL-2	*Ex vivo*	UTSO-H-MEL2 melanoma cells	IL-2	Retrovirus
Dranoff G. Dana-Farber Cancer Institute, Boston, USA	Vaccination with autologous-irradiated melanoma cells producing human GM-CSF	*Ex vivo*	Melanoma cells	GM-CSF	Retrovirus
Economou J. UCLA School of Medicine Los Angeles, USA	Vaccination with autologous-irradiated melanoma cells producing IL-2	*Ex vivo*	Melanoma cells	IL-2	Retrovirus
Economou J. UCLA School of Medicine Los Angeles, USA	Vaccination with autologous-irradiated melanoma cells producing IL-7	*Ex vivo*	Melanoma cells	IL-7/ HyTK	Retrovirus
Figlin RA. UCLA Medical Center Los Angeles, USA	Immunotherapy of metastatic cancer by direct gene transfer	*In vivo*	Renal carcinoma cells	IL-2	Lipid
Figlin RA. UCLA Medical Center Los Angeles, USA	HLA-B7 as an immunotherapeutic agent in renal cancer with IL-2 therapy	*In vivo*	Renal carcinoma cells	HLA-B7	Lipid
Fox BA. Providence Portland Medical Center, USA	Adoptive cellular therapy of cancer combining direct HLA-B7/β2 microglobulin gene transfer with autologous tumour vaccination for generation of vaccine primed anti-CD3 activated lymphocytes	*In vivo*	Irradiated autologous tumour cells	HLA-B7/β2 microglobulin	Plasmid
Gansbacher B. Memorial Sloan-Kettering Cancer Center, New York, USA	Immunization with HLA-A2 matched allogeneic melanoma cells that secrete IL-2 in patients with metastatic melanoma	*Ex vivo*	Irradiated HLA-A2 matched allogeneic tumour cells	IL-2	Retrovirus
Gansbacher B. Memorial Sloan-Kettering Cancer Center, New York, USA	Immunization with Il-2 secreting allogeneic HLA-A2 matched irradiated renal cell carcinoma cells in patients with advanced renal cell carcinoma	*Ex vivo*	Renal carcinoma cells	IL-2	Retrovirus
Gluckman JL. Univ. of Cincinnati, USA	Allovectin-7 in the treatment of squamous cell carcinoma of the head and neck	*In vivo*	Squamous cell carcinoma	Allovectin-7	Lipid
Gore M. Royal Marsden Hospital, London, U.K.	Treatment of metastatic malignant melanoma with melanoma cells genetically engineered to secrete IL-2	*Ex vivo*	Melanoma cells	IL-2	Retrovirus
Harris AL. Churchill Hospital, Oxford, U.K.	Cancer therapy of metastatic melanoma	*In vivo*	Melanoma cells	Tyrosinase, IL-2, β-Gal	Plasmid
Hersh E. Arizona Cancer Center, Tucson, USA	Study of gene transfer of IL-2 gene	*In vivo*	Tumour cells	Leuvectin	Lipid

Table 1A. (continued)

Principal Investigator	Protocol Title	Gene Transduction	Target	Vector Name	Delivery
Hersh E. Arizona Cancer Center, Tucson, USA	Study of gene transfer of HLA-B7 gene	*In vivo*	Tumour cells	Allovectin-7	Lipid
Hwu P. National Institute of Health, Bethesda, USA	Treatment of patients with advanced epithelial ovarian cancer using anti-CD3-stimulating peripheral blood lymphocytes transduced with chimaeric T cell receptor gene.	*Ex vivo*	PBLs	Chimaeric T cell receptor	Retrovirus
Ilan J. Case Western Reserve Univ., Cleveland, USA	Episome-based antisense cDNA transcription of IGF-I for brain tumours	*Ex vivo*	Glioblastoma cells	anti-IGF-I	Liposome
Lindemann A. Medizinische Universitätsklinik, Freiburg, Germany	Vaccination study with B7,1+IL-2 gene transfected allogeneic cell lines in renal cell carcinoma	*Ex vivo*	Renal carcinoma cell lines	B7,1/IL-2	Lipid
Lindemann A. Medizinische Universitätsklinik, Freiburg, Germany	Evaluation of vaccine preparations in melanoma patients	*Ex vivo*	Allogeneic fibroblasts + NATC	IL-2 or GM-CSF	Lipid
Link CJ. Human Gene Therapy Research Inst, Des Moines,USA	Adoptive immunotherapy for leukaemia: donor lymphocytes transduced with HSV-TK for remission induction	*Ex vivo*	Lymphocytes	HSV-TK	Retrovirus
Lotze MT. Univ. of Pittsburgh School of Medicine, USA	IL-4 gene-modified antitumour vaccines	*Ex vivo*	Irradiated autologous fibroblasts + NATC	IL-4	Retrovirus
Lotze MT. Univ. of Pittsburgh School of Medicine, USA	IL-12 gene therapy with genetically engineered autologous fibroblasts	*Ex vivo*	Autologous fibroblasts	IL-12	Retrovirus
Lyerly HK. Duke Univ. Durham, USA	Autologous human IL-2 lipofection gene-modified tumour cells in patients with refractory or recurrent metastatic breast cancer	*In vivo*	Metastatic breast cancer cells	IL-2	Lipid
Mackiewicz A. Great Poland Cancer Center, Poland	Immunogene therapy of malignant melanoma with autologous cells admixed with allogeneic cells engineered to secrete IL-6 and soluble IL-6R	*Ex vivo*	Autologous cells mixed with allogeneic cell lines	IL-6 and soluble IL-6R	Retrovirus
Marshall JL. Georgetown Univ. Washington, USA	Study of recombinant ALVAC virus that expresses CEA in patients with advanced cancers	*In vivo*	Autologous muscle cells	CEA	Pox virus
Mertelsmann R. Medizinische Univ.-klinik Freiburg, Germany	T cell-mediated immunotherapy by cytokine gene transfer in patients with malignant tumours	*Ex vivo*	Irradiated autologous fibroblasts + NATC	IL-2	Lipid

Table 1A. (continued)

Principal Investigator	Protocol Title	Gene Trans-duction	Target	Vector Name	Delivery
Nabel GL. Univ. of Michigan Medical Center, Ann Arbor	Immunotherapy of cancer by *in vivo* gene transfer into tumours	*In vivo*	Melanoma cells	HLA-B7, β2-micro-globulin	Lipid
Osanto S. Academisch Ziekenhuis Leiden, The Netherlands	Immunization with IL-2-transfected melanoma cells for patients with metastatic melanoma	*Ex vivo*	Melanoma cells	IL-2	Plasmid
Paulson DF. Duke Univ. Medical Center, Durham, NC, USA	Autologous IL-2 gene-modified tumour cells for locally advanced or metastatic prostate cancer	*Ex vivo*	Prostate cancer cells	IL-2	Lipid
Podack E. Antoni Van Leeuwenhoek Hospital, Amsterdam, The Netherlands	Small-cell lung tumour cells trans-duced with a vector expressing IL-2	*Ex vivo*	Small-cell lung cancer cells	IL-2	Lipid
Rankin EM. Antoni Van Leeuwenhoek Hospital, Amsterdam, The Netherlands	Vaccination with autologous GM-CSF-transduced and irradiated tumour cells in patients with advanced melanoma	*Ex vivo*	Melanoma cells	GM-CSF	Retrovirus
Rosenberg SA. National Cancer Institute, Bethesda, USA	Gene therapy of patients with advanced cancer using TILs trans-duced with gene coding for TNF	*In vitro*	TILs	TNF	Retrovirus
Rosenberg SA. National Cancer Institute, Bethesda, USA	Immunization of cancer patients using autologous cancer cells modi-fied by insertion of gene for IL-2	*In vitro*	Autologous tumour cells	IL-2	Retrovirus
Rosenberg SA. National Cancer Institute, Bethesda, USA	Immunization with autologous melanoma tumour cells transduced with gene for TNF	*In vitro*	Autologous tumour cells	TNF	Retrovirus
Rosenberg SA. National Cancer Institute, Bethesda, USA	Patients immunized with recombin-ant adenovirus containing the gene for the MART-1 tumour antigen	*In vivo*	Melanoma cells	MART-I	Adenovirus
Rosenberg SA. National Cancer Institute, Bethesda, USA	Recombinant adenovirus containing the gene for the gp 100 melanoma tumour antigen	*In vitro*	Melanoma cells	gp130	Adenovirus
Rosenblatt J. Univ. of California, Los Angeles, USA	Interferon gamma gene-transduced tumour cells in patients with neuroblastoma	*Ex vivo*	Neuroblastoma cells	INF-gamma	Retrovirus
Rubin J. Mayo Clinic. Rochester, USA	Interferon gamma gene-transduced tumour cells in patients with neuroblastoma	*Ex vivo*	Colorectal carcinoma cells	INF-gamma	Lipid
Schmidt-Wolf I. Insti-tut für Molekularbiolo-gie, Berlin, Germany	IL-7 gene therapy for lymphoma	*Ex vivo*	Lymphoma cells	IL-7	Plasmid
Seigler HF. Duke Univ. Medical Center, Durham, USA	Human interferon gamma-transduced autologous tumour cells for disseminated malignant melanoma	*Ex vivo*	Melanoma cells	INF-gamma	Retrovirus

Table 1A. (continued)

Principal Investigator	Protocol Title	Gene Trans-duction	Target	Vector Name	Delivery
Silver H. BC Cancer Center, Vancouver, BC Canada	Immunotherapy by direct gene transfer	*In vivo*	Melanoma/ renal/ lymphoma cells	VCL-1005-201	Lipid
Silver H. BC Cancer Center, Vancouver, BC Canada	Intralesional transfection with plasmid HLA-B7 in melanoma cells	*In vivo*	Melanoma cells	VCL-1005	Lipid
Simons J, Johns Hopkins Oncology Center, Baltimore, USA	Phase I study of nonreplicating tumour cells injections using cells prepared with or without GM-CSF gene transduction in patients with metastatic renal cell carcinoma	*Ex vivo*	Renal carcinoma cells	GM-CSF	Retrovirus
Sobol RE. San Diego Regional Cancer Center, USA	Injection of a glioblastoma patient with autologous tumour cells and irradiated fibroblasts genetically modified to secrete IL-2	*Ex vivo*	Autologous tumour cells and fibroblasts	IL-2	Retrovirus
Sobol RE. San Diego Regional Cancer Center, USA	Injection of colon carcinoma patients with autologous irradiated tumour cells and irradiated fibroblasts genetically modified to secrete IL-2	*Ex vivo*	Autologous fibroblasts	IL-2	Retrovirus
Sznol M. National Institutes of Health, Frederick, USA	Trial of B7-transfected lethally-irradiated allogeneic melanoma cells lines to induce cell-mediated immunity against tumour associated antigens	*Ex vivo*	Irradiated allogeneic melanoma cells	B7	Lipid
Vogelzang NJ. Univ. of Chicago Medical Center, USA	Immunotherapy of metastatic renal cell carcinoma by direct gene transfer: phase II study in kidney, colon, breast	*In vivo*	Renal cancer cells	HLA-B7	Lipid
Vogelzang NJ. Univ. of Chicago Medical Center, USA	Immunotherapy of metastatic cancer by direct gene transfer	*In vivo*	Cancer cells	HLA-B7	Lipid
Yee C,.Univ. of Washington, Seattle, USA	Adoptive immunotherapy using autologous CD8+ tyrosinase-specific T cells for metastatic melanoma	*Ex vivo*	Tyrosinase-specific T cells	HyTK	Retrovirus

Table 1. (continued)

B. Administration of "suicide genes" and activation of suicide mechanism for direct killing of cancer cells

Principal Investigator	Protocol Title	Gene Transduction	Target	Gene Transduced	Delivery
Albelda SM. Univ. of Pennsylvania Medical Center, Philadelphia, USA	Gene therapy for malignant mesothelioma with HSV-TK	*In vivo*	Malignant mesothelioma	HSV-TK	Adenovirus
Crystal RG. Cornell Medical Center, New York, USA	Administration of replication-deficient adenovirus vector containing the *Escherichia coli* cytosine deaminase gene to metastatic colon carcinoma of the liver with 5-fluorocytosine	*In vivo*	Liver cells	CD	Adenovirus
Curiel D. Univ. of Alabama, Birmingham, USA	Adenovirus intraperitoneal HSV-TK for ovarian and extra ovarian cancer patients	*In vivo*	Ovarian cancer cells	HSV-TK	Adenovirus
Eck SL, Univ. of Pennsylvania, Philadelphia, USA	Recombinant adenovirus for the treatment of CNS cancer	*In vivo*	Glioblastoma/ astrocytoma cells	HSV-TK	Adenovirus
Fetell MR. Columbia-Presbyterian Medical Center, New York, USA	Stereotactic injection of HSV-TK vector producer cells for treatment of recurrent malignant glioma	*In vivo*	Glioma cells	HSV-TK	Retrovirus
Finocchiaro G. Inst. Nazionale Neurologico C, Besta, Milan, Italy	Gene therapy of glioblastoma with HSV-TK	*In vivo*	Glioblastoma cells	HSV-TK	Retrovirus
Freeman SM. Tulane Univ. Medical Center, New Orleans, USA	Treatment of ovarian cancer with a modified HSV-TK cancer vaccine	*Ex vivo*	PA-1 ovarian tumour cells	HSV-TK	Retrovirus
Freeman SM. Tulane Univ. Medical Center, New Orleans, USA	Vaccination with HER/neu-expressing tumour cells and HSV-TK gene-modified tumour cells	*Ex vivo*	PA-1 ovarian/ MDA breast cancer cells	HSV-TK	Retrovirus
Grossman RG. Baylor College of Medicine, Houston, USA	HSV-TK for central nervous system tumours	*In vivo*	Brain tumour cells	HSV-TK	Adenovirus
Izquierdo M. Univ. Autonoma de Madrid, Spain	Gene therapy of glioblastoma with HSV-TK	*In vivo*	Glioblastoma cells	HSV-TK	Retrovirus
Klatzman D. Hopital Pitie Salpetriere, Paris, France	Gene therapy for metastatic melanoma with HSV-TK	*In vivo*	Melanoma cells	HSV-TK	Retrovirus
Klatzman D, Hopital Pitie Salpetriere, Paris, France	Gene therapy for glioblastoma with HSV-TK	*In vivo*	Glioblastoma cells	HSV-TK	Retrovirus

Table 1B. (continued)

Principal Investigator	Protocol Title	Gene Transduction	Target	Gene Transduced	Delivery
Kun LE. St. Jude Children's Research Hospital, Memphis, USA	Stereotactic injection of HSV-TK producer cells for progressive or recurrent primary supratentorial pediatric brain tumours	*In vivo*	Neoplastic glial cells	HSV-TK	Retrovirus
Link CJ. Human Gene Therapy Research Inst., Des Moines, USA	HSV-TK treatment of refractory or recurrent ovarian cancer	*In vivo*	Ovarian carcinoma cells	HSV-TK	Retrovirus
Mariani L. Neurochirurgische Klinik, Inselspital Bern, Switzerland	Gene therapy for glioblastoma with HSV-TK	*In vivo*	Glioblastoma cells	HSV-TK	Retrovirus
Mulder NH. Academisch Ziekenhuis Groningen, The Netherlands	Gene therapy for glioblastoma with HSV-TK	*In vivo*	Glioblastoma cells	HSV-TK	Retrovirus
Munshi NC. Univ. of Arkansas Medical Center, Little Rock, USA	TK-transduced donor leukocyte infusions for patients with relapsed or persistent multiple myeloma after bone marrow transplant	*Ex vivo*	Lymphocytes	HSV-TK	Retrovirus
Oldfield EH. National Institutes of Health, NINDS, Bethesda, USA	Gene therapy of brain tumours with HSV-TK	*In vivo*	Malignant glial tumours	HSV-TK	Retrovirus
Raffel C. Mayo Clinic, Rochester, USA	Gene therapy for treatment of recurrent pediatric malignant astrocytomas with *in vivo* tumour transduction with the HSV-TK gene	*In vivo*	Astrocytoma cells	HSV-TK	Retrovirus
Van Gilder JC. Univ. of Iowa Hospital, Iowa City, USA	Gene therapy for glioblastoma with HSV-TK	*In vivo*	Glioblastoma cells	HSV-TK	Retrovirus
Yla-Herttuala S. Univ. of Kopio, Finland	Gene therapy for glioma with HSV-TK	*In vivo*	Glioma cells	HSV-TK	Retrovirus

C. Inactivation of oncogenes or activation of tumour suppressor genes which regulate cell-cycle

Principal Investigator	Protocol Title	Gene Transduction	Target	Gene Transduced	Delivery
Bishop M. Univ. of Nebraska Medical Center, USA	Antisense p53 for ex vivo treatment of autologous peripheral blood stem cells with OL in patients with acute myelogenous leukaemia	*Ex vivo*	Myelogenous leukaemia cells	anti-p53	Oligos
Clayman GL. M.D. Anderson Center, Houston, USA	Modification of tumour suppressor gene expression in head and neck squamous cell carcinoma with an adenovirus expressing wildtype p53	*In vivo*	Squamous cell carcinoma of head and neck	anti-p53	Adenovirus

Table 1C. (continued)

Principal Investigator	Protocol Title	Gene Trans- duction	Target	Gene Trans- duced	Delivery
Habib N. Hammersmith Hospitals NHS Trust, Lonon, UK	p53 DNA injection in colorectal liver metastases	*In vivo*	Colorectal liver metastases	p53	Plasmid
Holt J. Vanderbilt Univ. Medical School, Nashville, USA	Retroviral antisense c-fos RNA for metastatic breast cancer	*In vivo*	Breast cancer cells in infu- sion	anti-fos	Retrovirus
Holt J. Vanderbilt Univ. Medical School, Nashville, USA	BRCA-1 retroviral gene therapy for ovarian cancer	*In vivo*	Ovarian cancer cells	BRCA1	Retrovirus
Hortobagyi GN. M.D. Anderson Cancer Center, Houston, USA	E1A gene therapy for patients with metastatic breast or epithelial ova- rian cancer that overexpresses HER- 2/neu	*In vivo*	Breast cancer	E1A gene	Lipid
Luger S. Hospital of the Univ. of Pennsyl- vania, Philadelphia, USA	Autologous bone marrow trans- plantation using c-myb antisense oligodeoxynucleotide-treated bone marrow in CML in chronic or accelerated phase	*Ex vivo*	Leukaemic cells in bone marrow	Anti-c- myb	Oligos
Luger S. Hospital of the Univ. of Pennsyl- vania, Philadelphia, USA	Infusional c-myb antisense oligode- oxynucleotides in chronic myelo- genous leukaemia and acute leukaemia	*Ex vivo*	Leukaemic cells	Anti-c- myb	Oligos
Roth JA. M.D. Ander- son Cancer Center, Houston, USA	Modification of tumour suppressor gene expression and induction of apoptosis in NSCLC with adeno- virus vector expressing wildtype p53 and cisplatin	*In vivo*	Lung cancer cells	p53	Adenovirus
Roth JA. M.D. Anders- on Cancer Center, Houston, USA	Modification of oncogene and tumour suppressor gene expression in NSCLC	*In vivo*	Lung cancer cells	p53, ras	Retrovirus
Steiner M. Univ. of Tennessee, Memphis, USA	Treatment of advanced prostate cancer by *in vivo* transduction with prostate-targeted retroviral vectors expressing antisense c-myc RNA	*In vivo*	Prostate cancer cells	c-myc	Retrovirus
Venook A. Univ. of California, San Francisco, USA	Adenovirus expressing p53 *via* hepatic artery infusion for primary and metastatic liver tumours	*In vivo*	Primary and metastatic liver cancers	p53	Adenovirus

Table 1. (continued)

D. Introduction of multidrug resistance genes (MDR) into patient bone marrow cells as a protection from massive chemotherapy

Principal Investigator	Protocol Title	Gene Trans-duction	Target	Gene Trans-duced	Delivery
Cowan K. National Institutes of Health, Bethesda, USA	Retroviral mediated transfer of MDR-1 into haematopoietic stem cells during transplantation after chemotherapy for metastatic breast cancer	*Ex vivo*	Haematopoietic stem cells	mdr-1	Retrovirus
Cowan K. National Institutes of Health, Bethesda, USA	Antimetabolite induction followed by high-dose single alkylating agent consolidation and retroviral transduction of the MDR-1 and NEO-R genes into peripheral blood progenitor cells	*Ex vivo*	Haematopoietic stem cells	mdr-1	Retrovirus
Deisseroth AB. Yale Univ., New Haven, USA	Use of retrovirus to introduce chemotherapy resistance sequences into normal haematopoietic cells for chemoprotection during therapy for breast cancer	*Ex vivo*	Haematopoietic cells	mdr-1	Retrovirus
Deisseroth AB. Yale Univ., New Haven, USA	Use of retrovirus to introduce retro-viral chemotherapy resistance se-quences into normal haematopoietic stem cells for chemoprotection during therapy for ovarian cancer	*Ex vivo*	CD34	mdr-1	Retrovirus
Hesdorfer C. Columbia Univ., New York, USA	MDR gene transfer in patients with advanced cancer	*Ex vivo*	Haematopoietic stem cells	mdr-1	Retrovirus
Mickioch C. Univ. Hospital Rotterdam, The Netherlands	Autologous reinfusion of haemato-poietic precursor cells genetically modified by retroviral gene transfer of the multidrug-resistance gene in patients with metastatic refractory bladder carcinoma	*Ex vivo*	Haematopoietic stem cells	mdr-1	Retrovirus
Sonneveld P. Univ. Hospital Rotterdam, The Netherlands	Autologous reinfusion of haemato-poietic stem cells derived from bone marrow and genetically modified by retroviral gene transfer of the multi-drug-resistance gene in patients with relapsed or primary refractory high-risk non-Hodgkin's lymphoma	*Ex vivo*	Haematopoietic stem cells	mdr-1	Retrovirus
Stoter G. Univ, Hospital Rotterdam The Netherlands	Reinfusion of autologous bone mar-row genetically modified by retro-viral gene transfer of the multidrug-resistance gene in patients with breast cancer refractory to first-line chemotherapy	*Ex vivo*	Haematopoietic stem cells	mdr-1	Retrovirus

Molecular Aspects of Cancer and its Therapy
A. Mackiewicz and P.B. Sehgal (eds)
© 1998 Birkhäuser Verlag Basel/Switzerland

Antisense strategy for cancer therapy

T. Skorski[1], C. Szczylik[2] and B. Calabretta[3]

[1]*Thomas Jefferson University, Kimmel Cancer Institute, Jefferson Alumni Hall, Rm. 372, 1020 Locust Street, Philadelphia, PA 19107, USA*
[2]*Cezary Szczylik, Department of Oncology, CSK WAM, Warsaw, Poland*
[3]*Thomas Jefferson University, Kimmel Cancer Instizute, Bluemle Life Sciences Bldg., Rm. 630, 233 South 10th Street, Philadelphia, PA 19107, USA*

Summary. Antisense oligodeoxynucleotides (AS-ODNs) are short nucleotide sequences of DNA synthesized as reverse complements of the target mRNA nucleotide sequence. On formation of the RNA-DNA duplex, gene expression is prevented. Delivery of AS-ODNs which target oncogene-encoded mRNAs to human cells in culture is associated with inhibition of cell proliferation and, in some circumstances, cell death. AS-ODNs, chemically modified to survive nuclease attack, have been used systematically in murine models of human malignancies. In some studies, a measurable anti-tumor effect has been observed. On the basis of these preclinical investigations, phase I clinical trials involving *ex vivo* and systemic administration of such compounds are now in progress at various institutions. Despite the remarkable progress of the past few years, much remains to be investigated: uptake, cellular distribution, mechanism(s) of action, and metabolism of AS-ODNs. Furthermore, the 'antisense effects' of the AS-ODNs might also be associated with nonspecific effects. Time, a great deal of effort, and patience will tell whether such compounds have a role as novel antineoplastic agents.

Introduction

Conventional chemotherapeutic agents for cancer are designed to inhibit enzymes or the nucleic acid functions necessary for cell growth. The most important limitation of these agents, and their primary source of side effects, derives from their lack of specificity, since they either block enzymatic pathways or interact randomly with DNA irrespective of the cell phenotype. Accordingly, any killing of neoplastic cells preferentially over normal cells by a particular drug exploits differences in biochemical or metabolic process (e.g., growth rate) between normal and cancer cells, rather than the specific effects of that drug on genetically defined characteristics that distinguish neoplastic cells.

The identification of genes that confer a growth advantage to neoplastic cells, and the understanding of the genetic mechanism(s) responsible for their activation, have made possible a direct genetic approach to cancer treatment, using nucleic acid therapeutics. The ability to block expression of individual disease-causing genes provides a powerful tool to explore the molecular basis of normal growth regulation, and the opportunity for therapeutic intervention when a particular gene is pathogenetically activated. Specific species of synthetic ODNs provide the biological tool and, in principle, the potential therapeutic agent.

Mechanisms of altered gene expression in cancer cells as a target for antisense strategy

Aberrant proto-oncogene or tumor suppressor gene expression is common in cancer cells and probably contributes to distinct steps of tumor development. Such altered expression is often due to a recognizable mechanism of gene activation (oncogene) or inactivation (tumor suppressor gene) such as amplification, translocation (with or without rearrangement), or point mutation.

Amplification

Proto-oncogene overexpression is in some cases due to gene amplification. This occurs rarely in normal cells [1], but appears to become more common as cells progress towards a malignant phenotype [2]. Many tumors carry abnormally amplified domains of DNA that can include proto-oncogenes and magnify their expression [3]. The most common examples of gene amplification include N-*myc* in neuroblastoma, L-*myc* in carcinoma of the lung, *erb*-B1 in astrocytoma and *erb*-B2 in adenocarcinoma of breast and ovary [3–5]. Proto-oncogene amplification is rarely detected in hematological malignancies, although c-*myc* amplification in HL-60 promyelocytic leukemia cells was one of the earliest cases described [6–7].

Translocation

Translocations are frequently detected in cancer cells and appear to contribute to tumorigenesis by activating proto-oncogenes to oncogenes [8]. Two of the most common translocations described in neoplastic cells occur in hematological malignancies: in Burkitt's lymphoma, the c-*myc* proto-oncogene on chromosome 8 is juxtaposed to the chromosomal sites of the immunoglobulin genes [9]; in the 9;22 translocation of chronic myelogenous leukemia (CML), the c-*abl* gene is translocated from chromosome 9 into the breakpoint cluster region (*bcr*) gene localized on chromosome 22 [10, 11].

In Burkitt's lymphoma, the involved c-*myc* allele is constitutively expressed, perhaps under the control of the B lymphocyte-specific immunoglobulin enhancer [12], whereas in CML, a chimeric gene is generated from the fusion of the truncated *bcr* gene with the translocated c-*abl* gene [13]; the chimeric gene has higher tyrosine kinase activity than that of the non-translocated c-*abl* gene [14]. The constitutive expression of the c-*myc* gene product and the enhanced tyrosine kinase activity of the *bcr-abl* fusion product are the most likely mechanisms for oncogenic activation of these two genes.

Point mutations

A large number and variety of human neoplastic cells contain consistent point mutations in *ras* proto-oncogenes that are responsible for oncogenic activation [15]. In many cases of acute myelogenous leukemia, N-*ras* carries nucleotide substitutions that mutate codon 13 [16]. The *ras* proteins belong to the GTPase superfamily, the members of which are involved in signal transduction [17]. The biochemical consequences of *ras* mutations in human malignancies could be maintenance of the protein in the GTP-bound form which is responsible for transformation of rodent fibroblasts [17].

Point mutations also cause inactivation of tumor suppressor genes such as p53 [18]. Mutated p53 acts as an oncogene by blocking the activity of the product of the remaining wild-type allele.

In summary, these three types of genetic aberration determine deregulated expression of either a normal proto-oncogene product (amplification and translocations which leave the affected gene intact) or synthesis of an abnormal gene product (point mutations or translocations which alter the gene product), and could be targeted by antisense strategy.

Mechanisms of the antisense effect

Oncogene expression can be disrupted by a variety of methods. The available technologies can be grouped according to whether they target the gene itself (e.g., homologous recombination), or the gene's transcriptional product, a messenger RNA. Among RNA-directed perturbation strategies, the most widely used are catalytic RNA molecules or ribozymes, and antisense oligodeoxynucleotides (AS-ODNs). The latter are short nucleotide sequences of DNA synthesized as exact reverse complements of the desired mRNA target's nucleotide sequence. In theory, the antisense DNA molecule can hybridize in a stable manner only with its mRNA target. Once the RNA-DNA duplex forms, translation of the message is prevented and/or destruction of the molecule by RNase H is promoted. The major appeal of the antisense approach is based on this apparent simplicity: a short sequence of DNA is synthesized, applied to a cell, taken up by the cell, and use of a specific mRNA molecule is inhibited. Viral delivery vectors are unnecessary, and because DNA is weakly immunogenic, tachyphylaxis theoretically never occurs. Of course, prediction and reality do not always coincide, but since the earliest attempts by Zamecnick and Stephenson to inhibit Rous sarcoma virus replication and cell transformation by a specific ODN [19], antisense DNA compounds have appeared to be an attractive tool not only for investigations of normal and pathological gene functions, but also as potential therapeutic agents in a spectrum of pathologic processes ranging from viral infections to neoplastic disorders.

The specificity of Watson-Crick base pairing provides the theoretical basis for AS therapeutics. AS sequences complementary to a target sequence can be designed with exquisite specificity: oligonucleotide sequences as short as 15 bases are likely to be unique in the mRNA pool of a eukaryotic cell and therefore, assuming that full homology is required for an AS effect, capable of specific interaction. However, a number of issues must be addressed before this strategy can be usefully employed [20–22]: the AS molecule must enter the cell efficiently and reach the appropriate compartment within the cell, it should resist breakdown by intra- and extracellular nucleases, it should not be toxic to the cell or interact with sequences other than the target, and the target sequence must be accessible to the AS molecule.

Chemical modifications can be introduced which confer nuclease resistance, whereas unmodified phosphodiester oligomers are very sensitive to endo- and exonucleases. They can also be synthesized in quantities sufficient for clinical use. However, chemical modifications may also have important effects on cellular distribution, toxicity and target specificity which must be taken into account. For example, phosphorothioate oligomers, which have a sulfur for oxygen substitution in the phosphate backbone to confer nuclease resistance, seem to be extensively trapped in the endosomal compartment [23] and bind avidly to a variety of intracellular proteins [24] which may contribute to the toxicity of these molecules. Table 1 briefly summarizes the characteristics of the most common ODN chemical derivatives.

Accessibility of a target sequence to the action of AS-ODNs appears, at least partly, to be a function of its secondary structure. DNA can be targeted by virtue of its ability to form triple helical structures *via* Hoogsteen base pairing in the major groove. More commonly, mRNA is the intended target, but not all sequences are equally accessible because of folding of the mRNA strand. Preferred target sites appear to be the initiation AUG region and hairpin loops, but their accessibility is largely dependent on the precise target sequences. For example, the 5' cap region of *MYC* mRNA is a better target than the AUG region [25].

The pioneering observations of the Weinberg, Barbacid and Wigler laboratories, on point mutations of the *ras* transforming genes isolated from epithelial neoplasia [26] and the subsequent elucidation of two other common modalities of oncogene activation in cancer cells, amplification (e.g., *erb*-B2 in breast and ovarian cancers) and translocation (e.g., juxtaposition of the *bcr* and *c-abl* genes in CML), have led to the realization that the tumor-specific abnormalities generated by the activation of proto-oncogenes can be exploited for nucleic acid-targeted therapy. Table 2 lists

Table 1. Biochemical characteristics of different ODN derivatives

AS-ODNs	Characteristics					
	Easy synthesis	Stability *in vivo*	Uptake	Half-life in the cells	Targeting	Non-antisense effect
Phosphodiester	+	−	+	−	+	−
Phosphorothioate	+	+	+	+	+	+
Phosphoramidate	−	+	+	+	+	?
Methylphosphonate	+	+	−	+	+	−

Table 2. Examples of targets for AS-ODN strategy

Disease	Gene
Breast carcinoma	c-*myb*, *erb*-B2, *ras* mutant
Chronic myelogenous leukemia	*bcr/abl*, c-*myb*, c-*myc*
Acute myelogenous leukemia	c-*myb*, *p53* mutant, *AML1/ETO*
Melanoma	c-*myb*, c-*myc*
Colon carcinoma	c-*myb*, *PKA/RJa*
Lung carcinoma	c-*kit*
Fibrosarcoma	NF-kB
Burkitt lymphoma	c-*myc*
Non-Hodgkin lymphoma	*bcl*-2
Neuroblastoma	c-*myb*, B-*myb*, N-*myc*

potential targets for AS-ODNs as antineoplastic agents. The potential for such highly specific targeting contrasts with the mechanism(s) of action of conventional anticancer chemotherapeutic agent which block enzymatic pathways or randomly interact with nucleic acids irrespective of cell phenotype. AS-ODNs exploit the presence of genetically defined characteristics that distinguish neoplastic cells and are responsible for their growth advantage over normal cells.

In recent years, the AS-ODNs strategy for cancer therapy has progressed from studies *in vitro* to animal models and now to clinical studies. We describe the current state of progress toward gene-directed AS-based cancer therapy primarily from the viewpoint of initial proof-of-concept studies in animal models of human leukemias and phase I clinical investigations.

Targeting of an oncogene in a SCID mouse model of human leukemia

The ideal strategy for the treatment of leukemia would selectively eliminate leukemic cells and restore normal hematopoiesis. An example of such rational drug design is the targeting of *bcr/abl* transcripts found in leukemic patients carrying the Philadelphia chromosome translocation [10, 13], which has attracted considerable attention as a paradigm uniquely suited to AS. The pathogenetic role of the *bcr/abl* gene in CML has been strongly suggested by the appearance of CML-like syndromes in mice bearing *bcr/abl* constructs [27–29]. Synthetic ODNs complementary to the junction of *bcr/abl* transcripts, produced from the splicing of either the second or the third exon of the *bcr* gene to the second exon of c-*abl*, were shown to suppress Philadelphia[1] leukemic cell proliferation *in vitro* and to spare the growth of normal marrow progenitors [30]. A prerequisite for the *in vivo* use of AS-ODNs as anticancer drugs is the development of animal models that mimic the natural course of the disease in humans. Unlike other types of human neoplasia, leukemic cells obtained directly from a patient's marrow can be transplanted into immuno-deficient SCID mice, where they show a pattern of leukemic spread similar to the natural course of the disease [31]. Initial *in vivo* findings in SCID mice, injected with Philadelphia[1] BV173 cells and systematically treated with a nuclease-resistant 26-mer b2/a2 phosphorothioate AS-ODNs at 1 mg/day for 9 consecutive days, have been very encouraging [32]. The treatment led to marked decrease in three different measures of leukemia burden: percent CALLA-positive cells, number of clonogenic leukemic cells, and amounts of *bcr/abl* transcript in mouse tissues. Similar studies in SCID mice carrying Philadelphia[1] cells obtained directly from CML patient in blast crisis confirmed the ability of *bcr/abl* phosphorothiate AS-ODNs to suppress the spread of leukemia temporarily [33].

Targeting of an oncogene and its downstream effector(s)

Although *bcr/abl* is clearly the most rational therapeutic target for patients with CML, theoretical considerations suggest it might be wise to explore other molecular targets as well. The most significant consideration is based on the possibility that some CML stem cells might persist after exposure to *bcr/abl*-targeted AS-ODNs because they do not express the bcr/abl mRNA [34]. For this reason, and because the usefulness of bcr/abl AS-ODNs is restricted to CML patients, other molecular targets are being sought. On the other hand, the partial antitumor effect of AS-ODNs *in vivo* may reflect their inadequate uptake by the leukemic cells, or an inefficient treatment schedule. Accordingly, repeated AS-ODN injections may prolong survival or even cure leukemic mice if the tumor burden is greatly diminished. Alternatively, a combination of these agents with low doses of conventional antitumor chemotherapeutic agents or a cocktail of ODNs might enhance the therapeutic effect. We have therefore been particularly interested in the c-*myc* gene.

c-*myc* was first associated with human malignancies because of its involvement in the chromosomal translocation of Burkitt's lymphoma [35, 36], and its amplification in tumor cell lines [37, 38]. Subsequently, the demonstration that c-*myc* expression is induced by mitogens and by platelet-derived growth factor [39], and that its constitutive expression partially abrogated growth factor requirements in growth factor-dependent cells [40, 41] formally established the relevance of this gene in the regulation of cell proliferation.

AS-ODNs targeted to the initiation codon and downstream sequences of the human c-*myc* mRNA inhibited proliferation of normal T lymphocytes and myelogenous leukemia line HL-60 [42–44]. Several pieces of evidence, such as the synergy of c-*myc* and v-*abl* in transgenic models of plasmacytomas [45], and the selective enhancement of c-*myc* expression in myeloid hematopoietic cell lines constitutively expressing v-*abl* [46], suggest cooperation between *bcr/abl* and c-*myc* in the transformation of hematopoietic cells. Recently it was shown that a dominant negative c-*myc* protein blocks the transformation induced by v-*abl* and *bcr/abl* [47], and that c-*myc* is required for the proliferation of CML cells [48], raising the possibility that c-*myc* is a downstream effector of *bcr/abl*. In addition, trisomy of chromosome 8 (on which c-*myc* is localized) has been detected in some CML patients in blast crisis [49]. Together, these findings suggest that the combined use of bcr/abl and c-myc AS-ODNs might lead to enhanced therapeutic effects in SCID mice injected with Philadelphia[1] leukemic cells. Indeed, preliminary evidence suggests that, bcr/abl and c-myc AS-ODNs in combination exert a synergistic antiproliferative effect *in vitro* and *in vivo*, on BV173 cells [50] and CML blast crisis primary cells [33], at concentrations at which individual ODNs were only partially effective or completely ineffective. The reasons for the synergistic effect are not fully understood. It seems likely, especially *in vivo*, that AS-ODNs reach a plateau in their ability to downregulate gene expression, insufficient to block cell proliferation completely. Targeting of a second oncogene involved in the disease process may arrest the growth of cells that escaped the inhibitory effect associated with individual gene targeting. Alternatively, the downregulation of gene expression by single AS-ODNs at the relatively low concentrations reached *in vivo* might be insufficient to inhibit cell proliferation, whereas partial inhibition of two cooperating oncogenes might induce a more permanent block in the ability to proliferate. Although the importance of c-*myc* for normal cell proliferation raises the issue of undesirable side effects associated with c-myc AS-ODN administration, use of such compounds at nontoxic concentrations together with, for example, bcr/abl AS-ODNs, which target leukemia-specific sequences, did not cause evident toxicity in mice [33, 50]. A similar strategy in humans might achieve enhanced therapeutic efficacy with minimal adverse effects.

Among the *bcr/abl* downstream effectors described thus far is phosphatidylinositol-3 kinase (PI-3k), which phosphorylates phosphoinositols at the D-3' position of the inositol ring and produces novel phosphorinosidides [51], that activate downstream effectors of PI-3k [52]. We focused on this molecule because inhibition of PI-3k function (but not of molecules such as RAS

[53], GAP [53] or RAF [54]), appears to induce a selective antileukemia effect, while sparing normal hematopoietic cells [52]. Wortmannin (WT), a specific PI-3k inhibitor when used at low concentrations, selectively eliminated CML cells from a mixture of leukemic and normal hematopoietic cells. Moreover, simultaneous inhibition of *bcr/abl* and PI-3k by AS-ODNs and WT, respectively, induced a synergistic and selective antileukemia effect by induction of apoptosis in CML cells (T. Skorski, unpublished data). Thus the targeting of *bcr/abl* and one of its downstream effectors might provide a unique opportunity for developing a selective antileukemia therapy.

Another strategy that might enhance the therapeutic potential of oncogene-targeted ODNs involves the combined use of these compounds with conventional antineoplastic drugs. It is becoming clear that the therapeutic effects of most of these drugs depend not only on interference with distinct aspects of tumor cell metabolism, but also on a more general ability to modulate the levels of proteins involved in regulating apoptosis. This raises the possibility of adjusting drug concentrations to limit the effects on metabolic processes (which are also toxic for normal cells), while preserving the apoptosis-inducing function. Specifically, the therapeutic potential of oncogene-targeted ODNs might be optimized by use in combination with conventional antineoplastic drugs, as indicated by the highly efficient *in vitro* killing of Philadelphia[1] cells exposed to a suboptimal concentration of mafosfamide and bcr/abl AS-ODNs [55].

The *in vivo* efficacy of such combination therapy and the mechanism(s) underlying the apparently synergistic effects of this treatment modality have recently been investigated. Systemic treatment with the bcr/abl AS-ODNs + cyclophosphamide combination was associated with a retardation of the disease process that correlated with an apparent cure of 50% of the leukemic mice and a much longer survival of the remaining mice [56]. This enhanced antileukemic effect appears to correlate with an increase in the induction of apoptosis associated with upregulation of p53 and bax and downregulation of bcl-2 protein levels in leukemic cells by the cytostatic and AS-ODNs, respectively. Furthermore, the uptake of bcr/abl AS-ODNs was 3 to 6 times higher in mafosfamide-pretreated CML blast crisis primary cells, as indicated by detection of cell-associated intact ODNs by blot hybridization, and of intracellular fluorescent ODNs by confocal microscopy. This increased ODN uptake correlated with a more profound downregulation of *bcr/abl* protein levels in cells pretreated with mafosfamide and exposed to relatively low b2/a2 AS-ODN concentrations. Thus, the combination of bcr/abl AS-ODNs and cyclophosphamide, at the concentration eliciting changes in the expression of genes involved in mediating apoptosis, is an effective treatment in SCID mice carrying a Philadelphia[1] leukemia, and might represent a rational strategy for treatment of human leukemias.

Oncogene-targeted AS-ODNs: potential clinical applications in hematological malignancies

AS-ODNs can, in principle, be used for *ex vivo* or systemic treatment of leukemia.

Among the various experimental applications of autologous cell therapy, bone marrow purging has had a definite place in the treatment of several neoplasms, including acute and chronic leukemias [57]. The marrow is cleansed of leukemic cells by a variety of agents, including immunological reagents [58] and chemotherapeutic drugs [59, 60], and is then reinfused in patients treated with ablative chemotherapy. Theoretically, AS-ODNs targeted against an oncogene that confers a growth advantage to leukemic cells should prove therapeutically useful and, most important, more selective than conventional chemotherapeutic agents in killing leukemic cells while sparing normal progenitor cells. However, several issues must be addressed before devising effective protocols for *ex vivo* use of AS-ODNs in therapy. One issue relates to the halflife of the mRNA target and, as a consequence, to the incubation time of marrow cells in the presence of ODNs. For example, the halflife of *myc* protein (10 to 30 min) is considerably shorter than that of *bcr/abl* protein (18–24 h), which suggests that a 24 to 48 h incubation of marrow cells might be adequate if the target is c-*myb* mRNA, but not *bcr/abl* mRNA. A second issue relates to the potential benefit of enriching hematopoietic progenitor cells before the *ex vivo* treatment, to compensate for the relatively low proportion of clonogenic cells in marginally manipulated marrows: the selection of such enriched progenitor cell populations (e.g., CD34[+] cells) could offset the probable differential uptake of ODNs among marrow cells, which might result in ineffective targeting of leukemic cells. Finally, and perhaps of equal or greater importance, the outcome of any purging approach for leukemia treatment is inextricably linked to the ability of the *in vivo* preparatory regimen to cleanse the patient of leukemic cells. Even the cleanest autograft will rapidly become contaminated by viable residual leukemic cells left alive in the host marrow. A protocol for *ex vivo* purging of CD34[+] -enriched CML marrow cells with bcr/abl AS-ODNs followed by autologous transplantation is now ongoing at the University La Sapienza, Institute of Hematology, Rome, Italy.

Oncogene-targeted AS-ODNs might also be used in combination with conventional purging agents under conditions that favor the killing of malignant cells and the sparing of a high number of normal progenitor cells. To this end, the bone marrow purging drug, mafosfamide, was used at low doses in combination with bcr/abl AS-ODNs, to eradicate Philadelphia[1] cells from a mixture of normal and leukemic cells. The full eradication of leukemic cells and the sparing of a significant number of normal progenitors was demonstrated by *in vitro* clonogenic assays and reconstitution experiments in immunodeficient mice [55]. Moreover, the combination of cyclophosphamide and bcr/abl AS-ODNs exerted synergistic and selective antileukemic effect in SCID mice bearing CML blast crisis cells [56]. The increase in AS-ODN uptake by cells penetrated with the drug and simultaneous induction of apoptosis by the drug and the AS-ODNs (using different mechanisms) are probably responsible for this effect.

Pharmacokinetics and biodistribution of phosphorothioate ODNs in animals

The *in vivo* efficacy (and toxicity) of any antisense agent is controlled not only by its ability to interact with a biologically relevant target, but also by its pharmacokinetics and biodistribution, which refer, respectively, to the time course of appearance in plasma and urine, and the percentage of dose found in an organ at any given time.

Initial pharamacokinetic measurements with phosphorothioates were conducted in either mice or rats given single intravenous (i.v.) injections and using either radioactivity (uniformly ^{35}S-labeled phosphorothioate backbone), gel electrophoresis, or high-performance liquid chromatography to monitor the amount and integrity of oligomer. This early work revealed that phosphorothioates of different lengths (20- to-27-mers) and base composition are excreted in urine largely intact and exhibit roughly comparable biphasic plasma kinetics, with relatively long $t_{1/2b}$ values of 40 to 72 h and slow urinary excretion (approximately 70% over about 48 h) [61, 62]. Inversen [61] found that this long $t_{1/2b}$ following single i.v. injection of phosphorothioate ODNs also occurs in rats, rabbits and monkeys. In the first studies with rhesus monkeys (*Macaca mullata*) a 20-mer phosphorothioate given single i.v. injections (50 to 150 mg) showed $t_{1/2b}$ of 5 minutes and $t_{1/2b}$ of 8 to 10 h. Urinary excretion and initial plasma concentrations were all proportional to dose: 13 to 27% of the dose was excreted within 6 days of injection and the organs with the highest concentrations were liver, kidney, heart, spleen and pancreas. Continuous i.v. infusion of rhesus monkeys with the 20-mer phosphorothioate at 0.5 to 2 g over 6 to 15 days gave peak plasma concentrations at 4 to 9 days, reaching values of 1.5 to 5.5 mmol/L, which is in the range of phosphorothioate concentrations reported to be effective in cell culture. Urinary excretion accounted for 25 to 75% of the material administered, and the same organs noted above showed the highest accumulation.

Distribution analysis of bcr/abl phosphorothioate AS-ODNs in mouse tissues by DNA hybridization with a ^{32}P-labeled oligomer complementary to the injected ODN revealed intact ODNs throughout the body, but accumulation in the liver at 24 and 72 h after the last ODN injection [32]. Intact ODNs were detected in the kidney and liver up to 14 days after the last injection. Accumulation of the bcr/abl phosphorothioate ODNs in various organs was also assessed by measuring the amount of ^{35}S-labeled material in weighed organ samples: tissue concentrations correlated with the relative levels of intact ODNs detected in the same tissues and ranged from 3 to 26 mmol/L. Because [S]ODNs undergo relatively slow degradation in mouse tissue [63], the 9-day treatment schedule in SCID mice appeared to achieve concentrations in every tissue (except brain) that would be sufficient to inhibit the growth of primary leukemic cells while sparing that of normal cells [30, 55].

Based on these data and the availability of a sufficient amount of compound, potentially therapeutic concentrations of phosphorothioate AS-ODNs in plasma and various organs of patients can be reached by continuous i.v. infusion. Analogous to the treatment of colorectal cancer patients with, for example, 5-fluorouracil, AS-ODNs can probably be administered with a portable, external, infusion device connected to a subcutaneously implanted venous catheter, thus allowing for outpatient treatment.

Safety studies in animals and humans

The only substantial body of data currently available on either tolerance or toxicity of AS agents is for phosphorothioate ODN analogues. Overall, these data indicate that phosphorothioates are relatively well tolerated and nontoxic in rodents, rabbits, monkeys and humans when administered either as single i.v. injections or continuous i.v. infusion for up to 10 days. For example, in the case of a 20-mer AS-ODN to p53, a 10 kg rhesus monkey given either a single i.v. dose of approximately 150 mg (15 mg/kg) or continuous i.v. infusion of about 2 g over 10 days (200 mg/day) showed no ill effects in behavior, food intake, excretion patterns, hematocrit, blood count, blood electrolytes, blood pressure, heart rate, or cardiac output. However, rapid i.v. administration of phosphorothioates in doses ≥5 to 10 mg/kg may lead to cardiovascular collapse and death. For this reason, phosphorothioates must be given by slow infusion with careful monitoring [63].

Other studies in rhesus monkeys (10 kg) using a different length (24-mer) phosphorothioate complementary to c-myb mRNA have used the same parameters to confirm the absence of side effects with repeated cycles of treatment, namely, approximately 1 g given by continuous infusion for 7 days (approximately 140 mg/d) repeated twice more at 21-day intervals (approximately 3 g total over 3 months). Evidently, higher doses need to be studied to define acute toxicities, which, if any, would probably be liver and kidney dysfunction, based on biodistribution and analogy to many other drugs. Unlike some oligopeptides/protein drug products, no detectable antigenicity is associated with administration of phosphorothioate ODNs, perhaps partly due to their relative similarity to natural DNA, which is a very poor antigen.

The first phase I safety study of any AS agent given systematically by i.v. infusion was performed at the University of Nebraska Medical Center in collaboration with Lynx Therapeutics. In this trial, which involved five dose groups of three patients each who received up to 4.5 g over 10 days for a body weight of 75 kg, no remarkable toxicities were found.

References

1. Wright JA, Smith HD, Watt FM, Hancock MC, Hudson DL, Stark GR (1990) DNA amplification rate in normal human cells. *Proc Natl Acad Sci USA* 87: 1791–1795.
2. Tlsty TD, Margolin BH, Lum K (1989) Differences in the rates of gene amplification in nontumorigenic and tumorigenic cell lines as measured by Luria-Delbruck fluctuation analysis. *Proc Natl Acad Sci USA* 86: 9441–9445.
3. Alitalo K, Schwab M (1986) Oncogene amplification in tumor cells. *Adv Cancer Res* 47: 235–282.
4. Slamon DJ, Clark GM, Wong SG, Levin WJ, Ulrich A, McGuire WL (1989) Human breast cancer: correlation of relapse and survival with amplification of the HER-2/neu oncogene. *Science* 235: 171–182.
5. Slamon DJ, Godolphin W, Jones LA, Holt JA, Wong SP, Keith DE, Levin WJ, Stuart SG, Udove J, Ollrich A et al. (1989) Studies of the HER-2/neu proto-oncogene in human breast and ovarian cancer. *Science* 244: 707–712.
6. Collins S, Groudine M (1982) Amplification of endogenous *myc*-related DNA sequences in a human myeloid leukemia cell line. *Nature* 297: 675–681.
7. Dalla-Favera R, Wong-Staal F, Gallo RC (1982) *Onc* gene amplification in promyelocytic leukemia cell line HL-60 and primary leukemic cells of the same patient. *Nature* 299: 61–63.
8. Bishop JM (1991) Molecular themes in oncogenesis. *Cell* 64: 235–248.
9. Haluska FG, Tsujimoto Y, Croce CM (1987) Oncogene activation by chromosome translocation in human malignancies. *Annu Rev Genet* 21: 321–347.
10. Rowley JD (1982) Identification of the constant chromosome regions involved in human hematologic malignant diseases. *Science* 231: 261–265.
11. Groffen J, Stephenson JR, Heisterkamp N, deKlein A, Bartram CR, Grosveld G (1984) Philadelphia chromosomal breakpoints are clustered within a limited region, *bcr*, on chromosome 22. *Cell* 36: 93–99.
12. Croce CM (1987) Role of chromosome translocations in human neoplasia. *Cell* 49: 155–156.
13. Shtivelman E, Lifshitz B, Gale RB, Roe BA, Canaani E (1986) Alternative splicing of RNAs transcribed from the human abl gene and from bcr-abl fused gene. *Cell* 47: 277–284.
14. Konopka JB, Watanabe SM, Witte DN (1986) An alteration of the human c-abl protein in K562 leukemia cells uumasks associated tyrosine kinase activity. *Cell* 37: 1035–1042.
15. Barbacid M (1987) *Ras* genes. *Annu Rev Biochem* 56: 779–827.
16. Bos JL, Toksoz D, Marshall CJ, de Vries MT, Beeneman GH, van der Eb AJ, Van Bloom JH, Janssen JHG, Steenvoorden ACM (1985) Amino-acid substitutions at codon 13 of the N-RAS oncogene in human acute myeloid leukemia. *Nature* 300: 186–188.
17. Bourne HR, Sanders DA, McCormick F (1991) The GTPase superfamily: conserved structure and molecular mechanisms. *Nature* 349: 117–127.
18. Kern SE, Pietenpol JA, Thiagalingam S, Seymour A, Kinzler KW, Vogelstein B (1992) Oncogenic forms of p53 inhibit p53-regulated gene expression. *Science* 256: 827–830.

19. Zamecnik P, Stephenson M (1988) Inhibition of Rous sarcoma virus replication and cell transformation by a specific oligodeoxynucleotide. *Proc Natl Acad Sci USA* 75: 280–284.
20. Stein CA, Cheng YC (1993) Antisense oligonucleotides as therapeutic agents – Is the bullet really magical? *Science* 261: 1004–1012.
21. Carter G, Lemoine NR (1993) Antisense technology for cancer therapy: does it make sense? *Brit J Cancer* 67: 869–876.
22. Ryte A, Morelli S, Mazzei M, Alama A, Franco P, Canti GF, Nicolin A (1993) Oligonucleotide degradation contributes to resistance to antisense compounds. *Anti-Cancer Drugs* 4: 197–200.
23. Geselowitz DA, Neckers LM (1992) Analysis of oligonucleotide binding, internalization, and intracellular trafficking utilizing a novel radiolabelled crosslinker. *Antisense Res Dev* 2: 17–25.
24. Gao WY, Storm C, Egan W, Cheng YC (1993) Cellular pharmacology of phosphorothioate homoligodeoxynucleotides in human cells. *Mol Pharmacol* 43: 45–50.
25. Bacon TA, Wickstrom E (1991) Walking along human c-myc mRNA with antisense oligodeoxynucleotides: maximum efficacy at the 5' cap region. *Oncogene Res* 6: 13–19.
26. Varmus H (1987) Cellular and viral oncogenes. *In*: Varmus H (ed.): *The Molecular Basis of Blood Diseases.* Philadelphia: Saunders.
27. Daley GR, Van Etten RA, Baltimore D (1990) Induction of chronic myelogenous leukemia in mice by the p120/*bcr/abl* gene of the Philadelphia chromosome. *Science* 247: 824–830.
28. Heisterkamp N, Jenster G, ten Hoeve J et al. (1990) Acute leukemia in *bcr/abl* transgenic mice. *Nature* 344: 251–253.
29. Elfanty AG, Hariharan IK, Cory S (1990) bcr/abl, the hallmark of chronic myeloid leukemia in man, induces multiple hematopoietic neoplasms in mice. *EMBO J* 9: 1069–1078.
30. Szczylik C, Skorski T, Nicolaides NC, Manzella L, Malaguamera L, Venturelli D, Gewirtz AM, Calabretta B (1991) Selective inhibition of leukemia cell proliferation by *bcr-abl* antisense oligodeoxynucleotides. *Science* 253: 562–565.
31. Kamel-Reid S, Letarte M, Sirard C, Doedens M, Grunberger T, Fulop G, Freedman MH, Phillips RA, Dick JE (1989) A model of human acute lymphoblastic leukemia in immunodeficient SCID mice. *Science* 246: 1597–1601.
32. Skorski T, Nieborowska-Skorska M, Nicolaides NC, Szczylik C, Iversen P, Iozzo RV, Zon G, Calabretta B (1994) Suppression of Philadelphia1 leukemia cell growth in mice by *bcr-abl* antisense oligodeoxynucleotides. *Proc Natl Acad Sci USA* 91: 4504–4508.
33. Skorski T, Nieborowska-Skorska M, Nicolaides NC, Szczylik C, Iverson P, Iozzo RV, Zon G, Calabretta B (1996) Antisense oligodeoxynucleotide combination treatment of primary chronic myelogenous leukemia blast crisis in SCID mice. *Blood* 88: 1005–1012.
34. Bedi A, Zehnhouer BA, Collector MI, Barber JP, Zicha MS, Sharkis SJ, Jones RJ (1993) BCR-ABL gene rearrangement and expression of primitive hematopoietic progenitors in chronic myeloid leukemia. *Blood* 81: 2898–2902.
35. Taub R, Kirsch I, Morton C, Lenoir G, Swan D, Tronick S, Aaronson S, Leder P (1982) Translocation of the c-myc gene into the immunoglobin heavy chain locus in human Burkitt lymphoma and murine plasmacytoma cells. *Proc Natl Acad Sci USA* 79: 7837–7841.
36. Dalla-Favera R, Wong-Staal F, Gallo RC (1982) Translocation and rearrangements of the c-myc oncogene locus in human undifferentiated B cell lymphomas. *Science* 219: 963–967.
37. Collins S, Groudine M (1982) Amplification of endogenous myc-related DNA sequences in a human myeloid leukemia cell line. *Nature* 299: 679–681.
38. Little CD, Nau MM, Carney DN et al. (1983) Amplification and expression of the c-myc oncogene in human lung cancer cell lines. *Nature* 306: 194–196.
39. Kelly K, Cochran BH, Stiles CD, Leder P (1983) Cell-specific regulation of the c-myc gene by lymphocyte mitogens and platelet-derived growth factor. *Cell* 35: 603–610.
40. Armelin HA, Armelin MC, Kelly K, Stewart T, Leder P, Cochran BH, Stiles CD (1984) Functional role of c-myc in mitogenic response to platelet derived growth factor. *Nature* 310: 655–660.
41. Kaczmarek L, Hyland JD, Watt R, Rosenberg M, Baserga R (1985) Microinjected c-myc as a competence factor. *Science* 228: 1313–1315.
42. Heikkila R, Schwab G, Wickstrom E, Loke SL, Pluznik DH, Watt R, Neckers LM (1987) A *c-myc* antisense oligodeoxynucleotide inhibits entry into S phase but not progress from G_0 to G_1. *Nature* 328: 445–449.
43. Wickstrom EL, Bacon TA, Gonzales A, Freeman DL, Lyman GH, Wickstrom E (1988) Human promyelocytic leukemia HL-60 cell proliferation and *c-myb* protein expression are inhibited by an antisense pentadecadeoxynucleotide targeted against c-myc mRNA. *Proc Natl Acad Sci USA* 85: 1028–1032.
44. Holt JT, Redner RL, Nienhuis AW (1988) An oligomer complementary to *c-myc* messenger RNA inhibits proliferation of HL-60 promyelocytic cells and induces differentiation. *Mol Cell Biol* 8: 963–973.
45. Rosenbaum H, Harris AW, Bath ML, McNeall J, Webb E, Adams JM, Cory S (1990) An Eμ-v-*abl* transgene elicits plasmacytomas in concert with an activated myc gene. *EMBO J* 9: 897–905.
46. Cleveland JL, Dean M, Rosenberg N, Wang JY, Rapp UR (1989) Tyrosine kinase oncogenes abrogate interleukin-3 dependence of murine myeloid cells through signaling pathways involving *c-myc*: Conditional regulation of c-myc transcription by temperature-sensitive v-abl. *Mol Cell Biol* 9: 5685–5695.

47. Sawyers CL, Callahan W, Witte ON (1992) Dominant negative MYC blocks transformation by ABL onco-genes. *Cell* 70: 901–910.
48. Nieborowska-Skorska M, Ratajczak MZ, Calabretta B, Skorski T (1994) The role of c-MYC in chronic myelogenous leukemia. *Folia Histochem Cytobiol* 32: 231–234.
49. Blick M, Romero P, Talpaz M, Kurzock R, Shtalrid M, Andersson B, Trujillo J, Beran M, Gutterman J (1987) Molecular characteristics of chronic myelogenous leukemias in blast crisis. *Cancer Genet Cytogenet* 27: 369–376.
50. Skorski T, Nieborowska-Skorska M, Iozzo RV, Campbell K, Zon G, Dazynkiewicz Z, Calabretta B (1995) Leukemia treatment in SCID mice by antisense oligodeoxynucleotides targeting cooperating oncogenes. *J Exp Med* 182: 1645–1653.
51. Carpenter CL, Cantley LC (1990) Phosphoroinositide kinases. *Biochemistry* 29: 11143–11152.
52. Skorski T, Kanakaraj P, Ku DH, Nieborowska-Skorska M, Ratzjczak ML, Wen SC, Zon G, Gewirtz A, Perussia B, Calabretta B (1995) Phosphatidylinosital-3 kinase activity is regulated by BCR/ABL and is required for the growth of Philadelphia chromosome-positive cells. *Blood* 86: 726–736.
53. Skorski T, Kamakaraj P, Ku DH, Nieborowska-Skorska M, Canaani E, Perussia B, Calabretta B (1994) Nega-tive-regulation of p120GAP promoting activity by p210[bcr/abl]: implication for RAS-dependent Philadelphia chromosome-positive cell growth. *J Exp Med* 179: 1855–1865.
54. Skorski T, Nieborowska-Skorska M, Szczylik C, Kanakavaj P, Perrotti D, Zon G, Gewirtz AM, Perussia B, Calabretta B (1995) c-RAF-1 serine/theonine kinase is required in BCR/ABL-dependent and normal hemato-poiesis. *Cancer Res* 55: 2275–2278.
55. Skorski T, Nieborowska-Skorska M, Barletta C, Malaguamera L, Szczylik C, Chen ST, Lange B, Calabretta B (1993) Highly efficient elimination of Philadelphia[1] leukemia cells by exposure to *bcr/abl* antisense oligode-oxynucleotides combined with mafosfamide. *J Clin Invest* 92: 194–202.
56. Skorski T, Nieborowska-Skorska M, Wlodarski P, Perrotti D, Hoser G, Kawiak J, Majewski M, Christensen L, Iozzo RV, Calabretta B (1997) Treatment of Philadelphia[1] leukemia in severe combined immunodeficient mice by combination of cyclophosphamide and bcr/abl antisense oligodeoxynucleotides. *J Nat Cancer Inst* 89: 124–133.
57. Santos GW (1990) Bone marrow transplantation in hematologic malignancies. *Curr Status* 65: 786–791.
58. Bell ED (1988) *In vitro* purging of bone marrow for autologous marrow transplantation in acute myelogenous leukemia using myeloid monoclonal antibodies. *Bone Marrow Transplant* 3: 387–393.
59. Yager AM, Kaizer H, Santos GW, Saral R, Calvin OM, Stuart RK, Braine HG, Burke PJ, Ambinder RF, Burns WH et al. (1986) Autologous bone marrow transplantation in patients with acute nonlymphocytic leukemia using *ex vivo* marrow treatment with 4-hydroperoxycyclophosphamide. *N Engl J Med* 315: 141–145.
60. Gorin NC, Douay L, Laporte JP, Lopez M, Mary JY, Najman A, Salmon O, Aegerter P, Stachowak J, David R et al. (1986) Autologous bone marrow transplantation using marrow incubated with Asta Z 7557 in adult acute leukemia. *Blood* 67: 1367–1373.
61. Iversen P (1991) *In vivo* studies with phosphorothioate oligonucleotides: Pharmacokinetics prologue. *Anti-cancer Drug Design* 6: 531–538.
62. Agrawal S, Temsamani J, Tang JY (1991) Pharmacokinetics, biodistribution, and stability of oligodeoxynu-cleotide phosphorothioates in mice. *Proc Natl Acad Sci USA* 88: 7595–7599.
63. Black LE, Farelly JG, Cavagnaro JA, Ahn CH, DeGeorge JJ, Taylor AS, DeFelice AF, Jordan A (1994) Regulatory considerations for oligonucleotide drugs: Updated recommendations for pharmacology and toxicology studies. *Antisense Res Dev* 4: 299–301.

Molecular Aspects of Cancer and its Therapy
A. Mackiewicz and P.B. Sehgal (eds)
© 1998 Birkhäuser Verlag Basel/Switzerland

Oligonucleotide therapeutics for human leukemia

M.Z. Ratajczak[1] and A.M. Gewirtz[1, 2]

[1]*Department of Pathology and Laboratory Medicine, University of Pennsylvania School of Medicine, Room 515 Stellar-Chance Building, 422 Curie Boulevard, Philadelphia, PA 19104, USA*
[2]*Department of Internal Medicine, University of Pennsylvania School of Medicine, Room 515 Stellar-Chance Building, 422 Curie Boulevard, Philadelphia, PA 19104, USA*

Introduction

In recent years, a large number of extracellular growth factors which regulate hematopoietic cell development have been molecularly cloned, expressed as active proteins, and used clinically. The intracellular events which are triggered when these growth factors interact with their receptors have also begun to be defined. Nevertheless, most of the molecular machinery which regulates blood cell development remains enigmatic and difficult to access. This is particularly so for normal blood cells because of the difficulty of applying modern molecular analytical techniques to the small numbers of cells usually available for such investigations.

To approach the problem of understanding gene function in hematopoietic cells, two main strategies have been applied. One involves infecting cells with a vector engineered to express the gene of interest at high levels [1–3]. If the cell's phenotype/behavior changes in the infected cell, but not a sham transfected cell, we can tentatively attribute the change in phenotype to the newly expressed gene. Function may therefore be inferred. This approach, while potentially informative, has a number of drawbacks. First, it is not certain that the changes observed are directly related to the gene's function, as any effect observed may be an indirect one. Second, the experiment is not really 'physiological' since overexpression of the gene may exaggerate its normal function or impart new functions by leading to an excess of the encoded protein. Finally, this approach is often limited to leukemic cell lines, since normal cells are often much more problematic in terms of both infection and expression of the vector.

An alternative experimental approach, and one which may yield more physiologically relevant data, is either to physically 'knock-out' the target gene, or to interfere with its function by perturbing the use of the gene's encoded mRNA. Homologous recombination remains the 'gold standard' for experiments of this type, since the methodology physically destroys the gene of interest [4–8]. However, because this strategy ultimately depends on selecting cells in which a rare crossover event has occurred, it would currently appear to have limited therapeutic practicality. Ribozymes, antisense RNAs and antisense DNAs, all of which interfere with use of the targeted mRNA, appear to have more immediate relevance from a therapeutic point of view. These approaches have therefore become an increasingly popular strategy for exploring gene function in cells of virtually any type.

For the past several years, we have been engaged in trying to develop an effective strategy of disrupting specific gene function with antisense oligodeoxynucleotides (AS-ODNs). We have also been actively engaged in attempting to use this strategy in the clinic. This latter pursuit has focused on finding appropriate gene targets for a successful antisense approach, and then scaling up the methods so that techniques developed in the laboratory could be applied clinically. It was our opinion that human leukemias would be particularly amenable to this therapeutic strategy. They can be successfully manipulated ex vivo, the tumor is 'liquid' *in vivo* and therefore more likely to take up ODNs successfully, and a great deal is known about their cell and molecular biology. The latter in particular facilitates choice of a gene target. Accordingly, if ODNs were to be developed as therapeutics, the hematopoietic system would seem an ideal model system.

The c-*myb* proto-oncogene

Of the genes we have targeted for disruption using the antisense AS-ODN strategy [9–13] one that has been of particular interest to our laboratory, and one where therapeutically motivated disruptions are now in clinical trial, is c-*myb* [14]. C-*myb* is the normal cellular homologue of v-*myb*, the transforming oncogene of the avian myeloblastosis virus (AMV) and avian leukemia virus E26. It is a member of a family composed of at least two other highly homologous genes, A-*myb* and B-*myb* [15]. Located on chromosome 6q in humans, c-*myb*'s predominant transcript encodes a ~75 kDa nuclear binding protein (Myb) which recognizes the core consensus sequence 5'-PyAAC(G/Py)G-3' [16]. Myb consists of three primary functional regions [17] (Fig. 1).

At the N-terminus is the DNA binding domain. This region consists of three imperfect tandem repeats (R1, R2, R3), each consisting of 51 to 52 amino acids. Three perfectly conserved tryptophan residues are found in each repeat. Together they form a cluster in the hydrophobic core of the protein which maintains the DNA binding helix-turn-helix structure. The mid-portion of the protein contains an acidic transcriptional activating domain. The DNA binding portion of the protein is required for these transcriptional effects to be observed. The protein also contains a negative regulatory domain which has been localized to the C-terminus. The C-terminus is deleted in v-Myb and this has been thought to contribute to v-Myb's transforming ability. Recently reported experiments have been among those to confirm this hypothesis and have further demonstrated that N-terminal deletions give rise to a protein with even more potent transforming ability [18]. Deletions of both the amino and C-termini create a protein with the greatest transforming ability, and one which induces the formation of hematopoietic cells more primitive than those produced

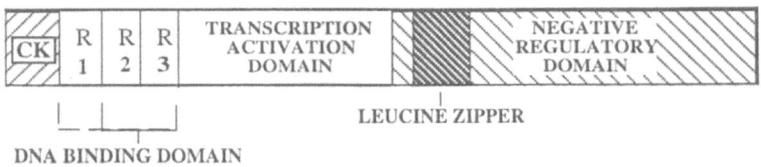

Figure 1. Functional map of the c-myb protein. See text for details

by N-erminal deletions alone [18]. These data suggest that simultaneous loss of Myb's ability to bind DNA and interact with as yet unidentified proteins are potent transforming stimuli. Nevertheless, this simple hypothesis is complicated by the observation that overexpression of the C-terminal portion of c-myb can also be oncogenic [19] whereas overexpression of the whole protein is not [18]. At least, we may conclude that sequestration of certain potential Myb binding proteins may also be an oncogenic event.

Recently, a putative leucine zipper structure was described within the amino terminal portion of Myb's C-terminal domain [20]. Leucine zippers, such as those found in the transcription factors Jun, Fos, and Myc are thought to facilitate the protein-protein interactions which permit hetero-dimerization of DNA binding proteins. Such dimerization is thought to play a key role in regulating the transcriptional activity of these factors. A Myb dimerizing binding partner has yet to be identified but Myb-Myb homodimerization, which probably occurs through its leucine zipper, does lead to loss of DNA binding and transactivation ability [21]. Accordingly, we could reasonably postulate that Myb-driven transactivation and/or transformation might be regulated by the binding of additional protein partners in the leucine zipper domain [20]. Alternatively, loss of the ability of Myb to dimerize with a putative regulatory partner might also contribute, directly or indirectly, to cellular transformation and leukemogenesis. Point mutations in the Myb negative regulatory domain might be one mechanism for bringing about such a loss [20]. Finally, interaction (not physical dimerization) with other nuclear binding proteins such as the CCAAT enhancer binding protein (C/BEP) [22], and the related myeloid nuclear factor NF-M [23] may also regulate Myb's transactivation or repressor functions.

The above discussion suggests that c-*myb* might play a role in leukemogenesis. Additional, albeit indirect, evidence also support this contention. For example, *c-myb* amplification in AML and overexpression in 6q⁻ syndrome has been reported [24]. The mechanism whereby overexpressed Myb might be leukemogenic is uncertain, but emphasizes the important difference of working with primary cells as opposed to cell lines. As noted above, it has been reported that over-expressing Myb is not by itself leukemogenic [18] but this work was carried out in cell lines which may give results that are valid only for the lines tested. As was also noted above, we could reasonably postulate that Myb-driven transformation might be regulated by the binding of additional protein partners in the leucine zipper domain [20]. Recent evidence demonstrating that Myb interacts with other nuclear binding proteins, and that Myb's carboxy terminus may interact with a cellular inhibitor of transcription supports this hypothesis [22, 25]. Other potential mechanisms might relate to Myb's ability to regulate hematopoietic cell proliferation [26], perhaps by its effects on important cell cycle genes including c-*myc* [27], and *cdc2* [28]. Finally, Myb also plays a role in regulating hematopoietic cell differentiation [29]. It functions as a transcription factor for several cellular genes including the neutrophil granule protein mim-1 [30], CD4 [31], IGF-1 [32], and CD34 [33] and possibly other growth factors [34], including *c-kit* [35]. The latter is of particular interest since it has been shown that when hematopoietic cells are deprived of *c-kit* ligand (Steel Factor) they undergo apoptosis [36]. Accordingly, *myb* is clearly an important hematopoietic cell gene which may, directly or indirectly, contribute to the pathogenesis or maintenance of human leukemias. For this reason it is a rational target for therapeutically motivated disruption strategies.

Targeting the c-*myb* gene

Our investigations were initially designed to elucidate the role of Myb protein in regulating hematopoietic cell development. Because the results obtained from these studies had obvious clinical relevance, more translationally oriented studies were also undertaken. These have now culminated in clinical trials presently being conducted at the Hospital of the University of Pennsylvania. Below I summarize the steps carried out in the clinical development of the c-*myb*-targeted AS-ODNs. In addition, I will also allude briefly to our initial clinical experience with the *myb*-targeted ODNs.

In vitro *experience in the hematopoietic cell system*

Role of c-myb encoded protein in normal human hematopoiesis: Attempts to exploit the c-*myb* gene as a therapeutic target for AS-ODNs began as an outgrowth of studies which were seeking to define the role of Myb protein in regulating normal human hematopoiesis [9, 26]. During the course of these studies it was determined that exposing normal bone marrow mononuclear cells (MNC) to c-myb AS-ODNs resulted in a decrease in cloning efficiency and progenitor cell proliferation. The effect was lineage indifferent since c-myb antisense DNA inhibited granulocyte-macrophage colony forming units (CFU-GM), CFU-E (erythroid), and CFU-Meg (megakaryocyte). In contrast, c-myb ODN with the corresponding sense sequence had no consistent effect on hematopoietic colony formation when compared to growth in control cultures. Finally, inhibition of colony formation was also dose related. Inhibition of the targeted mRNA was also demonstrated. Sequence-specific, dose-related biological effects, accompanied by a specific decrease or total elimination of the targeted mRNA, were strong pieces of evidence to suggest that the effects we were observing were due to an 'antisense' mechanism. It should be added that the effects we observed were largely confirmed using homologous recombination [37]. In other investigations, it was also determined that hematopoietic progenitor cells appeared to require Myb protein during specific stages of development, in particular when they were actively cycling [38], as might be expected given the above functional description of Myb protein.

Myb protein is also required for leukemic hematopoiesis: Since the c-myb AS-ODNs inhibited normal cell growth, we were also interested to determine their effect on leukemic cell growth. While we could reasonably postulate that aberrant c-*myb* expression or Myb function might play a role in carcinogenesis, demonstrating this was another matter. To address this question, we employed a variety of leukemic cell lines, including those of myeloid and lymphoid origin. In addition, we also employed primary patient material. We first determined the effect of myb sense and antisense ODNs on the growth of HL-60, K562, KG-1, and KG-1a myeloid cell lines [39]. The AS-ODN inhibited the proliferation of each leukemia cell line, although the effect was most pronounced on HL-60 cells. Specificity of this inhibition was demonstrated by the fact that the sense ODN had no effect on cell proliferation, nor did 'antisense' sequences with two or four nucleotide mismatches. To determine whether the treatment with myb AS-ODNs modified cell cycle distribution of HL-60 cells, we measured the DNA content in exponentially growing cells exposed to either sense or antisense myb ODNs. Control cells, and cells treated with c-myb sense ODN, had twice the DNA content of HL-60 cells exposed to the AS-ODNs. The majority of these cells appeared either to reside in the G1 compartment, or were blocked at the G1/S boundary. To examine the effect of the c-myb ODNs on lymphoid cell growth, we employed a lymphoid leukemia cell line, CCRF-CEM. As we noted in the case of normal lymphocytes [26], the CCRF-CEM cells were extremely sensitive to the antiproliferative effects of the c-myb AS-ODNs. When exposed to the sense ODN, we found negligible effects on CEM cell growth in short-term suspension cultures. In contrast, exposure to c-myb antisense DNA resulted in a daily decline in cell numbers. Compared to untreated controls, antisense DNA inhibited growth ~ 2 logs. Growth reduction was not a cytostatic effect since cell viability was reduced only ~70% after exposure to the AS-ODNs, and CEM cell growth did not recover when cells were left in culture for an additional nine days.

Results obtained from primary patient material were equally encouraging (Tab. 1) [40]. We began by attempting to determine if CFU-L from AML patients could be inhibited by exposure to

Table 1. Effect of c-myb oligomers on primary AML cell colony/cluster formation

Colonies – % Control			Clusters – % Control		
Case	Sense	Antisense	Sense	Antisense	
1	86	18 (0.058)	60	37 (0.080)	
4	NG	NG	90	28 (0.036)	
5	NG	NG	70	22 (0.101)	
6	NG	NG	79	22 (0.026)	
7	170	100 (0.423)	76	128 (0.502)	
8	92	11 (0.008)	96	46 (0.020)	
10	NG	NG	190	216 (0.034)	
11	45	14 (0.021)	58	21 (0.084)	
14	68	01 (0.152)	90	53 (0.071)	
15	66	81 (0.736)	100	100 (0.896)	
16	NG	NG	66	24 (0.001)	
17	NG	NG	16	8 (0.023)	
18	NG	NG	110	77 (0.164)	
19	113	116 (0.717)	91	91 (0.763)	
20	92	09 (0.051)	100	50 (0.009)	
21	94	00 (0.006)	90	06 (0.004)	
22	80	13 (0.001)	103	11 (0.015)	
23	63	06 (0.001)	74	27 (0.004)	
24	87	17 (0.002)	91	26 (0.018)	
25	100	00 (0.019)	107	38 (0.364)	
26	76	00 (0.009)	89	00 (0.001)	
27	79	21 (0.014)	59	18 (0.043)	
28	88	20 (0.009)	94	152 (0.096)	

Blast cells were isolated from the peripheral blood of AML patients and exposed to sense or antisense oligomers. Colonies and clusters were enumerated and values were compared with growth in control cultures, which contained to oligomers. For each case, the number of colonies or clusters arising in the untreated control dishes was assumed to represent maximal (100%) growth for that patient. The numbers of colonies or clusters arising in the oligomer-treated dishes are expressed as a percentage of this number. NG=No growth. The statistical significance (determined by Student's t test for unpaired samples) of the change observed in the antisense-treated dishes relative to the untreated control is given as a P value in parentheses.

c-myb AS-ODNs. Of the 28 patients we initially studied, colony and cluster data were available in 16 and 23 cases respectively. After exposure to relatively low doses of c-myb AS-ODNs (60 µg/ml) colony formation was inhibited in a statistically significant manner in 12/16 (~75%). Inhibition of cluster formation fell in a similar range. Of equal importance the numbers of residual colonies in the antisense-treated dishes was ~10%.

An obvious problem with interpreting these results, was determining the nature of the residual cells, i.e., were they the progeny of residual normal CFU or CFU-L? To try to answer this question in a rigorous manner we turned out attention to CML, where the presence of the t(9:22) or *bcr/abl* neogene provided an unequivocal marker of the malignant cells [41]. Exposure of CML cells to c-myb AS-ODN resulted in inhibition of CFU-GM derived colony formation in >50% cases evaluated and so far we have studied more than 40 patients. Representative data are shown in Figure 2, and are presented as a function of oligomer effect on cells with 'greater' cloning effi-

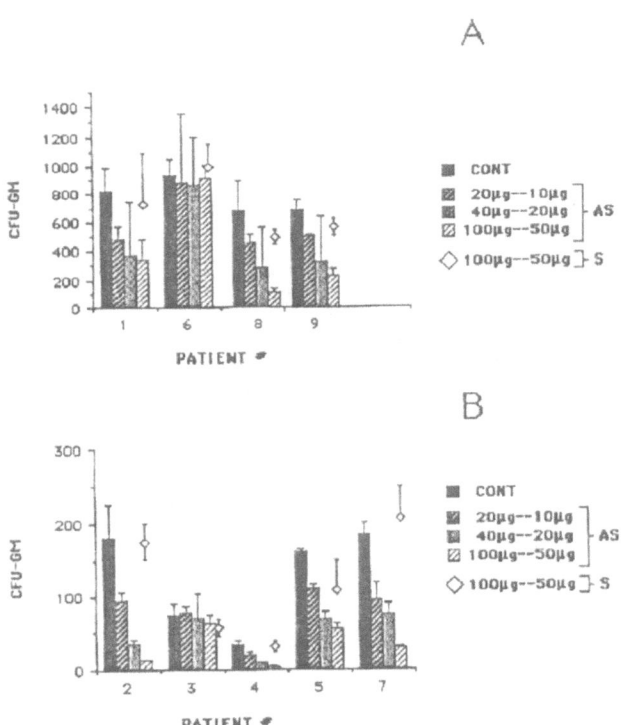

Figure 2. Effect of c-myb oligomers on chronic myeloid leukemia cell colony formation by cells with 'high' (A) and 'low' (B) cloning efficiency. Colony-forming cells were enriched from patient peripheral blood or bone marrow and exposed to oligomers. At 24 h cells were plated and resulting colonies were enumerated in plates containing untreated control cells [■]; antisense (▨-20 µg/ml then 10 µg/ml; ▦-40 µg/ml then 20 µg/ml; ▨-100 µg/ml then 50 µg/ml); and sense (◇-100 µg/ml then 50 µg/ml) treated cells. Values plotted are mean±SD of actual colony counts compared to growth in control cultures which contained no oligomers.

ciency (control colonies >250/plate) (Fig. 2A) *versus* 'lesser' cloning efficiency (control colonies <250/plate) (Fig. 2B). In this particular study, colony formation was observed in eight of eleven cases evaluated and was statistically significant ($p \leq 0.03$) in seven. The amount of inhibition seen was dose-dependent and ranged between 58% and 93%. In two cases the effect of the c-myb oligomers on CFU-GEMM colony formation was also determined to assess the effect of the oligomers on progenitors more primitive than CFU-GM. In each case, significant inhibition of CFU-GEMM derived colony formation was noted. It is also important to note that colony inhibition was sequence specific. For example, as shown in the graphs below, c-myb sense sequence ODN fails to inhibit colony formation significantly when employed at the highest antisense doses used.

Normal and leukemic progenitor cells rely differentially on c-myb function
In order to be useful as a therapeutic target, leukemic cells would have to be more dependent on Myb protein than their normal counterparts. To examine this critical issue, we incubated phagocyte and T cell depleted normal human marrow mononuclear cells (MNC), human T lymphocyte leukemia cell line blasts (CCRF-CEM), or 1:1 mixtures of these cells with sense or antisense ODNs to codons 2–7 of human c-myb mRNA [40]. ODNs were added to liquid suspension cultures at Time 0 and at Time +18 h. Control cultures were untreated. In controls, or in cultures to which 'high' doses of sense ODNs were added, CCRF-CEM proliferated rapidly, whereas MNC numbers and viability decreased <10%. In contrast, when CCRF-CEM were incubated for four days in c-myb antisense DNA, cultures contained $4.7 \pm 0.8 \times 10^4$ cells/ml (mean $\pm$ SD; n = 4) compared to $285 \pm 17 \times 10^4$/ml in controls. At the effective AS dose, MNC were largely unaffected. After four days in culture, remaining cells were transferred to methylcellulose supplemented with recombinant hematopoietic growth factors. Myeloid colonies/clusters were enumerated at day ten of culture inception. Depending on cell number plated, control MNC formed from 31 ± 4 to 274 ± 18 colonies. In dishes containing equivalent numbers of untreated or sense ODN exposed CCRF-CEM, colonies were too numerous to count. When MNC were mixed 1:1 with CCRF-CEM in AS oligomer concentrations ≤ 5 µg/ml, only leukemic colonies could be identified by morphological, histochemical and immunochemical analysis. However, when antisense oligomer exposure was intensified, normal myeloid colonies could now be found in the culture, while leukemic colonies could no longer be identified with certainty using the same analytical methods. Finally, at antisense DNA doses used in the above studies, AML blasts from 18 of 23 patients exhibited ~75% decrease in colony and cluster formation compared to untreated or sense oligomer treated controls. When 1:1 mixing experiments were carried out with primary AML blasts and normal MNC, we were again able preferentially to eliminate AML blast colony formation while normal myeloid colonies continued to form.

Use of c-myb ODN as bone marrow purging agents
The above experiments suggested that leukemic cell growth could be preferentially inhibited after exposure to c-myb AS-ODNs. In contemplating a clinical use for our findings, application in the area of bone marrow transplantation seemed compelling. In this application, exposure conditions are entirely under the control of the investigator. In addition, the patient's exposure to the antisense DNA is minimal. This circumstance would also make approval by regulatory agencies less

difficult. We therefore determined whether the AS-ODNs could be used as ex vivo bone marrow purging agents.

Normal MNC were mixed (1:1) with primary acute myelogenous leukemia (AML) or chronic myelogenous leukemia (CML) blast cells and then exposed to the ODNs using a slightly modified protocol designed to test the feasibility of a more intensive antisense exposure. With this in mind, an additional ODN dose (20 µg/ml) was given just prior to plating the cells in methylcellulose. In control growth factor-stimulated cultures leukemic cells formed 25.5 ± 3.5 (mean $\pm$ SD) colonies and 157 ± 8.5 clusters (per 2×10^5 cells plated). Exposure to c-*myb* sense ODN did not significantly alter these numbers (19.5 ± 0.7 colonies and 140.5 ± 7.8 clusters; $p > 0.1$). In contrast, equivalent concentrations of AS-ODN totally inhibited colony and cluster formation by the leukemic blasts. Colony formation was also inhibited in the plates containing normal MNCs, but only by ~50% in comparison to untreated control plates (control colony formation, 296 ± 40 per 2×10^5 cells plated; treated colony formation, 149 ± 15.5 per 2×10^5 cells).

To assess the potential effectiveness of an antisense purge, we carried out co-culture studies with cells obtained from CML patients in blast crisis and in chronic phase of their disease [11]. CML was a particularly useful model because cells from the malignant clone carry a tumor-specific chromosomal translocation which can be easily identified in tissue culture by looking for bcr-abl, the mRNA product of the gene produced by the translocation [42]. RNA was therefore extracted from cells cloned in methylcellulose cultures after exposure to the highest c-myb AS-ODN dose. The RNA was then reverse transcribed and resulting cDNA amplified. For each patient studied, mRNA was also extracted from a comparable number of cells derived from un-

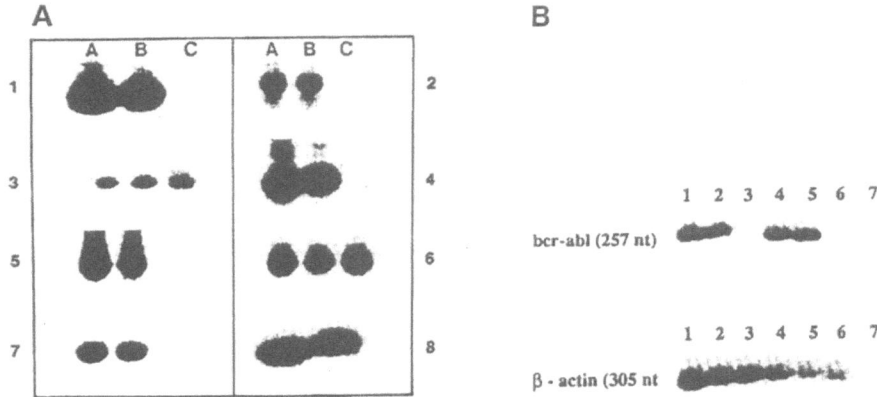

Figure 3. (A) Detection of *bcr/abl* transcripts in CFU-GM derived colonies from marrow of eight patients (#s 1-8) whose marrow was unexposed to c-myb AS ODN (A), to c-myb sense ODN (B), or to c-myb antisense ODN. All colonies present in the variously treated methylcellulose cultures were harvested and subjected to analysis. Colony selection bias was therefore avoided. (B) Detection of *bcr/abl* transcripts in CFU-GM (lanes 1–3), and CFU-GEMM (lanes 4–6) derived colonies obtained from reseeded primary colonies of patient #8. Note that while b-actin transcripts are clearly detected in all colony samples, *bcr/abl* in only detectable in colonies derived from untreated control colonies (lanes 1 & 4) and colonies previously exposed to Myb sense ODN (lanes 2 & 5). Cells derived from colonies originally exposed to c-myb AS ODN do not have detectable bcr/abl expressing cells. Lane 7 is a control lane for the PCR reactions and is appropriately empty.

treated control colonies using the same technique. Eight cases were evaluated and in each case bcr-abl expression as detected by RT-PCR correlated with colony growth in cell culture. In cases which were inhibited by exposure to c-myb AS-ODNs (7/11), bcr-abl expression was also greatly decreased or non-detectable (Fig. 3A). These results suggested that bcr-abl expressing CFU might be substantially or entirely eliminated from a population of blood or marrow mononuclear cells by exposure to the AS-ODNs. To explore this possibility further, replating experiments were carried out on samples from two patients (Fig. 3B). We hypothesized that if CFU belonging to the malignant clone were present at the end of the original 12-day culture period, but not detectable because of failure to express bcr-abl, they might re-express the message upon regrowth in fresh cultures. Accordingly, cells from these patients were exposed to ODN and then plated into methylcellulose cultures formulated to favor growth of either CFU-GM or CFU-GEMM. As was found with the original specimens, untreated control cells and cells exposed to sense ODN had RT-PCR detectable bcr-abl transcripts. Those exposed to the c-myb AS-ODNs had none. One of the paired dishes from these cultures was then solubilized with fresh medium, and all cells in it were washed, disaggregated, and replated into fresh methylcellulose cultures *without* re-exposing the cells to ODN. After 14 days, CFU-GM and CFU-GEMM colony cells were again probed for bcr-abl expression. Control and sense-treated cells had RT-PCR detectable mRNA but none was found in the antisense-treated colonies. These results suggest that elimination of bcr-abl expressing cells and CFU was highly efficient and perhaps permanent.

Efficacy of c-myb oligodeoxynucleotides in vivo: *development of animal models*

The studies described above were carried out primarily with unmodified DNA. Such molecules are subject to endo- and exonuclease attack at the phosphodiester bonds and are therefore of little use *in vivo*. We therefore needed to address two questions. First, we had to know if a more stable, chemically modified ODN would give similar results. Second, we needed to know if these materials would have effectiveness in an *in vivo* system against human leukemia cells. Since we could not give this material to patients we established a human leukemia/SCID mouse model system which would allow us to address both questions simultaneously [11]. To carry out these experiments, SCID mice were injected IV with K562 chronic myeloid leukemia cells after cyclophosphamide conditioning. K562 cells express c-myb, the AS-ODN target, and the tumor-specific *bcr\abl* oncogene which was used for tracking the human leukemia cells in the mouse host. After tumor cell injection, animals developed blasts in the peripheral blood within 4 to 6 weeks. After peripheral blood blast cells appeared, mean ($\pm$SD) survival of untreated mice (n=20) was 6$\pm$3 days. Dying animals had prominent central nervous system infiltration, marked infiltration of the ovary, and scattered abdominal granulocytic sarcomas. Infusion of either sense or scrambled sequence c-myb phosphorothioate ODN (24 bp; codons 2–9) for 3, 7 or 14 days had no statistically significant effect on sites of disease involvement, or animal survival in comparison to control animals. In contrast, animals treated for 7 or 14 days with c-myb AS ODN survived 3.5 to 8 times longer (p<.001) than the various control animals (n=60) (Fig. 4). In addition, animals receiving c-myb AS DNA had either rare microscopic foci or no obviously detectable CNS disease (Fig. 3), and a >50% reduction of ovarian involvement. A 3-day infusion of myb AS

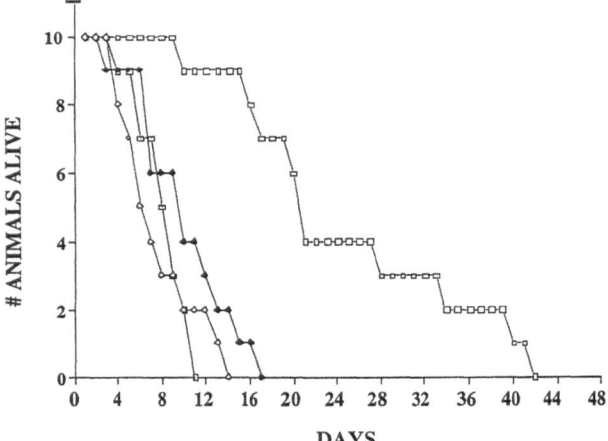

Figure 4. Survival curves of SCID – human chimeric animals transplanted with K562 chronic myelogenous leukemia cells. Animals received a 14 day infusion of oligomers at a dose of 100 µg/day. Legend – [———□———
CONTROL, ———◆——— SENSE, ———■——— ANTISENSE, ———◇——— SCRAMBLED].

(100 µg/d) was without effect. Infusing mice (n = 12) with AS ODN (200 µg/day × 14 days)
complementary to the c-*kit* protooncogene (which K562 cells do not express), also had no effect
on disease burden or survival (n = 12). These results suggested that phosphorothioate modified c-
myb antisense DNA might be efficacious for the treatment of human leukemia *in vivo*.

Why does downregulating Myb kill leukemic cells preferentially?

Our initial studies on the function of the c-*kit* receptor in hematopoietic cells suggested that c-*kit*
might be a Myb-regulated gene [11]. Since c-*kit* encodes a critical hematopoietic cell tyrosine kinase receptor [43], we hypothesized that dysregulation of c-*kit* expression may be an important
mechanism of action of Myb AS ODN. In support of this hypothesis, it has been shown that
when hematopoietic cells are deprived of c-kit R ligand (Steel Factor) they undergo apoptosis
[36]. It has also recently been shown that when CD56[bright] NK cells, which express c-*kit*, are
deprived of their ligand (Steel Factor), they too undergo apoptosis, perhaps because *bcl-2* is
downregulated [44]. Malignant myeloid hematopoietic cells, in particular CML cells, also express
c-*kit* and respond to Steel Factor. Accordingly, we postulate that perturbation of Myb expression
in malignant hematopoietic cells may force them to enter an apoptotic pathway by downregulating
c-*kit*. Preliminary studies of K562 cells exposed to c-myb antisense ODN demonstrates that such
cells do in fact undergo nuclear degenerative changes characteristic of apoptosis.

Use of AS-ODN in a clinical setting

CML seemed to us to be an excellent disease model for the purpose of developing an AS-ODN therapeutic. CML is relatively common, and it has a convenient marker chromosome and gene for objectively following potential therapeutic efficacy of a test compound [45]. In addition to these considerations, CML is uniformly fatal except for individuals who are fortunate enough to have an allogeneic bone marrow donor. Picking a gene target in CML was actually somewhat problematic. An obvious target was the *bcr/abl* gene encoded mRNA [46]. However, because *bcr/abl* is not expressed in primitive hematopoietic stem cells [47], and because it is uncertain if transient interruption of *bcr/abl* signalling actually results in the death of CML cells, we felt that an alternative target might be of greater use in treating this disease. Based on the type of data presented above, a favorable therapeutic index in toxicology testing, and more detailed knowledge of the pharmacokinetics of oligonucleotides, we have begun to evaluate the myb-targeted AS-ODN in the clinic [48].

To this end, we initiated clinical trials to evaluate the effectiveness of phosphorothioate modified AS-ODN to the c-*myb* gene as marrow purging agents for chronic phase (CP) or accelerated phase (AP) chronic myelogenous leukemia (CML) patients, and a Phase I intravenous infusion study for blast crisis (BC) patients and patients with other refractory leukemias. ODN purging was carried out for 24 h on CD34+ marrow cells. Patients received busulfan and cytoxan, followed by re-infusion of previously cryopreserved P-ODN purged MNC. In the pilot marrow purging study seven CP and one AP CML patients have been treated. Seven out of eight engrafted. In 4/6 evaluable CP patients, metaphases were 85–100% normal 3 months after engraftment, suggesting that a significant purge had taken place in the marrow graft. Five CP patients have demonstrated marked, sustained, hematological improvement with essential normalization of their blood counts. Follow-up ranges from 6 months to ~2 years. In an attempt to increase purging efficiency further we incubated patient MNC for 72 h in the P-ODN. Although PCR and LTCIC studies suggested a very efficient purge had occurred, engraftment in five patients was poor. In the Phase I systemic infusion study, 18 refractory leukemia patients (two patients were treated at two different dose levels; 13 had AP or BC CML). Myb AS-ODN was delivered by continuous infusion at dose levels ranging between [0.3 mg/kg/ day ×7 days] to [2.0 mg/kg/day ×7 days]. No recurrent dose-related toxicity has been noted though idiosyncratic toxicities, not clearly drug related, were observed (1 transient renal insufficiency; 1 pericarditis). One BC patient survived ~14 months with transient restoration of CP disease. These studies show that ODN may be administered safely to leukemic patients. Whether patients treated on either study derived clinical benefit is uncertain, but the results of these studies suggest to us that ODN may eventually be useful in the treatment of human leukemias.

Prospects for future development are dependent on solving important problems today

The power of the antisense approach has been demonstrated in experiments in which critical biological information has been gathered using AS technology, and has been subsequently verified by other laboratories using other methodologies [9, 37, 49]. However, this technology, in spite of its successes, has been found to be highly variable in its efficiency. To the extent that many have tried to employ ODNs and have been perplexed and frustrated by results that were non-informative at best, or at worst, misleading or unreproducible, it is easy to understand why this approach has become somewhat controversial. We believe that progress on two fronts would help address this problem.

First, in order for an ODN to hybridize with its mRNA target, it must find an accessible sequence. Sequence accessibility is at least in part a function of mRNA physical structure which is dictated in turn by internal base composition and associated proteins in the living cell. Attempts to describe the *in vivo* structure of RNA, in contrast to DNA, have been fraught with difficulty [50]. Accordingly, mRNA targeting is largely a hit or miss process, which accounts for many experiments where the addition of an ODN has no effect on expression. Hence, the ability to determine which regions of a given mRNA molecule are accessible for ODN targeting is a significant impediment to the application of this technique in many cell systems. We have begun to approach this issue by developing a footprinting assay to determine which physical areas of an RNA are accessible to the oligonucleotide. We have proceeded under the assumption that a sequence which remains accessible to single-stranded RNases in a more physiological environment may also remain accessible for hybridization with an ODN. Preliminary experiments performed in our laboratory, in which a labeled RNA transcript is allowed to hybridize with an oligonucleotide, in the presence or absence of nuclear extracts from the cells of interest along with RNase T1, suggest that footprinting of this type is feasible. Of more interest, our preliminary results suggest that this approach may be of use in designing oligonucleotides.

Second, the ability to deliver ODN into cells and have them reach their target in a bioavailable form also remains problematic [51]. Without this ability, it is clear that even an appropriately targeted sequence is not likely to be efficient. Native phosphodiester ODNs, and the widely used phosphorothioate modified ODNs, which contain a single sulfur substituting for oxygen at a non-bridging position at each phosphorus atom, are polyanions. Accordingly, they diffuse across cell membranes poorly and are only taken up by cells through energy dependent mechanisms. This appears to be accomplished primarily through a combination of adsorbtive endocytosis and fluid phase endocytosis, which may be triggered in part by the binding of the ODN to receptor-like proteins present on the surface of a wide variety of cells [52, 53]. After internalization, confocal and electron microscopy studies have indicated that the bulk of the ODNs enter the endosome/lysosome compartment. These vesicular structures may become acidified and acquire other enzymes which degrade the ODNs. Biological inactivity is the predictable result of this process. Recently described strategies for introducing ODNs into cells, including various cationic lipid formulations, may address this problem [54–56].

Conclusions

The ability to block gene function with AS-ODNs has become an important tool in many research laboratories. Since activation and aberrant expression of proto-oncogenes appears to be an important mechanism in malignant transformation, targeted disruption of these genes and other molecular targets with ODNs could have significant therapeutic use as well. In this regard, the potential therapeutic usefulness of ODNs has been demonstrated in many systems and against a number of different targets including viruses, oncogenes, proto-oncogenes, and an increasing array of cellular genes. These studies in aggregate suggest that synthetic ODNs have the potential to become an important new therapeutic agent for the treatment of human cancer. Nevertheless, it is clear that considerable optimization will be required before antisense oligonucleotides will emerge as effective agents for treating human disease. Progress will need to occur on several fronts. These include issues related to the chemistry of the molecules employed. For example, how chemical modification impact on uptake, stability and hybridization efficiency of the synthetic DNA molecule. A clearer understanding of the mechanism of AS-mediated inhibition, including where such inhibition takes place, will also be required. Finally, cellular 'defense' mechanisms, such as increasing transcription of the targeted message, may also be factors to consider in planning effective treatment strategies with these agents. Choice of target is also an important issue. Nevertheless, while many issues remain to be resolved, we remain optimistic that this approach will one day prove useful for the treatment of patients with a variety of hematological malignancies.

Acknowledgements
Supported by grants from the NIH and the Leukemia Society of America

References

1. Clarke MF, Kukowska-Latallo JF, Westin E, Smith, M Prochownik EV (1988) Constitutive expression of a c-myb cDNA blocks Friend murine erythroleukemia cell differentiation. *Mol Cell Biol* 8: 884–892.
2. Liebermann DA, Hoffman-Liebermann B (1989) Proto-oncogene expression and dissection of the myeloid growth to differentiation developmental cascade. *Oncogene* 4: 583–592.
3. Prochownik EV, Smith MJ, Snyder K, Emeagwali D (1990) Amplified expression of three jun family members inhibits erythroleukemia differentiation. *Blood* 76: 1830–1837.
4. Galli-Taliadoros LA, Sedgwick JD, Wood SA, Korner H (1995) Gene knock-out technology: a methodological overview for the interested novice. *J Immunol Methods* 181: 1–15.
5. Heyer WD, Kohli J (1994) Homologous recombination. *Experientia* 50: 189–191.
6. Morrow B, Kucherlapati R (1993) Gene targeting in mammalian cells by homologous recombination. *Curr Opin Biotechnol* 4: 577–582.
7. Osman F, Tomsett B, Strike P (1994) Homologous recombination. *Prog Ind Microbiol* 29: 687–732.
8. Willnow TE, Herz J (1994) Homologous recombination for gene replacement in mouse cell lines. *Meth Cell Biol* 43: Pt A: 305–334.
9. Gewirtz AM, Calabretta B (1988) A c-myb antisense oligodeoxynucleotide inhibits normal human hematopoiesis *in vitro. Science* 242: 1303–1306.
10. Luger SM, Ratajczak J, Ratajczak MZ, Kuczynski WI, DiPaola RS, Ngo W, Clevenger CV, Gewirtz AM (1996) A functional analysis of protooncogene Vav's role in adult human hematopoiesis. *Blood* 87: 1326–1334.
11. Ratajczak MZ, Hijiya N, Catani L, DeRiel K, Luger SM, McGlave P, Gewirtz AM (1992) Acute- and chronic-phase chronic myelogenous leukemia colony-forming units are highly sensitive to the growth inhibitory effects of c-myb antisense oligodeoxynucleotides. *Blood* 79: 1956–1961.
12. Small D, Levenstein M, Kim E, Carow C, Amin S, Rockwell P, Witte L, Burrow C, Ratajczak MZ, Gewirtz AM et al. (1994) STK-1, the human homolog of Flk-2/Flt-3, is selectively expressed in CD34+ human bone marrow cells and is involved in the proliferation of early progenitor/stem cells. *Proc Natl Acad Sci USA* 91: 459–463.
13. Takeshita K, Bollekens JA, Hijiya N, Ratajczak M, Ruddle FH, Gewirtz AM (1993) A homeobox gene of the Antennapedia class is required for human adult erythropoiesis. *Proc Natl Acad Sci USA* 90: 3535–8.
14. Lyon J, Robinson C, Watson R (1994) The role of Myb proteins in normal and neoplastic cell proliferation. *Crit Rev Oncogen* 5: 373–588.

15. Nomura N, Zu YL, Maekawa T, Tabata S, Akiyama T, Ishii S (1993) Isolation and characterization of a novel member of the gene family encoding the cAMP response element-binding protein CRE-BP1. *J Biol Chem* 268: 4259–66.
16. Biedenkapp H, Borgmeyer U, Sippel AE, Klempnauer KH (1988) Viral myb oncogene encodes a sequence-specific DNA-binding activity. *Nature* 335: 835–837.
17. Sakura H, Kanei-Ishii C, Nagase T, Nakagoshi H, Gonda TJ, Ishii S (1989) Delineation of three functional domains of the transcriptional activator encoded by the c-myb protooncogene. *Proc Natl Acad Sci USA* 86: 5758–5762.
18. Dini PW, Eltman JT, Lipsick JS (1995) Mutations in the DNA-binding and transcriptional activation domains of v-Myb cooperate in transformation. *J Virol* 69: 2515–2524.
19. Press RD, Reddy EP, Ewert DL (1994) Overexpression of C-terminally but not N-terminally truncated Myb induces fibrosarcomas: a novel nonhematopoietic target cell for the myb oncogene. *Mol Cell Biol* 14: 2278–2290.
20. Kanei-Ishii C, MacMillan EM, Nomura T, Sarai A, Ramsay RG, Aimoto S, Ishii S, Gonda T J (1992) Transactivation and transformation by Myb are negatively regulated by a leucine-zipper structure. *Proc Natl Acad Sci USA* 89: 3088–3092.
21. Nomura T, Sakai N, Sarai A, Sudo T, Kanei-Ishii C, Ramsay RG, Favier D, Gonda TJ, Ishii S (1993) Negative autoregulation of c-Myb activity by homodimer formation through the leucine zipper. *J Biol Chem* 268: 21914–21923.
22. Burk O, Mink S, Ringwald M, Klempnauer KH (1993) Synergistic activation of the chicken mim-1 gene by v-myb and C/EBP transcription factors. *EMBO J* 12: 2027–2038.
23. Ness SA, Kowenz-Leutz E, Casini T, Graf T, Leutz A (1993) Myb and NF-M: combinatorial activators of myeloid genes in heterologous cell types. *Genes Dev* 7: 749–759.
24. Barletta C, Pelicci PG, Kenyon LC, Smith SD, Dalla-Favera R (1987) Relationship between the c-myb locus and the 6q-chromosomal aberration in leukemias and lymphomas. *Science* 235: 1064–1067.
25. Vorbrueggen G, Kalkbrenner F, Guehmann S, Moelling K (1994) The carboxyterminus of human c-myb protein stimulates activated transcription in trans. *Nucl Acids Res* 22: 2466–2475.
26. Gewirtz AM, Anfossi G, Venturelli D, Valpreda S, Sims R, Calabretta B (1989) G1/S transition in normal human T-lymphocytes requires the nuclear protein encoded by c-myb. *Science* 245: 180–183.
27. Cogswell JP, Cogswell PC, Kuehl WM, Cuddihy AM, Bender TM, Engelke U, Marcu KB, Ting JP (1993) Mechanism of c-myc regulation by c-Myb in different cell lineages. *Mol Cell Biol* 13: 2858–2869.
28. Ku DH, Wen SC, Engelhard A, Nicolaides NC, Lipson KE, Marino TA, Calabretta B (1993) c-myb transactivates cdc2 expression *via* Myb binding sites in the 5'-flanking region of the human cdc2 gene [published erratum appears in *J Biol Chem* (1993) 268(17): 13010]. *J Biol Chem* 268: 2255–2259.
29. Weber BL, Westin EH, Clarke MF (1990) Differentiation of mouse erythroleukemia cells enhanced by alternatively spliced c-myb mRNA. *Science* 249: 1291–1293.
30. Ness SA, Marknell A, Graf T (1989) The v-myb oncogene product binds to and activates the promyelocyte-specific mim-1 gene. *Cell* 59: 1115–1125.
31. Nakayama K, Yamamoto R, Ishii S, Nakauchi H (1993) Binding of c-Myb to the core sequence of the CD4 promoter. *Int Immunol* 5: 817–824.
32. Travali S, Reiss K, Ferber A, Petralia S, Mercer WE, Calabretta B, Baserga R (1991) Constitutively expressed c-myb abrogates the requirement for insulinlike growth factor 1 in 3T3 fibroblasts. *Mol Cell Biol* 11: 731–736.
33. Melotti P, Ku DH, Calabretta B (1994) Regulation of the expression of the hematopoietic stem cell antigen CD34: role of c-myb. *J Exp Med* 179: 1023–1028.
34. Szczylik C, Skorski T, Ku DH, Nicolaides NC, Wen SC, Rudnicka L, Bonati A, Malaguarnera L, Calabretta B (1993) Regulation of proliferation and cytokine expression of bone marrow fibroblasts: role of c-myb. *J Exp Med* 178: 997–1005.
35. Ratajczak MZ, Luger SM, Gewirtz AM (1992) The c-kit proto-oncogene in normal and malignant human hematopoiesis. *Int J Cell Cloning* 10: 205–214.
36. Yu H, Bauer B, Lipke GK, Phillips RL, Van Zant G (1993) Apoptosis and Hematopiesis in Murine Fetal Liver. *Blood* 81: 373–384.
37. Mucenski ML, McLain K, Kier AB, Swerdlow SH, Schreiner CM, Miller TA, Pietryga DW, Scott WJ Jr, Potter SS (1991) A functional c-myb gene is required for normal murine fetal hepatic hematopoiesis. *Cell* 65: 677–689.
38. Caracciolo D, Venturelli D, Valtieri M, Peschle C, Gewirtz AM, Calabretta B (1990) Stage-related proliferative activity determines c-myb functional requirements during normal human hematopoiesis. *J Clin Invest* 85: 55–61.
39. Anfossi G, Gewirtz AM, Calabretta B (1989) An oligomer complementary to c-myb-encoded mRNA inhibits proliferation of human myeloid leukemia cell lines. *Proc Natl Acad Sci USA* 86: 3379–3383.
40. Calabretta B, Sims RB, Valtieri M, Caracciolo D, Szczylik C, Venturelli D, Ratajczak M, Beran M, Gewirtz AM (1991) Normal and leukemic hematopoietic cells manifest differential sensitivity to inhibitory effects of c-myb antisense oligodeoxynucleotides: an *in vitro* study relevant to bone marrow purging. *Proc Natl Acad Sci USA* 88: 2351–2355.

41. Ratajczak MZ, Kant JA, Luger SM, Hijiya N, Zhang J, Zon G, Gewirtz AM (1992) *In vivo* treatment of human leukemia in a scid mouse model with c-myb antisense oligodeoxynucleotides. *Proc Natl Acad Sci USA* 89: 11823–11827.
42. Witte ON (1993) Role of the BCR-ABL oncogene in human leukemia: fifteenth Richard and Hinda Rosenthal Foundation Award Lecture. *Cancer Res* 53: 485–489.
43. Ratajczak MZ, Luger SM, DeRiel K, Abrahm J, Calabretta B, Gewirtz AM (1992) Role of the KIT protooncogene in normal and malignant human hematopoiesis. *Proc Natl Acad Sci USA* 89: 1710–1714.
44. Carson WE, Haldar S, Baiocchi RA, Croce CM, Caligiuri MA (1994) The c-kit ligand suppressess apoptosis of human natural killer cells through the upreguation of bcl-2. *Proc Natl Acad Sci USA* 91: 7553–7557.
45. Gale RP, Grosveld G, Canaani E, Goldman JM (1993) Chronic myelogenous leukemia: biology and therapy. *Leukemia* 7: 653–658.
46. Melo JV (1996) The molecular biology of chronic myeloid leukaemia. *Leukemia* 10: 751–756.
47. Bedi A, Zehnbauer BA, Collector MI, Barber JP, Zicha MS, Sharkis SJ, Jones RJ (1993) BCR-ABL gene rearrangement and expression of primitive hematopoietic progenitors in chronic myeloid leukemia. *Blood* 81: 2898–2902.
48. Gewirtz AM, Luger S, Sokol D, Gowdin B, Stadtmauer E, Reccio A, Ratajczak MZ (1996) Oligodeoxynucleotide Therapeutics For Human Myelogenous Leukemia: Interim Results. *Blood* 88: Supplement 1: 270a.
49. Metcalf D (1994) Blood. Thrombopoietin – at last. *Nature* 369: 519–520.
50. Baskerville S, Ellington AD (1995) RNA structure. Describing the elephant. *Curr Biol* 5: 120–3.
51. Gewirtz AM, Stein CA, Glazer PM (1996) Facilitating oligonucleotide delivery: helping antisense deliver on its promise. *Proc Natl Acad Sci USA* 93: 3161–3163.
52. Beltinger C, Saragovi HU, Smith RM, LeSauteur L, Shah N, DeDionisio L, Christensen L, Raible A, Jarett L, Gewirtz AM (1995) Binding, uptake, and intracellular trafficking of phosphorothioate-modified oligodeoxynucleotides. *J Clin Invest* 95: 1814–1823.
53. Loke SL, Stein CA, Zhang XH, Mori K, Nakanishi M, Subasinghe C, Cohen JS, Neckers LM (1989) Characterization of oligonucleotide transport into living cells. *Proc Natl Acad Sci USA* 86: 3474–3478.
54. Bergan R, Hakim F, Schwartz GN, Kyle E, Cepada R, Szabo JM, Fowler D, Gress R, Neckers L (1996) Electroporation of synthetic oligodeoxynucleotides: a novel technique for ex vivo bone marrow purging. *Blood* 88: 731–741.
55. Lewis JG, Lin KY, Kothavale A, Flanagan WM, Matteucci MD, DePrince RB, Mook RA Jr, Hendren RW, Wagner RW (1996) A serum-resistant cytofectin for cellular delivery of antisense oligodeoxynucleotides and plasmid DNA. *Proc Natl Acad Sci USA* 93: 3176–3181.
56. Spiller DG, Tidd DM (1995) Nuclear delivery of antisense oligodeoxynucleotides through reversible permeabilization of human leukemia cells with streptolysin O. *Antisense Res Dev* 5: 13–21.

Molecular Aspects of Cancer and its Therapy
A. Mackiewicz and P.B. Sehgal (eds)
© 1998 Birkhäuser Verlag Basel/Switzerland

Genetic instability and tumor cell variation

G.P. Hemstreet, III

Department of Urology, University of Oklahoma Health Sciences Center, P.O. Box 26901, Oklahoma City, OK 73190, USA

Introduction

It has been a provocative experience to share my thoughts on tumor heterogeneity. This is not a subject I previously pondered in specific terms, but when I began to review the subject, it was apparent that the problem of tumor heterogeneity is one of the fundamental problems of cancer therapy [1–12]. Treating cancer is analogous to shooting at a continuously moving target. As our comprehension of cancer improves through scientific advances, the more scientific strategic approaches to control this devastating disease appear to be akin to Don Quixote throwing our national resources at the windmills in the fields outside Barcelona [13]. This is not to suggest that the expenditures have not resulted in remarkable scientific achievements but rather a successful conclusion has not been reached.

The importance of genetic instability was immediately apparent when a karyotype of a malignant melanoma was presented by Charles Balch during one of John Durant's multi-disciplinary conferences at the University of Alabama in 1976. Karyotypic analysis identified the presence of genetic instability well before the current thrust in molecular biology revealed its importance at the molecular level. A review of age-adjusted cancer mortality from 1972 to 1990 and in the four year interval (1990–1994) revealed that, in spite of some limited though impressive gains, we have been remarkably unsuccessful in reducing cancer mortality, given the national resources provided for this effort since 1972 [14]. The improvement in cancer survival over the four most recent years (1992–1995) was due to changing incidence or early detection. A recent report from the National Cancer Institute confirms a 5% decrease in breast cancer and a 6% reduction in colon cancer deaths. A reduction was also observed in prostate cancer deaths; the reason for this is unknown. (Source: *National Center for Health Statistics, Public Use Tapes*: 1995, preliminary data)

The complexities of the cancer problem have been vastly underestimated, as were the complexities of the networks of the central nervous system, the immune system, and signaling- pathways within single cells. In addition to these multiple complex signaling networks are the contributions of stromal-epithelial interactions, not to mention the relationship between the entire organism and its environment, all of which affect genetic instability. It seems each breakthrough promises to lead to success, but instead, we find another layer of complexity beneath the surface. This discussion examines tumor heterogeneity from a different point of view. Basic science has been extremely fruitful in understanding what happens in tumors and, in fact, most of our cancer research efforts have been directed at understanding and treating clinical cancers. By the time a tumor reaches this stage of development, tumor heterogeneity will generally defeat our efforts. An alternative approach is to redirect our basic research efforts toward understanding events which lead to the emergence of genetically unstable tumors. We can thereby hope to deal with tumor heterogeneity before it becomes a problem. What cancer research needs to illuminate is carcinogenesis itself. Ultimately we should treat the premalignant field prior to genetic instability and the expression of the metastatic phenotype. Consequently, I shall discuss tumor heterogeneity in the epithelial field [15–17] and biomarkers as they relate to genetic instability. Based on our experiences, utilizing biomarkers to unravel the complexities of genetic instability is both multifaceted and informative.

The primary goal of this chapter is not only to provide an overview of tumor heterogeneity and genetic instability as it relates to the current understanding of the molecular nature of the development of cancer but also to lend special credence to using biomarkers of effect on cells in the premalignant cancer field as a reliable means of identifying individuals who are at risk for developing biologically active cancer. It is my opinion that by using these markers alone or in combination with genetic markers of susceptibility to identify cancer in its premalignant stages, the inherent problems of treating cells that are both unstable and variable genetically would be obviated. For these reasons it is important to know when specific biomarkers of effect are expressed in the cascade of tumorigenesis. Knowing when markers are expressed early or late will assist in monitoring the effect of chemopreventive agents that can be tested in patients at risk, as well as in determining at what point genetic instability becomes a therapeutic problem. To accomplish these objectives, it is first necessary to review past perspectives on tumor heterogeneity, then to a discuss biomarkers of genetic instability. Finally, a biomarker study in an occupationally exposed cohort at risk for bladder cancer will be presented to illustrate the salient concepts and power of this approach.

General historical perspectives on genetic instability

Prior to attempting to relate current perspectives on tumor heterogeneity, it is useful to reflect on the concepts and scientific advances of the past 15 years. In 1982, a closed state-of-the-art meeting was held in Saskatchewan, Canada [18]. One important session was specifically related to tumor heterogeneity. Particularly germane to the discussions and this manuscript was a presentation by Dr. Victor Ling discussing genetic instability, clonality, and the metastatic phenotypes [18]. In general, the presentations consisted of descriptive data, reflecting the significant advances made in cell biology, and virtually excluded molecular biology and the signaling pathways defined since the conference was held. It is now apparent that concepts pertaining to heterogeneous clones resulting in a metastatic phenotype were correct. Epigenetic alterations or genetic mutations from within the cloned cells contributed to metastatic diversity. The "Summary" failed to mention the mechanisms of signaling pathways related to tumor heterogeneity and a discussion of biomarkers pertaining to genetic instability was conspicuously absent.

Discussions by Gloria Heppner brought into focus that the cellular heterogeneity of subpopulations within a solitary tumor could be defined by the tumor's metastatic potential and karyotypic analysis [19]. A glimpse of the importance of growth factors was supplied by the observation that supernatant from one clone enhanced the growth of slower growing clones [6]. These concepts were extended to observations related to drug sensitivity testing, explaining the importance of interactive ecosystems [7]. However, the general themes derived from the presentations clearly demonstrated that, although our insight into the mechanisms involved in tumor heterogeneity were progressing, there was a paucity of discussion pertaining to the mechanism leading to tumor heterogeneity. A search continued for "magic bullets" to enhance the effectiveness of various treatment modalities, including radiation therapy, chemotherapy, and immunotherapy [20].

Tumor heterogeneity – the clinical cancer problem

Since President Nixon's war on cancer commenced, there has been cautious optimism that current scientific advances would give an effective therapeutic result. In the intervening years, there has been optimism that *in vitro* drug sensitivity assays would be effective in identifying active chemotherapeutic agents, the problems of drug resistance would be understood and overcome, and immunotherapy would be successful. Now, 25 years later, all therapeutic modalities including radiation therapy, chemotherapy, and immunotherapy are still ultimately thwarted by genetic instability. I shall illustrate this point by drawing on my personal research experience to bring an immunological perspective to this issue. Similar points could be made for radiation and chemotherapy.

   Although McFarland Burnett's theory on immune surveillance may be correct, the enthusiasm for manipulating the immune system in the early 1970s has not been translated into widely applicable therapies [21]. By contrast, immune surveillance is highly effective in animal models with chemically induced tumors [22]. These positive results are not to be confused with earlier studies where transplantation antigens were responsible for perceived tumor immunity. Critical experiments by Peter Gore resolved this confusion [23]. In spite of animal studies, the effectiveness of immune surveillance in controlling spontaneous human neoplasms remains a point of speculation. A balanced perspective on this subject was realized when I heard Richmond Prehn's presentation at an International Cancer Congress in Houston, Texas, in the early 1970s.

   Although not totally optimistic, the discussion confirmed my decision to pursue a fellowship in immunology at Duke University with Bernard Amos, a world class transplantation immunologist ,and H.F. Seigler [24], his creative clinical arm and colleague who has spent his professional career studying the immunobiology of malignant melanoma. Caught in the enthusiasm of tumor biology, I decided to pursue a doctoral degree to master the rigors of the discipline. My objective was to develop an *in vitro* assay to detect cellular immunity in patients with renal cell carcinoma, utilizing the mixed lymphocyte tumor reaction [25]. These basic science-clinical studies confirmed that renal cell tumor plasma membranes would stimulate autologous peripheral blood lymphocytes in what was then termed a "mixed lymphocyte tumor reaction" [26]. The stimulating membrane antigens were shown to be glycolipids, and confidence abounded [27]: a major scientific advance had been made, and my research was on the pathway to autologous vaccines. The autologous vaccines would address the problems of tumor heterogeneity, particularly if adequate tissue could be obtained. At this time, awareness of antigenic heterogeneity was reaching new heights of awareness and was, subsequently, elegantly reviewed in a number of scholarly articles [1, 10, 20, 28].

Tumor antigens, expressed on precancerous lesions, were hypothesized to be clonal in origin with the later development of antigenic diversity. After reviewing the current literature, it is the author's impression that tumors may arise as clonal neoplasms and form a tumor, developing from an expanding field change, or arise as multifocal heterogenous neoplasms from a premalignant field. This is not to suggest that premalignant field changes do not occur in organs where they arise as a single focus. These concepts support the earlier observations of Nowell, Poste, and others regarding antigenic diversity [29–35]. Consolidation of my thinking occurred when I read a study of Y-chromosome expression in prostatic cancer, where multiple patterns of cellular expression were clearly documented in an area of glandular prostate intra-epithelial neoplasm (PIN) [36]. Another fallacy of the vaccine concept was the lack of appreciation for continued immunological diversity developing at the distant tumor site [37]. Grant support was evasive, but the research evolved in an attempt to isolate a T cell growth factor to expand activated tumor infiltrating lymphocytes (TILs). While a very bright graduate student was working on this project, the Cetus Corporation commercialized genetically engineered IL-2, and the lymphocyte activated killer cell concept spawned new enthusiasm because of the non-selective but specific affinity of these cells for the transformed phenotype [38, 39]. This work of Elizabeth Grimm and Steve Rosenberg was logical, and brought the clinical trials in the area of biological response modifiers to a new level [40–43].

Basic and clinical research efforts facilitated our contract with Cetus to define the pharmacokinetics of subcutaneous IL-2 in patients with renal cell carcinoma [44, 45]. It was our impression that the clinical responses with subcutaneous IL-2 were not nearly as impressive as the responses following a protocol with moderate doses of IL-2 and lymphocyte activated killer (LAK) cells developed at Oklahoma, although randomized trials have not been performed to confirm this impression. There was a sense of regret and a wish that our group had been allowed to administer high doses of IL-2 [42, 46]. The subcutaneous pharmacokinetics studies, however, did establish the fundamental pharmacological data for the subcutaneous route of IL-2 today [45]. Interestingly the response of malignant melanoma and renal cell carcinoma to IL-2 paralleled the high rate of spontaneous regression of these neoplasms [47].

Paradoxically, other tumors responding to IL-2 *in vitro* were clinically unresponsive *in vivo*, suggesting the more immunogenic nature of renal cell carcinoma (RCC) and melanoma may be relevant. A more specific immune mechanism may be involved, such as cell-mediated lysis induced by IL-2 [47]. Whatever the mechanism, it was rather spectacular to document the regression of 100 grams of RCC metastatic to the liver in a patient receiving IL-2 and LAK cells [48]. I never witnessed such a response in a patient with renal cancer treated with chemotherapy or radiation. The press was caught in the enthusiasm, and misquoted our results in a headline on the front page of *The Daily Oklahoman*. The patient subsequently refused further therapy and died of her metastatic disease. However, another patient who had a large bulky tumor compressing his spinal cord was treated with IL-2 and multimodality therapy, including surgery, and is still alive 10 years later. Because of cases such as these, most admire the rigor of the FDA who facilitated approval of this drug but not without considerable debate because of the associated toxicity and the marginal efficacy of the biological response modifiers as single agents.

Optimism for the clinical efficacy of natural killer (NK) cells, [41, 43, 49–52] activated macrophages or, more recently, LAK cells persists, as they are perceived as the potentially effective "Pac-Man" killers. Effective therapeutic progress has been made in this arena in selected patients and the mean duration of response now exceeds 15.4 months [53]. Patients are undoubtedly living longer when treated with biological response modifiers in combination with other modalities, including radiation and surgery and, more recently, growth factors(N.J. Vogelzang, personal communication). However, most clinical results are defined in terms of months rather than years, and tumor heterogeneity ultimately foils the system.

Although the majority of therapeutic advances with biological response modifiers have not been curative, what has evolved is an appreciation for the complexities of the immunological signaling pathways and the problem of tumor heterogeneity [28]. Our inability to achieve clinical cures routinely relates to the complexities of signaling pathways present in an unstable state, perturbated by unidentified exogenous and endogenous risk factors. One approach to solving the cancer problem is to identify the final common signaling pathways pertinent to the development of the metastatic phenotypes and manipulate them within the context of the organism's unstable epithelial ecosystem [54]. An alternative and logical solution to these complexities is to address the cancer problem at its earliest stages of perturbation, defined by quantitative alterations of biomarkers, specifically related to the common pathways of tumorigenesis. For the past ten years, this has been the primary direction and focus of our research laboratory, having abandoned IL-2 research with the exception of treating clinically ill patients.

Chronologically prior to clinical research with IL-2, Bacillus Calment Guerin (BCG) was reported to be an effective treatment for superficial bladder cancer [55]. Subsequent to the initial report on BCG therapy for the treatment of non-invasive bladder cancer, the effectiveness of this vaccine has been confirmed by a Southwest Oncology Group trial [56]. One usually thinks of vaccine therapy as eliciting a specific immune response against tumor-associated antigens; however, data suggest that nonspecific immune mechanisms may be relevant. Because BCG's efficacy is related to nonspecific immunological mechanisms, it is particularly effective in a closed compartment like the bladder [57]. Other therapies, including genetic engineering with retrovirus vectors which deliver gene products such as cytokines, may also be delivered effectively to the lining of the hollow vesicle. BCG vaccine therapy is not without considerable toxicity and, consequently, great attention to detail is required during its administration to prevent unexpected death [58]. A "take home" message from years of research is that BCG is effective because it circumvents the problem of tumor heterogeneity by seemingly nonspecific mechanisms. Total success is elusive because genetic instability persists or recurs, but deaths from bladder cancer in this century are slowly decreasing [59], in part because of these rather remarkable scientific advances.

Curative therapeutic results with immunotherapy have been limited, and tumor heterogeneity imposes limitations on chemotherapy and radiation therapy as well. In Heppner's review of tumor heterogeneity, she mentions the problems associated with effective chemotherapy and multidrug resistance [1]. One key to successful chemotherapy is solving the problems of multidrug resistance (MDR). There are two types of MDR. One is due to high levels of P-glycoprotein. The other is due to a failure of cells to die of apoptosis, even when exposed to drugs. P-glycoprotein is a specific transport glycoprotein that can export a drug as fast as it enters cells, a key to phenotypic markers for MDR. A consensus conference report in 1996 emphasized that the principal problem even with establishing reliable assays for multidrug resistance, is tumor heterogeneity [60]. If reliable assays could be established, the variable expression of P-glyco-protein on cellular heterogeneity and expression at the single cell level would prevail. More recently, chemotherapy-induced upregulation of the apoptosis-inducing protein Fas with the subsequent interaction of its complementary ligand (Fas ligand) has been implicated as a common mechanism underlying drug sensitivity [61, 62]. Again, however, tumor cells containing a mutated or deleted p53 are unable to upregulate Fas and die in response to the chemotherapeutic agent, allowing outgrowth of a p53 mutant chemoresistant tumor cell subpopulation [61, 63]. The summarized consensus confirms the need for reliable assays and in a sense, recapitulates some of the principles we have expressed [64].

Radioimmunotherapy

One area of research and clinical investigation that shows promise for the future is radioimmu-notherapy, particularly for nonsolid neoplasms. Antibody targeting of cell membrane-associated epitopes, e.g. CD20 B-lymphocyte cell surface antigen, shows some promise in B cell non-Hodgkin's lymphomas, [65] and remissions have been observed 16 to 31 months following treatment. Cell surface membrane antigens are expressed in these malignancies, and there appears to be less genetic instability and antigenic diversity. Based on the effectiveness of anti-T cell anti-sera for transplant immunosuppression, one can anticipate that this therapy might be at least partially effective. The promise of the treatment of solid tumors, such as of the breast has been a focus of research for many years, and currently there is little progress in this area [66]. Attempts to improve treatment efficacy involve the incorporation of new immunoconjugates, but they may be more immunogenic [67]. Complete remission responses as high as 30% to 50% have been reported. Wilder recently reviewed this topic and summarized the problems associated with radioimmunotherapy [68]. In this review, he suggested solutions for of many of the problems and remains optimistic, but no solution was offered for antigenic tumor heterogeneity, antigenic modulation, or the lack of antigenic expression high enough to elicit an immune response. A similar multiplicity of problems also relate to oncologic antibody imaging. The use of human antibody fragments isolated from bacteriophage filaments have improved penetration and are not trapped in the liver, should enhance the resolution of imaging and radionucleotide therapy [69–71]. Overall, the power of radioimmunotherapy probably resides in combination with more conventional chemotherapeutic approaches [72].

General concepts about biomarkers and tumor variability

From the work of several special study groups, a paradigm for understanding biomarkers in relation to the pathogenesis of disease and chemoprevention has evolved [73, 74] (Fig. 1). A brief synopsis of the various classes of biomarkers is reviewed in the context of genetic instability. Biomarkers of susceptibility are genotypic, i.e. DNA, and contain the genetic code of life and, ultimately, the *code* of death [75, 76]. Alterations in the genotype are genetically determined

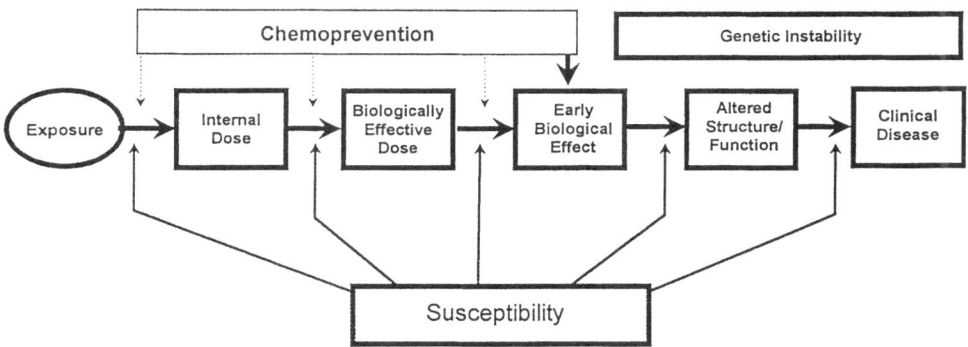

Figure 1. Flow chart depicting the classes of biological marker (indicated by boxes). Solid lines reflect the progression, if it occurs, to the next class of marker. Dashed lines represent the potential susceptibility and chemopreventive influences on the rates of progression. Biological markers reflect a continuum of change. Adapted from the *Committee on Biological Markers of the National Research Council*, 1986, and the *Committee on Biological Markers in Urinary Toxicology*, 1993.

(biomarkers of susceptibility) or may be altered by endogenous or exogenous exposures by either genetic (mutational) or epigenetic mechanisms which promote or retard genetic instability and carcinogenesis. Mutated genes are biomarkers of effect. Mutations or deregulations of biomarkers of susceptibility which modulate metabolic variants that impair an organism's ability to regulate cell cycle arrest, proliferation, apoptosis, the metastatic phenotype or repair DNA damage, may contribute to individual risk assessment. Other genes classified as biomarkers of susceptibility include the *p53* gene associated with Li-Fraumeni syndrome, *Rb* associated with retinoblastoma, and the *BRC1* gene associated with breast cancer in 10% to 13% of women with no family history [77, 78]. Many genetic mutations reported in cancers are not inherited, but are a result of genetic instability or mutations. These are then classified as biomarkers of effect, and should be distinguished from genetically inherited markers.

Epigenetic events are inferred from biological observations, such as those of Pilot, Rubin, and others [79–84]. Table 1 summarizes important biological observations which support the importance of epigenetic mechanisms in carcinogenesis. In contrast to mutagenic biomarkers or chromosomal aberrations, documentation of phenotypic biomarkers requires precise quantitative changes in normally expressed phenotypic biomarkers that may exist in the absence of genetic alterations. Only recently have techniques been developed which can accurately determine quantitative differences at the single cell level [76, 85–88].

Innumerable cellular biomarkers have been identified, but few have been integrated into longitudinal controlled trials or have met the standards of quality control necessary for clinical implementation. Currently, our knowledge of markers and their potential utility needs to be expanded, and there is a paucity of support for well-constructed clinical trials to evaluate biomarkers to define the precancerous condition. Given the changes in health care delivery and the demands on clinicians, it is highly unlikely these issues will be solved shortly. Aggressive approaches are needed to resolve this problem. Clinicians without a strong basic scientific knowledge are not

Table 1. Epigenetic mechanisms of carcinogenesis

Mechanism	Reference
Morphological transformation of cultured cells.	80
Microfilament network is one of the earliest targets of oxidative stress.	247
Oxidant injury products dramatic changes in cytoskeleton organization and cell shape.	251–253
Inhibiting the assembly of actin monomers.	334
Ionizing radiation induces several ongoing processes that involve altered gene function without known changes in DNA base sequences and which are widespread among exposed cell populations.	344, 345
Increased transcription of a variety of genes.	346
Altered DNA methylation patterns.	347
Increased somatic recombination.	348
NIH3T3 line- neoplastically transformed foci when they are maintained at high density for more than one week.	349
Hepatocellular carcinomas result from the overproduction of hepatitis B virus large envelope polypeptide in transgenic mice. Non-genetic mechanism for carcinogenesis that could involve the production of oxygen-free radicals.	350
Changes in cell shape or architecture can regulate gene expression.	351
Alteration of cytoskeletal and nuclear matrix proteins is related to the process of transformation.	244
Self-perpetuating changes in patterns of gene expression are a plausible mechanism for an epigenetic component of carcinogenesis.	336
Non-mutational nature of cancer initiation: of 262 compounds listed by the U.S. National Toxicological Program, 162 were rodent carcinogens of which only 90 (56%) were mutagens. Of the 100 non-carcinogens, 25 (25%) were mutagens. Mutagenicity is neither necessary nor sufficient for carcinogenicity.	94

equipped to address such problems, particularly if one is interested in determining when genetic instability develops in the cascade of tumorigenesis. Biomarkers of instability may be defined by the gene, message or protein product. Which of these is the most clinically useful depends on a variety of complex factors, including sample type, cost, instrumentation, specificity, sensitivity, and many other parameters [89].

Endogenous or exogenous exposures may either promote or prevent genetic instability. Nutritional and environmental exogenous exposures have, historically, been difficult to quantify, and their biological effects are often variable and indefinite. Epidemiological reconstruction of exposure history is at best an approximation, and is particularly complex as it relates to disease outcome because many more individuals are exposed than actually progress to pathological disease. Consequently, statistical correlations are frequently weak when analyzed in epidemiological studies. As a result, when one attempts to relate weak exposure factors, i.e. nutritional, environmental or occupational exposures, large expensive studies are required and usually exclude interesting, unknown, confounding variables.

To correlate and determine the relevance of exogenous exposures more accurately, such as nutritional factors or xenobiotics, analysis in relation to early biomarkers of effect may be significantly more informative and require smaller sample sizes. The relevance of exogenous and endogenous exposures to cancer development is clearly illustrated by the increased incidence of prostate cancer in second generation Chinese-Americans compared to Asian Chinese [90]. The importance of nutritional factors and primary cancer prevention has recently been reviewed [91]. Analysis of nutritional factors in relation to early biomarkers of effect rather than disease and susceptibility factors may show a better correlation because not all initial events progress to disease. Defining exposures, linking them to susceptibility, and analyzing them in terms of early biomarkers of effect should markedly enhance the statistical power of analyses. Biomarkers of effect, when analyzed and linked to susceptibility, enhance our ability to analyze the importance of biomarkers of toxic exposure. This defines a significant opportunity for basic science and molecular epidemiological research. However, other factors including complex interactions such as environment, nutrition or confounding genetic polymorphisms and equilibrium of reactions, further confound interpretation.

Jones and others have hypothesized that mutational patterns found in specific genes can serve to predict the effects of occupational exposures [92]. For those with a focus on the precision of base pair analysis and the powerful computer microchip's array analysis, the results may well contribute to individual risk assessment [93]. These techniques are conceptually attractive but fail to consider the complex networks of signaling pathways and post-translational events and regulatory signals associated with epigenetic mechanisms that are not an integral part of the model. Support for the importance of epigenetic mechanisms is given by the fact that only two-thirds of carcinogens are mutagenic. The general applicability of this approach is, thus, understandably limited [94]. A recent chapter review by Feinberg on *Genomic Imprinting and Cancer* provides an elegant up-to-date review [94b]. He states loss of imprinting (LOI) is "one of the most common alterations in human cancer".

Biomarkers of effect, by definition, may be phenotypic or genotypic; an issue which is frequently confused. Inherited DNA base pairs are genotypic markers of susceptibility, in contrast to mutational alterations, chromosomal deletions, translocations, or amplifications detected by fluorescence *in situ* hybridization (FISH) or by comparative genomic hybridization. All of the latter are genetic biomarkers of effect. Quantitation of these rather complex genetic alterations gives clues to the mechanisms of carcinogenesis and may, in many instances, reflect genetic instability. How biomarkers function and when they are expressed or altered in the cascade of tumorigenesis are two important considerations [64, 89]. Perhaps more importantly, epigenetic mechanisms and the genetic mutations and chromosomal aberrations affect the messages and protein products, all biomarkers of effect. Our research has primarily focused on biomarkers of effect related directly to phenotypic pathways of disease. One important observation is that cancers, with their tumor heterogeneity, do not develop in isolation. Instead, tumors develop within an epithelial field of cells which are phenotypically altered by the presence of the tumor cells and by epigenetic events which act as promoters [15].

This view resulted from the rather remarkable research of Dr. Seymour West, who proved that with appropriate instrumentation, biophysical cytochemical measurements could be made at the single cell level using fluorescence microscope-based systems [86]. His concepts built on the fundamental theories of T. Casperson, the father of quantitative microscope-based data acquisition [95]. His work served to emphasize that all disease starts in the cell, as proclaimed by Virchow. Our research group has built on these concepts and developed quality control methods for automated instrumentation [96]. What I have come to appreciate is that most diseases are subtle, quantitative perturbations of normal cellular functions [97]. West suggested that a cell can function as a microcuvette (S. West, personal communication) and with appropriate controls, quantitative analysis may be performed on single cells. Their communication is a very powerful tool for understanding the chemistry of single cells and one to another, i.e. "cell talk", in relation to disease. Precise quantification of biomarkers in individual cells establishes a unique means to understand tumor heterogeneity. Traditional techniques for biomarker analysis relied on conventional biochemical methods using extraction techniques for protein, DNA and RNA analysis with the hope that the biomarker changes of interest occurring in a minority of cells would be sufficiently strong to detect them. Microdissection techniques have facilitated the study of DNA and RNA at the cellular level by applying the polymerase chain reaction and RT-PCR. Flow cytometry with fluorescence can be achieved, but correlation with cellular morphology, e.g. nuclear *vs.* cytoplasm, is more difficult [76]. Moreover, the precise detection of the gene or message does not necessarily correlate with the protein product [98, 99]. Current conventional immunohistochemical techniques quantify measurements as dichotomous variables based on the number of positive cells. Increased sensitivity is obtained by quantifying data as threshold count markers or by quantifying precise average values for a population of cells [64]. Critical to the success of defining when tumor heterogeneity occurs is defining of normal biomarker values at the cellular level considering normal cellular senescence, independent of or associated with the aging process and cell cycle expression.

The complexities of the clinical implementation of related biomarkers is illustrated by the biomarker prostate specific antigen (PSA). Even the lay community has some idea of the complexity of interpreting this simple test. It is not uncommon for a physician (urologist) to be confronted with a 20 page print-out from the Internet, provided by the patient, to assure the physician's knowledge base. The print-out may contain the details of the test, the pros and cons of cancer screening, and a discussion related to the complex issue of the desirability of radical prostatectomy. To improve the test, age-adjusted values have been defined because of the high false-positive rate in older men and missed tumors in younger men [100]. New baseline PSA values for African-American men may be another refinement [101, 102]. Other attempts to improve the sensitivity have included PSA density and velocity [103]. This is a subject I have reviewed earlier, and perhaps the free *versus* total PSA will contribute to enhanced specificity and sensitivity of the PSA test [73, 104].

Since patients with an elevated PSA frequently undergo biopsy, an alternative approach is to incorporate cellular biomarkers expressed in the normal appearing cells in the cancer field to define the probability that an elevated PSA is cancer associated. Several markers which might be evaluated include G-actin and transglutaminase or DNA 5-CER [27, 105]. Others not quantitatively evaluated at the single cell level, could include telomerase or glutathione transferase II. Both show a high correlation with the malignant phenotype. The frequency of patients with biochemical failures, e.g. increased PSA, following radical prostatectomy supports the notion that PSA is a late biomarker of effect. Furthermore, it is frightening that only 30% of the positive PSAs (4–10 ng/ml) have prostate cancer, requiring a large number of unnecessary biopsies. Inaccuracy of biopsy, and other confounding variables such as benign growth of the prostate and prostatitis contribute to the dilemma. Thus, cellular biomarkers might be used, for example, to determine the necessity for a repeat biopsy. A major factor in assessing biological potential is the degree of tumor heterogeneity and whether specific metastatic phenotypes are expressed. Other biomarkers are needed for preventing, detecting, and predicting the biological potential of this neoplasm. The historical problems associated with a simple marker such as PSA clearly illustrate the complexity of integrating a biomarker into clinical practice and the enormous effort required to optimize its utility. This same rigor would be required for bringing biomarkers of genetic instability to the clinical arena.

Previously, I was asked to present approaches for the selection of biomarkers. This was recently summarized in a review and there is no need to pollute the literature with duplication [64, 106]. Several points related to this discussion deserve emphasis. (1) Biomarkers of genetic instability may be most useful for knowing that the initiation of therapy is too late, or that very aggressive therapy is indicated. (2) Functional biomarkers of effect may be the most informative if they herald risk of developing the metastatic phenotype. (3) The use of surrogate intermediate endpoint markers of effect and the point at which they are expressed in the cascade of tumorigenesis may be the most informative for directing therapy. (4) Identification of early markers prior to the onset of genetic instability may be the most informative for cancer prevention. Table 2 summarizes an approach for identifying biomarkers and testing them in a variety of clinical assessment schemes [64]. A rational approach to eliminating the problem of genetic instability is to treat clinical cancer prior to its onset.

Targeting normal cell receptors that are upregulated during carcinogenesis but are not affected by tumor heterogeneity provides an alternative approach. J. Folkman has devoted his research career to defining and identifying angiogenic factors and crucial signaling pathways demonstrating that tumor proliferation requires angiogenesis [107–110]. Several molecules including VEGF and basic FGF are active in the network of signaling pathways that control endothelial cell proliferation associated with neovascularity. Attempts to neutralize the signals mediating neovascularity to date have not been totally effective, probably due to the redundancy of signals. An

Table 2. Summary of the various types of studies that can be used to evaluate a biomarker to determine its clinical utility alone or in combination with other biomarkers. Adapted from Hemstreet [2].

Paradigm for clinical evaluation of biomarkers
Pilot study
Stratified risk study
The "simple" trial
The field disease model
Evaluate biomarkers in patients undergoing tumor progression or regression

alternative approach is to attack a normal upregulated cellular component relevant to neovascularity such as the $\alpha_5\beta_3$ integrin glycoprotein associated with normal endothelial proliferation [111]. Interestingly, a specific cyclic peptide containing arginine, glycine, and aspartate (RGP) binds with high affinity to the proliferating endothelial cell receptors [111]. Attacking the more stable upregulated receptors on a normal cell not plagued by genetic instability makes sense, providing the reagent can be delivered and antigenic modulation is not a concurrent problem. Thus, using biomarkers of effect to define premalignant changes prior to the onset of genetic instability or to target cancer prevention or therapeutic treatments to target genetically stable cells participating in the carcinogenesis process are two viable options.

Biomarkers for monitoring genetic instability

A discussion of biomarkers of genetic instability is complicated because the multiple mechanisms and the complexity of the signaling pathways leading to this undesirable state have not been fully elucidated. A summary of candidate biomarkers which may reflect tumor heterogeneity is provided. For those actively involved in this area of research, I trust that they will not be offended if their area of expertise is not represented, but given the complexity of the network of signaling pathways I am sure that this will occur. A summary of this topic is relevant because our hypothesis is that once genetic instability has occurred, clinical treatment of the malignant neoplasm is profoundly complicated. Therefore, it is logical to use biomarkers of instability to define when this salient event occurs. Although this is intuitively obvious, the concept did not become an integral part of my thinking until I met Karl Bergey, an aerospace engineer, trained at the Massachusetts Institute of Technology. Bergey designed the Cherokee Piper aircraft, and now builds wind machines. His wind machines are in demand worldwide because they seldom fail, and because of their durability. A joint venture has just been initiated with the People's Republic of China. While working together on a biopsy gun to obtain FNA single cells for biomarker analysis automatically, Bergey kept stressing the concept of reducing the design to its least degree of complexity to minimize instrument failure and costs. Cancer should also be defined and prevented during its least complex state for the very same reasons.

Biomarkers of genetic instability may be attributed to genetically inherited susceptibility factors. Genes involved in DNA repair may contribute directly because of inherited defects or be secondary to genetic or epigenetic exogenous or endogenous risk factors. Other proto-oncogenes or suppressor genes, such as *p53*, which regulate cell cycle arrest, facilitate DNA repair, or regulate apoptosis or cellular proliferation, participate more indirectly in the genetically unstable state.

Establishing thresholds for biomarkers of genetic instability is not a simple issue and by definition must include quantitation of apoptosis and proliferation. For example, it is recognized that a small number of cells with greater than 5C DNA (aneuploid cell) may be present in the urine of smokers, presumably reflecting a clastogenic effect. Clastogenic cells are incapable of clonal expansion because of decreased proliferation or increased apoptosis. Thus the genetically unstable cell expressing a defined biomarker must be capable of clonal growth for some prescribed interval or until a new clone develops. A number of theoretical models have been proposed, all of which lead directly or indirectly to the metastatic phenotype [112–114]. My personal bias is that the process is not necessarily linear, but may have an unstructured order because of the pre-existing gene expression in a given organ or cell, undefined and defined exogenous factors, and genetic instability.

Faulty DNA repair

Genetic instability may be caused by faulty DNA repair. Faulty DNA repair results from a number of potential causes, including inherited and mutational genetic and epigenetic factors. Although the primary cause may be attributed to inherited DNA repair genes such as those associated with right-sided hereditary non-polyposis colorectal carcinoma (HNPCC), other mechanisms such as cell cycle arrest, quantity of telomerase, degree of DNA methylation, alteration in the cytoskeleton, or oxidative stress, may lead to faulty DNA repair. Bohr concisely summarized the various DNA repair mechanisms that maintain the normal integrity of the genome as illustrated in Figure 2 [115]. Most faulty DNA repair is probably not due to mutated DNA repair genes, but is the result of multiple genetic polymorphism with DNA repair resulting from exogenous and endogenous factors. The organism is uniquely set to correct most of these genetic defects. Current research is directed at identifying functional biomarkers regulating cell cycle arrest or DNA repair genes which are the functional cause in a specific neoplasm(s). Depending on the method, i.e., single cell *vs.* homogenate or mixed sample, the results may only reflect the average change in a population and not the relevant clone, i.e. functional metastatic phenotype.

Microsatellite DNA is a phenotypic marker for genetic instability resulting from replication errors attributed to mismatched repair genes. Four human genotypic mismatched repair genes

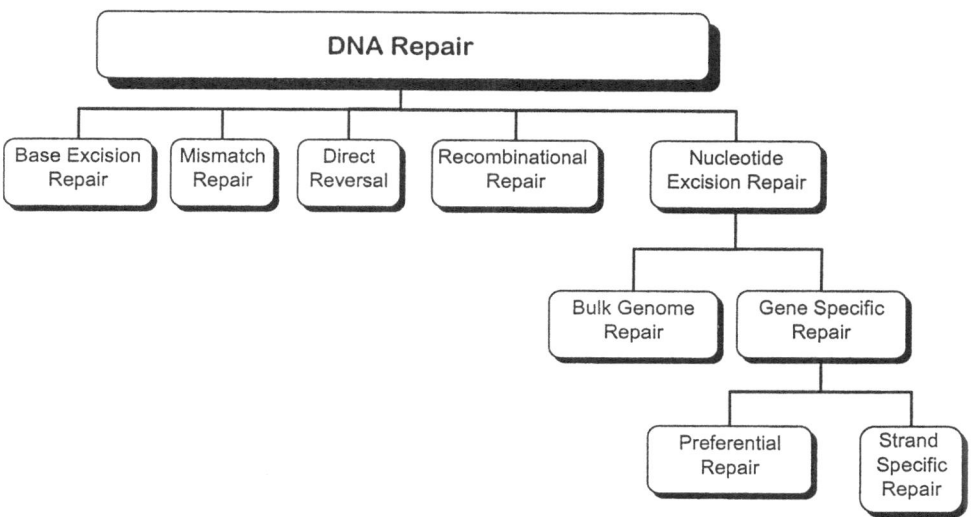

Figure 2. Different mechanistic pathways for mammalian DNA of repair. Adapted from [1].

have been designated as *hMSH2*, *hMLSH1*, *hPMS1*, and *hPMS2* [116–124]. As the sensitivity for detecting microsatellites increases with additional probes, what functionally defines a genetically unstable ecosystem with immortality will require scientific validation. Cells with microsatellites could also reflect a clastogenic event, analogous to that observed with 5C DNA ER. Perhaps cells with microsatellites and increased telomerase or with hypomethylation will be highly indicative of genetic instability. The accurate identification of faulty DNA repair at the phenotypic level may require developing a biomarker profile at the cellular level to exclude rare event clastogenic changes.

Cervical cancer serves as a useful model for documenting and observing the molecular biomarker changes, i.e. microsatellite formation and loss of heterozygosity (LOH) associated, with malignant transformation because of the defined orderly histopathological dedifferentiation. There is a need for defining individuals at risk for cervical cancer, because a large number of women with cervical dysplasia unnecessarily undergo surgical or laser intervention who would not necessarily progress to the malignant phenotype. The incurred cost approaches $6 billion annually. Biomarkers which more precisely define individuals at risk for dysplasia progress would be a significant improvement over the weak association with papilloma virus now thought to perturb cell cycle G arrest *via* E 6 and E7 proteins [125, 126]. Based on our studies with bladder cancer, we suggest G or F actin or 5C DNA ER could potentially be useful, but other markers remain to be investigated [105, 127]. An interesting technique using a modification of DNA sequence analysis is to increase the specificity of the PCR-based assay, eliminating the number of stutter repeats. This study served to show that in 89 cervical cancers, the mismatch repair and the microsatellite formation with RER was relatively infrequent [128]. The authors conclude that the function was primarily due to tumor suppressor genes, and not to genetically acquired defects in mismatched repair genes, confirming that microsatellite function is not primary in cervical cancer. They suggest that lack of cell cycle arrest may be attributed to *p53* or aberration of some other genes in the cell cycle arrest pathway [128]. What is currently unknown is what is the threshold or the cut-off points, or the combination of biomarkers which constitute genetic instability in cervical cancer and other diseases.

Telomerase

Telomerase is a nuclear protein complex, functioning as an internal guide to the maintenance of chromosomal telomeres [129]. Telomeres are the truncated end of the chromosomes with repeat 5'TTAGGG3' arrays. In humans, they are 15 kb in length and protect the chromosome from exonuclease and ligases, and prevent the activation of DNA damage check points. With cellular senescence, there is a shortening of the telomeres with resultant chromosomal deletions and eventual cell death [130]. Immortalized cells are programmed to produce increased amounts of telomerase and, consequently, the cell achieves a state of immortality; although not without genetic and epigenetic drift in its unstable state [131]. Somewhat paradoxically, an enzyme expressed at low levels in untransformed eukaryotic cells becomes a marker of genetic instability at increased levels. A number of methods are available for measuring telomerase and telomeres. Many of these involve functional assays or RT-PCR techniques to assay the message [132]. Detera

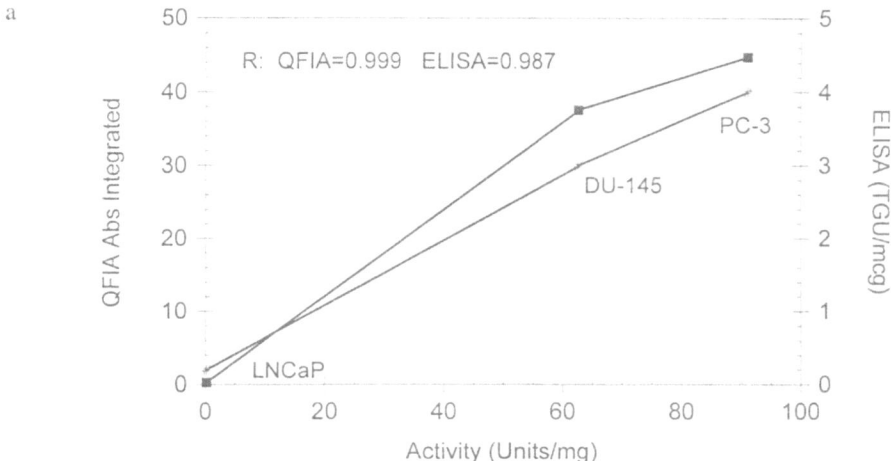

b

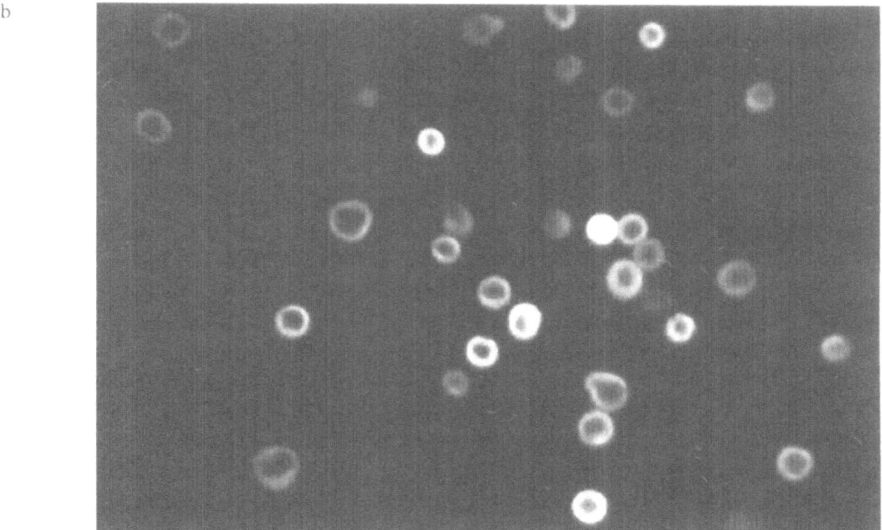

Figure 3. (a) Correlation of transglutaminase of human prostate cell lines by three methods. Cells were harvested and assayed for transglutaminase activity, amount of transglutaminase by ELISA or amount of transglutaminase by quantitative fluorescence image analysis. X-axis, transglutaminase activity; Y1-axis, quantitative fluorescence image analysis (#—#); Y2-axis, ELISA (■—■). Based on the QFIA and ELISA data for these cells, the lower limit of QFIA detection is approximately 10^{-19} moles of 10^5 molecules of transglutaminase per cell. (Provided by Paul Birckbichler). (b) Immunofluorescent staining of human prostate PC-3 cell line for transglutaminase. Cells were harvested, fixed, and assayed for transglutaminase by quantitative fluorescence image analysis, using a monoclonal antibody to tissue transglutaminase and a biotin-Texas Red detection system. Magnification 32X. (Provided by Paul Birckbichler)

mination of the protein sequence will facilitate production of antibodies to the telomerase which can then be assayed at the single cell level as demonstrated for transglutaminase (Fig. 3a). The heterogeneous expression of the enzyme is clearly documented in the photograph (Fig. 3b).

However, quantification of the protein does not necessarily translate to functionality because of other components contributing to the reaction such as binding proteins. Quantitative antibody assays at the single cell level may result in methods with clinical utility. Thus, with this biomarker, as with other biomarkers, a number of parameters contribute to genetic instability and the utility of a biomarker. How early the biomarker is perturbated in carcinogenesis may be reflected by slightly increased levels in the cancer field [15]. Coffey reported on increased telomerase in 12% of normal appearing cells in the adjacent field in three of 25 prostate cancer cases [133]. These observations should stimulate more precise studies in the future. The potential exists to use this marker in combination with other markers to predict which patients will develop biologically active disease and genetic instability. Initial studies indicated telomerase was expressed only in transformed cells, but more recent studies confirm it is expressed at low levels in peripheral (normal samples) blood lymphocytes and stem cells. Thus, it may be quantitatively up regulated during the cell cycle. There is a debate related to its quantitative expression during the cell cycle [134].

Since telomerase appears to be a late marker associated with transformation, some have suggested it as a target for cancer therapy. Quite frankly, Sharma's review of the subject was one of the most objective reviews of potential new cancer therapy I have read [135]. Sharma emphasized that telomerase is not expressed in all cancer cases and, therefore, alternate pathways must exist. (Genetically unstable cells are likely to find these pathways.) Secondly, he predictably raises the question that anti-telomerase agents might be toxic to stem cells and germ cells and other viable cells expressing telomerase at low levels. Additional studies quantifying this biomarker at the single cell level should provide further insight into its mechanisms of action, its influence on the microecosystem, and its relationship to genetic instability.

DNA methylation

DNA methylation represents a common functional mechanism for controlling gene expression and is important in invertebrates. Methylation of cytosine within CpG dinucleotides by the enzyme methyltransferase serves to control gene transcription. The mechanisms whereby this occurs are only now being elucidated. DNA methylation may be quantified by specific and nonspecific assay techniques [136].

Studies of methylation patterns indicate that punative suppressor genes, such as *Rb* and *p53*, and oncogenes may initially be involved in a variety of tumors, and the degree of methylation is variable [137]. Somatic hybridization experiments and cell culture experiments clearly reveal increased DNA methylation with aging, and in association with carcinogenesis [138]. DNA methylation is clearly an epigenetic mechanism for controlling suppressor gene function during carcinogenesis and embryogenesis [139]. The field of methylation research was advanced with an improvement in chromatographic techniques and with ligation-mediated PCR techniques developed by Müller in 1989 [136]. Conversion of the unmethylated cytosine to uracil facilitates the amplification of uracil and 5-methylcytosines with strand-specific primers using a PCR reaction.

With this technique, the amount of DNA required for methylation studies has been substantially reduced [136]. The specificity whereby one gene is hypermethylated by methyltransferase and the other is not involved in the regulatory events, requires further elucidation.

Methylation of DNA promoter regions presumably makes them inaccessible to the transcriptional apparatus [140]. Other studies indicate that feedback autoregulation pathways are related to the density of methylation of the promoter region [141]. The regulation of transcription by DNA methylation in some systems may depend on the phosphorylation on the interacting histones [142]. There is also evidence to suggest that the trace metal arsenic may affect the methylation of the promoter controlling suppressor genes such as *p53* [143]. This is potentially important because low levels of arsenic are ubiquitous in our environment.

DNA methylation is not only a mechanism for controlling gene expression, but has diagnostic and therapeutic implications as well. These include the detection of residual leukemic cells and by the inhibition of DNA methyltransferase in patients with acute leukemias. Particularly germane to this discussion is the observation that hyper-methylation precedes LOH or mutations on the *p53* gene in renal cell carcinomas. These results strongly suggest that DNA methylation is an epigenetic mechanism which may contribute to genetic instability [144].

DNA aneuploidy

Although aberrant ploidy has long been used as a marker for bladder cancer, the presence of cells with >5C DNA is not synonymous with aberrant ploidy [76], and is a useful marker of genetic instability. One immediate difference is that in measuring ploidy, one is attempting to extract a signal in the form of an aberrant cell population from the region where the DNA content of normal cells, which are usually in a large majority, is expressed [76]. In contrast, normal cells do not contain more than 5C DNA. The signal from abnormal cells, then, is separated from the normal signal, thereby greatly improving the signal to noise ratio. Cells with >5C DNA are generated by the genetic instability of transformed or transforming cells, exposure to clastogenic substances (e.g. smoking), or the presence of dividing aneuploid cell populations [64, 87, 105, 145]. Several studies have documented the clinical utility of DNA ploidy to improve the sensitivity of exfoliated urinary cytology [86–88, 96, 146, 147]. New techniques such as fluorescence *in situ* hybridization (FISH) are redefining ploidy to include gain or loss of one or more chromosomes, or even segments of a single chromosome or virus DNA [148–151]. This is possible because of the increased optical resolution of fluorescence and the implementation of new fluorescence probes, and combinations of probe assayed on multiple chromosomes simultaneously [152]. One can anticipate there will be an operational threshold wherein a correlation exists with genetic instability. It seems a threshold of aberrations occur prior to the onset of a transformed phenotype. This is clearly indicated in FISH studies in individuals who have previously had bladder cancer and who are at risk for recurrence [148, 149]. Perhaps the biomarker combination of upregulated telomerase and LOH defined by FISH will provide insight into the relationship between chromosomal aberrations and the nuclear matrix. Assaying these alterations at the single cell level may be most instructive.

Other potential phenotypic markers of genetic instability

Microsatellites, LOH, and gross chromosomal aberrations detected by comparative genomic hybridization are phenotypic biomarkers of effect, while DNA repair genes and their associated mutations are genotypic markers of genetic instability. The current dilemma is which biomarkers, or combination of biomarkers, reflect functional genetic instability. Genetic instability occurs when a cell is at least transiently immortalized, with uncontrolled growth associated with continued perturbation of the genetic machinery. It eventually forms a neoplasm that acquires the metastatic phenotype and circumvents therapeutic intervention. If the scientific community is to address genetic instability then a precise definition seems appropriate. From a clinical perspective, patients' tumors that express early biomarkers of effect should receive chemopreventive agents prior to the development of genetic instability. Monitoring biomarkers expressed at different intervals in the carcinogenic process during chemoprevention may be extremely useful for validating more precisely when genetic instability develops and what the thresholds of biomarkers are that determine genetic instability.

LOH has been observed in a number of neoplasms as specific chromosomes and are preferentially affected in a given neoplasm. For specific cancer types, LOH appears to occur preferentially in a number of chromosomes. In bladder cancer, LOH has been observed in chromosomes 9 and 17 [153, 154]. LOH has been summarized for a number of tumors [155–158]. An important concept emphasized by Field is that "LOH may not necessarily be indicative of a tumor suppressor gene," because the presence or absence is defined by the relative imbalance in the staining of two bands and thus, may reflect an amplification or a deletion on the contralateral chromosome [159]. Thus, the methods themselves are limited in their accuracy. Fractional allelic loss (FAL) is another approach which has been used as a marker for genetic instability. FAL has been correlated with genetic instability by correlating FAL with the grade and stage of disease in a variety of tumors [159]. In general, more severe perturbations are observed with increasing FAL.

Mechanisms of genetic instability

Somatic hybridization changes in biomarker profiles provide clues to their relative importance and highlight the relevance of the previous discussion on biomarkers. Their relative contributions of genetic and epigenetic mechanisms to carcinogenesis remain to be defined and may be different for each individual tumor. Defining or determining epigenetic factors must be integrated with an understanding of genetically regulated signaling pathways. The ultimate functionality must also occur at the protein level and the mechanisms are likely to be highly variable.

Establishing contributing factors requires the ability to quantify the effects of mutational and nonmutational events in cells, and this includes alterations in epigenetic signaling pathways and specific gene products which herald the metastatic phenotype. Molecular biology techniques including DNA sequencing have contributed to precise base-pair analysis and as mentioned previously, microchip array technology provides a means to screen for DNA sequence changes, but these do not facilitate measurements at the single cell level. Negatively regulated changes may be missed. Proto-oncogenes, tumor suppressor genes and, more recently, DNA repair genes contribute to the process. What is less clear are the mechanisms contributing to the more gross chromosomal aberrations such as DNA translocations, deletions, amplifications, and factors contributing to DNA repair or strand scissors such as the nuclear matrix and other factors that effect the mitotic spindle. Many of the known carcinogens such as oxidative stress affect both the cytoskeleton and the DNA. Improved methods are needed for quantifying nonmutational effects.

When I began to review the subject of biomarkers of the genitourinary tract in relation to our own research on the cytoskeleton, I questioned the relative contributions of genetic and epigenetic mechanisms for the first time [15]. Previously, I had fully accepted Knudson's hypothesis of suppressor and proto-oncogenes in carcinogenesis as the driving primary force in cancer development [160–162]. The foundation for the mutational events was seemingly supported by inherited disorders such as those attributed to the Li Fraumeni syndrome [163–166] and retinoblastoma [167], or genetically acquired thyroid cancer. However, this obviously was not the total story, because of the occurrence of gross chromosomal translocations [168] and deletions [155, 169, 170], and the marked genetic polymorphism, which contribute to the cancer process.

Even in the case of breast cancer, one gene (*BRCA1*) predicts breast cancer development only in 50% to 90% of those with the abnormal gene and a family history [171, 172]. Although certainly a major advance, the single gene is important in only 10% to 13% of total patients with breast cancer [173]. One cannot question that there are specific genes which control the balance of proliferation, apoptosis, gene repair, and growth control, all of which contribute to the evolution of the carcinogenic process. Richmond, Prehns' article, "Do mutations beget cancer or does cancer beget mutations?" emphasizes a number of salient points which others have failed to address, and now must be countered by evolving new concepts in models for carcinogenesis [174].

Addressing the mechanism of carcinogenesis in humans is a highly complex issue. Most *in vitro* models of carcinogenesis have utilized cell culture systems which severely limit the facets of stromal and epithelial paracrine interactions, not to mention endocrine influences on the integrated system [83, 175]. The use of animal models to study carcinogenesis, although informative, is artificial in the dose, and lacks the subtle background of human genetic susceptibility and associated polymorphisms. Patients with clinical disease, cancer families and alternatively occupationally-exposed cohorts who are at increased cancer risks provide a unique opportunity to detect the molecular mechanisms of carcinogenesis in longitudinal follow-up studies. However, the mechanisms may not be the same in nonoccupational cancers, and occupational cancers are estimated to cause 10%–20% of all malignancies [176, 177].

Several observations drive me to consider that epigenetic factors are more important in the perturbation of the functioning signaling network of normal growth control. The first is the fact that all spontaneous morphological models have not fit the conventional theories of carcinogenesis. Secondly, gross chromosomal karyotypic analysis reveals that there are gross chromosomal alterations in the peripheral blood lymphocytes in patients with bladder cancer and carcinogen-exposed individuals which are different from controls [178]. One might hypothesize that patients who develop occupational bladder cancer develop the disease because the carcinogen is present in higher quantities in the bladder than the blood. However, an alternative explanation is there is a balanced network of signaling pathways which makes the bladder more perturbated by the specific gross chromosomal aberration, or a generalized defect may exist in DNA repair [179, 180].

This, in many respects, parallels the concept that very diverse creatures in the hierarchy of evolutionary development have common genes. This is not surprising, given that organs with the same genes are profoundly different. There are quantitative differences in the phenotypic expression of functional molecules that contribute to the differential development of an individual or an organ. Arguments concerning the epigenetic mechanisms of carcinogenesis are quite convincing and parallel the thinking we favored several years earlier and those of others before that. To obtain convincing evidence of epigenetic mechanisms will require the careful documentation of the genetic and epigenetic forces during the precancerous process prior to the onset of genetic instability [181]. Finally, it should be remembered that at any particular point along an evolutionary process, looking backward the process appears to be linear and direct. In our own family trees, a straight line can be drawn to any particular ancestor, but this ignores the contributions of all the other forbears. The same is true with a tumor cell and its potentially numerous progeny. It is possible that tumors appear to be clonal only because genetic instability and selection lead to the extinction of all but a single tumor cell lineage.

p53 – the cancer gene: A model for mutagenic mechanisms

Elegant research has recently evolved regarding the postulated functional mechanisms of p53 activity, and there is a growing scientific support for the importance of this and other genes in the carcinogenic process [182, 183]. Part of the reason for this enthusiasm are the advances in the understanding of molecular biology and new techniques that facilitate defining specific mutations in this gene, and correlating these mutations with phenotypic expression of the protein product in relation to the gene's function. An insightful appreciation has evolved regarding signaling pathway expression [184–186], and correlation with the risk for cancer and response to therapy. The discussion which follows will relate to the functional role p53 signaling pathways, DNA repair; genetic instability, proliferation and apoptosis. As an example the mutagenic alterations which affect the signaling pathways in bladder and prostate cancer will be discussed, and the differences between low and high-grade pathways will be considered. Throughout the course of the discussion, an attempt will be made to relate general concepts pertinent to clinical problems of individual risk assessment and strategic therapeutic options, and overall concepts pertinent to mutational events in carcinogenesis leading to genetic instability.

The p53 gene is located on chromosome 17-p 13.1, and codes for a phosphoprotein consisting of 393 amino acids, with a molecular weight of 53 kd [182]. Although the discussion will focus on the mutational events in p53, it is important to recognize that the function of this gene may be affected not only by mutations, but by LOH, translocations, deletions, and amplifications as reflected by microsatellite formation [187–189]. Which of these is most relevant to a specific tumor remains to be defined by a variety of molecular methods and is extremely complex because of the genetic or epigenetic mechanisms and the complex network of signaling pathways. Mutations in the p53 gene may affect any one of four functional domains which can be correlated with protein functional phenotypes. Critical to cell-cycle regulation and DNA repair and apoptosis is the N-terminus domain consisting of 42 amino acids [190]. p53 protein targets CDKN1/p21, inhibiting cyclin-dependent kinase Cdk [191, 192] and GADD45. During DNA repair, the p21 protein is upregulated and binds to cyclin-dependent kinases, which then inhibit the phosphorylation of Rb, arresting the cell in G-1 [193, 194]. An integral part of the signaling pathways are p21 and GADD45 which bind to PCNA and block cellular proliferation [195, 196]. These interactions serve to illustrate a linkage between increased cellular proliferation, DNA repair and apoptosis, all related to carcinogenesis. Other portions of the p53 molecule include the specific DNA binding domain, associated with exons 5–8, a tetramerization domain, and a C-terminus domain, which regulates p53 binding to specific DNA sequences [182]. When DNA damage occurs by any one of a variety of mechanisms, the normal functioning wild-type p53 will induce programmed cell death by upregulating BAX while reciprocally downregulating *bcl2* expression, thus linking p53 functional phenotype to apoptosis [197–199]. The point is that any one of a number of mutations in any one of five or six proteins in the immediate network of signaling pathways may result in the same fundamental functional phenotypic deficit. There are a variety of pathways whereby the overall functional phenotype may be altered and the most important one will be related to its frequency of expression. The final common pathways of genetic and epigenetic alterations result in a process of altered "functional genomics." Functional genomics may be the result of gain or loss of function. It is clear from this discussion that there are multiple signaling pathways affecting multiple genes, and an array of relevant and irrelevant mutations making a complex network of regulation analogous in many respects to a neural network.

Two pathways have been hypothesized for bladder cancer. One involves mutations in *p53*. This pathway is generally related to high grade disease and carcinoma *in situ*. The high and low grade pathways involve potential tumor suppressor genes in both the long and the short arm of chromosome 9 [200–204] and chromosome 17 [205, 206]. However the pathways may not be nearly as clear-cut as hypothesized, since only 60% of the high grade tumors have mutational or more gross genetic abnormalities identified on chromosome 17p.1 [205, 206]. Given the complex set of genetic interactions discussed above with *Cdk*, *GADD45* and *Rb* [207], one can immediately hypothesize that a constellation of other mutagenic events could be affecting the network of signaling pathways. The Hubert Humphrey case, demonstrating *p53* genetic abnormalities early in the history of his disease, suggests *p53* may be an early cancer genetic alteration in high grade disease [208]. The frequency with which this occurs is unknown, but if it correlated with genetic instability associated with 5C DNA ER, then one would anticipate greater than 20% of all tumors to have genetic alterations in this gene or other associated genes.

Czernick mapped *p53* alterations by microsatellite analyses in chromosome 17 in five bladder cases [209]. Three-fifths of the bladders had abnormalities in *p53* with focal or plaque-like areas suggesting a clonal origin, while others were intermittently dispersed. The fundamental observation is that many of the abnormalities are clonal, while others are more sporadic. A gene vector of chromosome 17 summarized a list of tested markers [210]. Allelic and mutational losses were both observed early in carcinogenesis. These results support the hypothesis that both mutagenic and epigenetic mechanisms occur and may be related or independent of one another. One might speculate that low grade tumors may be more frequently associated with epigenetic alterations than high grade tumors.

p53 mutations have also been studied in prostate cancer, and it is estimated that 35% of localized prostate cancers have *p53* mutations [211]. While *p53* mutations are more common in hormone-refractory prostate cancer [212], the question to be addressed is, "Are these mutations a result of genetic instability or do they contribute to it?" Analysis of *p53* mutations in PIN lesions (prostatic intra-epithelial neoplasia) or in normal appearing epithelial cells in prostate glands with PIN or with cancer, will assist in clarifying this issue. When multiple studies are combined, gene vectors confirm that there are certain "hot spot" base-pair sequences at which specific repeated base pair mutations occur [213]. It is not surprising that when the functionality of genetic mutations is analyzed, there is gain or loss of functional genetic effects [190, 214–216]. Because of the network of signaling pathways, and without knowing the constellation of network genetic and epigenetic changes, both quantitative and qualitative, one cannot be sure a specific mutation is a result of the mutational event, not to mention the possibility that an epigenetic factor mediated through a new energy level could be contributing to the ultimate functional phenotype. Now *p53* is not only a major contributing factor to the final stages of carcinogenesis because its inactivation represents one means to escape apoptotic death [217, 218], it also allows genetic instability to develop. Mutations are therefore not removed. With a loss of DNA repair, the stage is set for the development of malignant instability [219, 220].

Given these complexities, some have suggested correcting the *p53* defect. Once again, in my opinion, we are naive because we have fallen into the trap of attempting to modulate a presumed functional genetic defect which occurs against the background of a complex network of genetic instability and tumor heterogeneity. This is the latest mousetrap which defies scientific logic. Numerous start-up companies have been founded expending precious resources with limited success, based on similar faulty logic. Nature has provided us with inherited mistakes in our genetic machinery which provide clues to the eventual appreciation of a system's complexity; *p53* and its related signaling networks fall into this category. In many respects, the complexities which have evolved in the study of this gene are similar to the complexities of T and B cell function that evolved following the discovery of the bursa of Fabricius and thymus-derived T cell immunity. These anatomical observations triggered our interest in T and B cell-deficiency states associated with cellular and humoral immunity, not to mention the intricacies of the cytokine networks. Understanding the complexities of the immune system has been tedious and is still continuing twenty years later. Any attempt to correct a system which is in a continuous state of networking plagued by genetic instability is *not* cost-effective. This is unlike the AIDS problem which, intuitively, I have always felt we would eventually solve because it is perpetrated by an infectious process. But like cancer, its escape of therapeutic measures resides in the mutational capacity of the AIDS active and latent virus [152, 221–223]. Thus, it is logical to treat it in its early stages to avoid the complexities of the mutating virus and in this respect it parallels the cancer problem. Genetic engineering for AIDS and cancer are more likely to be successful prior to genetic instability.

The great genius of Watson and Crick led to the unraveling of the genetic code and the structure of the double helix, all of which resulted in the birth of molecular biology and an enhanced understanding of genetic signaling. It is a double helix containing intons and exons with signaling starts and stops. Although insightful, it opens up a Pandora's box of the complex signals required to read the basic genetic code. It fails to emphasize post-transcriptional and post-translational alterations in the complex network of signaling pathways. It has "diverted" our attention from proteins which are the actual functional molecules that respond to the network signaling pathways and control DNA synthesis, both in homeostatic regulation and metastasis. However, the potential exists that understanding these signaling pathways will lead us to a new level.

Strohman has summarized the Kuhnian revolution as paradigm shifts concerned with the rise and fall of major physical science modes guiding scientific thought [224]. In his article, Strohman challenges Adam Wilkin's conclusion that paradigm shifts may be over in biology, specifically as they relate to the Watson-Crick era where the proper theory of the gene has evolved into a molecular form of genetic determinism [224]. Many scientists have been enamoured with the concepts and tools of modern molecular biology which have served us well in comprehending the functional mechanisms of gene regulation and protein synthesis. The Watson-Crick model has provided us with a framework for interpreting and thinking conceptually about biomarkers, and relates specifically to the inter-relationship between DNA and markers of susceptibility, but does not encompass the exogenous and endogenous environment that subtly perturb the organism as a whole. In order to develop a new model to explain the relationship between genetic determinism and our environment, it is useful to reflect on the past. Then, and currently, much emphasis is placed on the importance of the Human Genome Project, particularly as it relates to biomarkers of susceptibility. A limitation of the Watson-Crick model with its emphasis on molecular biology, is that it does not explain the network of protein interactions which may be altered by their environment. Even when considering genetic instability driven by alterations in DNA, there are inter-related proteins and enzymes so important to DNA repair processes that control functional evolution. My personal view is that cancer, and other diseases as well, are related primarily to quantitative alterations in normal proteins, driven by both genetic and epigenetic mechanisms that perturb the complex network of signaling pathways.

Oxidative stress in carcinogenesis and genetic instability

The relevance of oxidative stress to carcinogenesis is not fully understood and the importance of oxidative stress to tumor cytoxicity and carcinogeneses requires clarification. Both genetic and epigenetic mechanisms of carcinogenesis may be affected by oxidative stress. The purpose of this section is to present the fundamental mechanisms of oxygen free radical generation and describe the actions of oxygen free radicals in biologic systems. Literature is cited to relate key points but is not all inclusive. In aerobic eukaryotic cells, oxygen free radicals are an integral component of the endogenous multiple mitochondrial metabolic pathways, as well as NADP-oxidase in cellular membranes. Directly related to the production of the oxygen free radicals are iron (Fe) and copper (Cu). The bioavailability of these metals is dependent on compartmentalization and binding proteins such as metallothionein [225]. Leukocytes generate reactive oxygen species (ROS), as a part of an organism's defense against tumor development and bacterial invasion, and are another endogenous source of oxygen free radicals.

Exogenous generation of ROS may result from xenobiotic exposure, chemotherapy, and foreign bodies. All of these, including generation of ROS from lipids frequently generate $\cdot OH$ or $RO\cdot$ and $HOCl\cdot$ products. These exogenous factors form oxygen free radical intermediates. Detection of oxygen free radicals *in vivo* is not a simple issue, but significant advances have been made with spin-trap techniques using salicylates and nitrone-based free radical traps (NRTs) [226]. A balance of ROS is maintained *in vivo* by cellular catalase, superoxide dismutase,

Table 3. Oxidative stress in carcinogenesis and genetic instability

Oxidative process	Products	Possible influence	References
Lipid oxidation	Aldehydes	Reacts with proteins and nucleic acid and may be mutagenic	235 236
	General oxidized protein ADF. GST-n, GHS ↑ Oxidized LDL	Chemotherapy resistant, tumor heterogeneity	239 235 236 234 233 232
Protein oxidation	Protease inhibitor damage α_1-proteinase inhibitor α_2-macroglobulin	Proteinase activity increase - Invasion and metastasis	244 247 248 249 250 240 251 252
	Cytoskeleton and nuclear cytoskeleton alterations, microfilament network	Malignant transformation, Tumor heterogeneity	
	ATP depletion Oxidation of actin SH group Cross linking of actin		253 254
Nucleic acid oxidation	Conformational change in DNA template mutations Strand breaks	Replication errors May contribute to Carcino-genesis	255 256 236 239 232 237 257 256
	Altered bases 8-Hydroxyguanine Oncogene activation DNA protein cross-links DNA damage Double-strand RNA protein interactions	Chromosome aberration Genomic instability DNA lesions Malignant transformation	
Signal transduction pathway	c-*myc* c-*fos* c-*jun* hMTH1 BCl-2, Fas TNF-α NF-$_\kappa$B Protein kinases Phosphorylation	Cell proliferation Malignant transformation Overexpression of mRNA HIV-1 gene expression Transcriptional activation Overexpression of wild-type HSP27 Apoptosis Tumorigenic conversion	230 231 258 229 228 259 260 261 262 232 229

Abbreviations used: LDL, low-density lipoprotein, TNF, tumor necrosis factor, HIV, human immunodeficiency virus, NF-$_\kappa$B, transcription factor nuclear factor-kappa B, ADF, adult T cell leukemia - derived factor, GST-P, glutathione-S-transferase II hMTH1, human homologue of the *E. coli mutT* gene, HSP27, heat shock protein 27.

glutathione reductase, and glutathione peroxidase. These enzymes may also be used to detect ROS in biological systems.

Specific enzymes are upregulated with transformation, such as glutathione transferase II in prostate cancer and kidney cancers. Furthermore, the type of polymerase in the cell may influence the type of mutation which ultimately results from oxidative DNA damage. Other more indirect controls on the effects of oxygen free radicals involve heat shock proteins. Huot showed an increase in heat shock proteins protected against actin fragmentation by the phosphorylation of HSP27, known to regulate micro- filament dynamics through the activation of MAP-KAP kinase-2 [227]. What is apparent from this review is that signaling pathways of reactive oxidative stress (ROS) are complex and that sorting out the relevance in each system is not a trivial issue. Jacobson stressed the importance of these complex pathways as they relate to apoptosis (programed cell death) [228]. The mechanisms related to inflammation or peroxidation occur through multiple biochemical pathways, including direct effects on cellular proteins [229–235].

The development of sensitive new techniques for measuring oxidative stress provides new information pertaining to the mechanisms of carcinogenesis and other diseases. Floyd reviewed the various mechanisms by which oxygen free radicals can damage DNA and potentially promote carcinogenesis [236] (see Tab. 4). Oxygen free radicals may occur at the tumor site as a result of a number of specific and nonspecific immunological mechanisms which attract a variety of leukocytes. In the enriched cytokine environment leukocytes and macrophages release oxygen free radicals. Activated macrophages are cellular scavengers that amplify the cytotoxic potential of the immune system, but paradoxically may promote genetic instability by affecting the cytokines or by producing direct DNA damage (e.g., formation of 8-OH-guanine). For example, oxygen

Table 4. Mechanisms and biological effects of oxidative stress

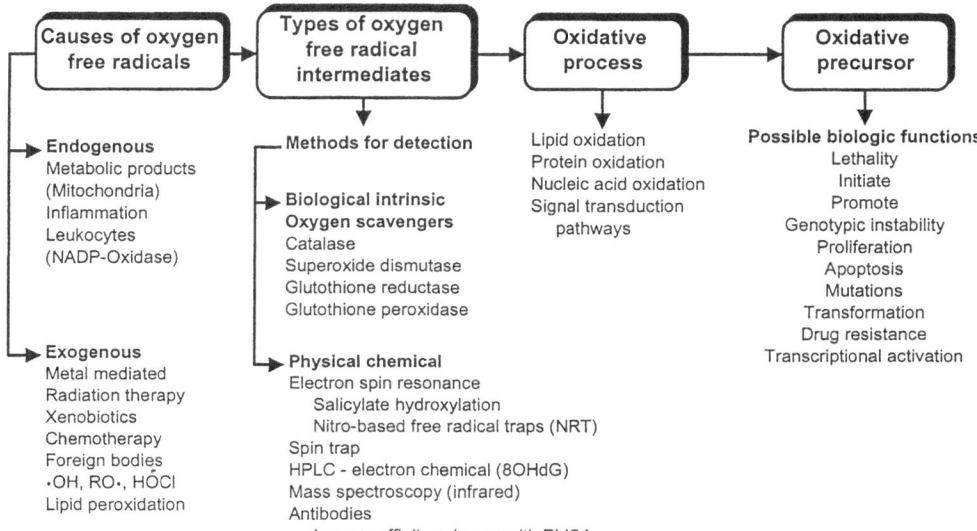

free radicals may be cytotoxic or stimulate cellular proliferation just as chemotherapeutic agents may promote carcinogenesis and genetic instability [237, 238].

In support of a paradoxical role of potentially cytotoxic activated macrophages is the observation that in some experimental systems they are more often associated with metastasis and malignant transformation, presumably through the oxygen free radical mechanism [239]. Supporting this view, tumor-activated macrophages were mutagenic when assayed in the Ames test and embryocyte mammalian tumor systems, indicating the potential for epigenetic mechanism. These biological effects were abrogated by a variety of active oxygen free radical scavengers, confirming the specificity of the oxygen free radical mechanism. To investigate the potential dual function (tumor promotion or regression) of active oxygen species, the effect of various concentrations of oxygen free radicals was investigated. Because of our interest in bladder cancer, we initially investigated the cytotoxic affects of methylene blue as a potential therapy for bladder cancer. This seemed like a logical approach because methylene blue is FDA approved for clinical use. When injected intravenously, the dye is excreted in the urine and identifies the ureteral orifices at the time of cystoscopy, which occasionally are difficult to visualize because of a variety of pathological conditions. When HUC-BC cells (human urothelial cells, an untransformable clone developed by C.A. Reznikoff) are exposed to methylene blue and white light, a constellation of events

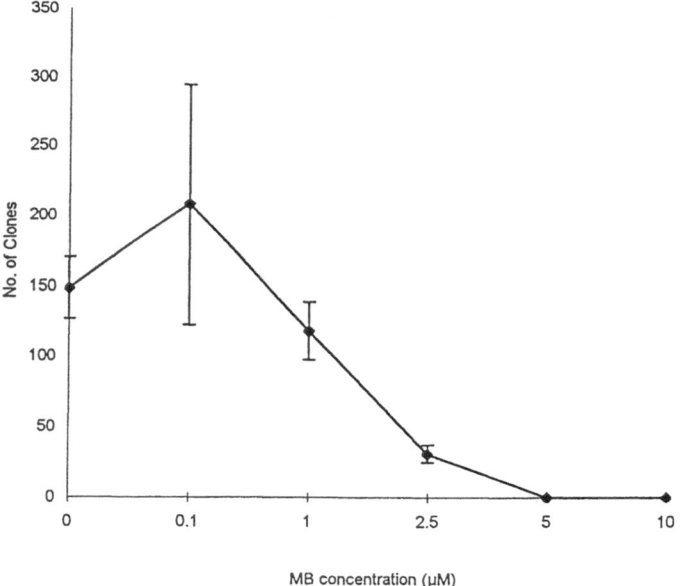

MB concentration (μM)

Figure 4. HUC-BC cells were seeded at 1000 cells/dish (60 mm) in triplicate, and were treated with methylene blue at the indicated concentration. Following 24 h of culture, methylene blue was added by diluting 1 mM stock solution by serum free medium. Following exposure to light for 30 minutes, the dye was decanted twice with PBS. The treated cells were then grown in complete medium for 10–14 days. Clones were stained by Giemsa and counted. The biphasic curve demonstrates the variable affects of oxidative stress that may stimulate cell growth, i.e. proliferation and cell death.

occur. The multiple effects include the formation of 8-0H guanine and protein cross-linking (Y. Liang-Hemstreet, unpublished data). The differential effect of oxidative stress on proliferation and cell death is illustrated in the dose response of methylene blue treatment of HUC-BC cells in a clonogenic assay (see Fig. 4). At low doses increased proliferation occurs and at high doses, it is decreased and cell death is predominant. These results clearly illustrate the dichotomous effects of oxygen free radicals.

The importance of the cytoskeleton and the nuclear matrix, both substrates for oxygen free radicals, in relation to genetic instability is a novel new area for research. Alterations in the cytoskeleton by epigenetic or genetic mechanisms may affect both the cytoplasmic and nuclear cytoskeleton, including nuclear matrix proteins [240, 241]. Oxygen perturbation of the cytoskeleton affects key functions, such as cellular differentiation, proliferation, and apoptosis, and can contribute to malignant transformation. Stimulation of HL-60 cells with phorbol esters results in a decrease in F-actin and an increase in cytoplasmic G-actin when assayed by quantitative fluorescence image analysis [242]. Treatment of HL-60 cells with DMSO or cis-retinoic acid retinoids corrects this response and normalizes the F-actin [240]. Interestingly, quantification of the cytoplasmic changes in F-actin paralleled the risks for recurrent bladder cancer [105]. Treatment of patients with non-invasive bladder cancer with BCG corrected the DNA 5C ER rate, a marker of genetic instability, but did not correct the early dedifferentiation defect [105]. Instillation of DMSO into the bladder weekly for six weeks corrected the defect in cytoskeleton G- and F-actin [243]. These clinical results confirm the perturbation of cytoplasmic actin during malignant transformation, both *in vitro* and *in vivo*. In addition to the effects of oxidative stress on gene activation, it may directly affect actin polymerization by epigenetic effects perturbing signaling pathways.

Barboro and Patrone have suggested the nuclear matrix may be a key to malignant transformation, serving as a scaffold for organizing the DNA during transcription [244]. Almost simultaneously, we were focusing our attention on nuclear actin in association with malignant transformation in the HUC-BC and HUC-PC tissue culture model, the rat hepatocellular malignant transformation model, and in human bladder cancer. Barboro reported changes in more than nine nuclear matrix proteins associated with transformation [244]. We have clearly demonstrated changes in the nuclear actin during transformation, using quantitative fluorescence image analysis. The results in Table 5 clearly demonstrate changes in nuclear actin in association with transformation in the three different tumor model systems, including human bladder cancer. These observations are intriguing, because the nuclear cytoskeleton can be perturbed both by genetic and epigenetic mechanisms, including oxidative stress (Tabs 1 and 3). Consequently,

Table 5. Nuclear actin changes in transformation

	In vitro Huc-RE cell line		*In vivo* AAF-induced rat liver tumor		Human samples bladder tumor		
	Control	Transformed	Control	Transformed	Normal	Control	Tumor
Nuclear G	19.2±2	28±2	77.0±33.3	158.3±767	3.17±0.45		5.53±0.68
Nuclear F	32±4	13±2	210.7±114.7	102.3±42.3	48.1±5.3		38.9±2.2

quantitative changes in the nuclear and cytoplasmic actin may reflect common pathways in carcinogenesis, leading to genetic instability and tumor heterogeneity.

High concentrations of oxygen free radicals are mutagenic and cytotoxic, whereas lower doses, which probably more closely parallel *in vivo* conditions, stimulate cellular proliferation. The disease of carcinogenesis includes cellular initiation and promotion, both of which are enhanced by proliferation. Proliferation is balanced by apoptosis [245]. It has recently been shown that the molecular machinery for apoptotic cell death involves a family of ICE (interleukin converting enzyme)-related proteases or caspases [246]. Inhibition of ICE proteases reduces apoptosis and may act through a molecular cascade event. However, the precise mechanisms of action for the ICE proteases are not clear. Recent observations suggest cytoskeletal networks such as actin may function, as the G-actin binds to DNAase1 inhibiting apoptotic DNA degeneration. Consequently, a decrease in G-actin will, thereby, increase the bioavailability of DNAase1 to participate in apoptosis (manuscript in preparation). Using zymography and QFIA (quantitative fluorescence image analysis) techniques, we have demonstrated that the polymerization agent jasplakinolide (JAS) decreases G-actin by polymerizing to F-actin and increases DNAase1 in HL-60 cells. This leads directly to apoptosis. In K562 cells, the jasplakinolide induced a transient actin polymerization and membrane bleb formation followed by a predominant F-actin disruption with G2/M arrest. The differential response of these cell lines reflects a difference in the cell lines' signaling pathways and, in a sense, reflects tumor heterogeneity. This study confirms that all three major morphometric features of apoptosis (apoptotic body formation, membrane blebbing and DNA fragmentation) are regulated by the cytoskeletal network. Thus, the complex signaling pathways for both proliferation and apoptosis may be orchestrated through the cytoskeletal network by a common functional phenotypic pathway. Similar arguments can be made for regulation through genetically regulated signaling pathways. Whatever the mechanisms of oxygen free radical scavengers, whether nutritional or therapeutic, are germane to cancer prevention and may promote or retard genetic instability [232]. Current epidemiological studies support the importance of both vitamins D and E in prostate carcinogenesis, as well as in other malignancies. The duality of effects of vitamins may be related to the quantitative differential effects of oxygen free radicals in the biological system. Enzymes such as GST-Π (glutathione-S-transferase-Π) in prostate are more directly implicated as an inhibitors of oxygen free radicals and may explain the exogenous effects of selenium, an antioxidant in preliminary studies.

Tumor heterogeneity, genetic instability, and the organs' cellular ecosystem

Understanding an organ's ecosystem is instructive for unraveling the complex factors that contribute to genetic instability. It is not enough to study biomarkers in transformed cells or even pretransformed cells, unless it is in the context of their microecosystem. Both the bladder and the prostate are derived from the same genome. Both reside in the pelvis, and both are embryologically derived from mesoderm and endoderm. Each organ's biological potential and predetermined signaling pathways are driven by genetically programmed DNA, and cytoplasmic factors (mitrochondrial DNA), and their microecosystem. Understanding the functional regulation within each of these two systems is quite intriguing, and should facilitate defining biomarkers for risk and therapeutic approaches for treating individuals at risk. If the ecosystem's regulation system could be comprehended at the protein level with the same precision that mutations and base pairs code for gene transcription and RNA translation, a number of therapeutic approaches might be possible. This is not a simple task. We recognize that most diseases, such as cancer and heart disease, are determined by multiple factors. Over 200 molecules or enzymes affect heart disease, and most of these were initially appreciated at the protein level. Yet, some have searched for and suggested that a single gene may be responsible for the malignant metastatic phenotype in prostate cancer. To illustrate these concepts, the similarities and differences in the bladder and prostate will be discussed because these are familiar subjects.

The bladder is a specialized hollow vessel embryologically derived from the hindgut and consisting of a neuromuscular component shielded by an impermeable epithelial layer. The muscularis is lined by a basal layer consisting of overlying transitional cells capped by an umbrella cell layer capable of expansion and contraction mediated by voluntary and involuntary neurological signaling pathways. Most transitional cells within the bladder are in a resting state, but during carcinogenesis they may proliferate more rapidly and respond to growth stimulation. The increased number of exfoliated cells in a patient's urine with premalignant disease, compared to the normal bladder, supports this statement.

Specialized histopathological features of the transitional epithelium maintain membrane impermeability to solutes, bacteria infection, and potential chemical toxicants. Contributing to the protection of the bladder epithelium are desmosomes, specialized ion pumps and proteoglycans [263]. All are vital elements that contribute to the biochemical and morphological architecture relevant to stromal epithelial interactions. Within the bladder cells, a number of metabolic pathways includ-

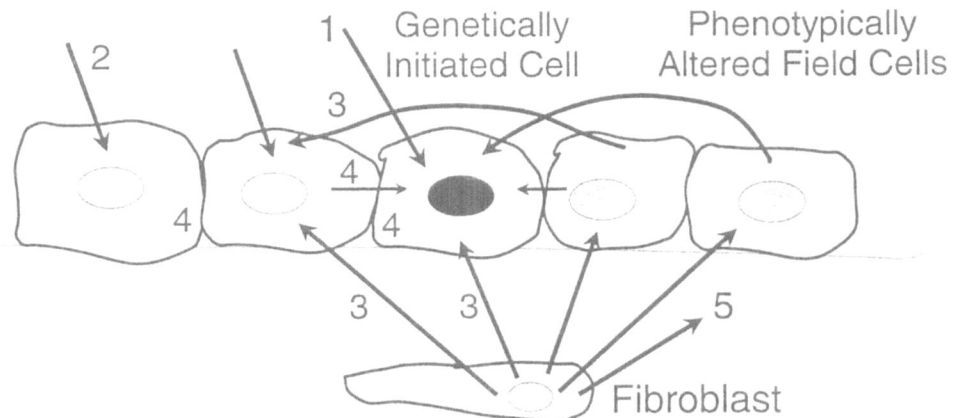

Figure 5. Chemoprevention in the bladder can function through a variety of signaling pathways, as well as act directly in a cell: (1) Can induce apoptotic death in initiated cells; (2) Can induce differentiation in field cells; (3) Paracrine interactions through stromal or other epithelial cells can suppress malignant phenotype; (4) Juxtacrine interactions and cell surface-mediated interactions with neighboring cells can suppress malignant phenotype; (5) Restore extracellular matrix to differentiation-promoting form.

ing genetically controlled acetylation and P-450 oxidative enzymes may biologically alter exogenous exposures [264, 265]. A constellation of genetic polymorphism affects the metabolism of most toxicants, related to the general health of the host [266–268].

Figure 5 represents a diagram of the bladder and the potentially complex categories of signaling pathways which contribute to the homeostatic mechanisms. Variable expression of biomarkers in the transitional epithelium is normal, reflecting alterations in the organ's biochemical ecosystem and, in a sense, illustrates normal cellular heterogeneity. For instance, Messing showed EGF is normally expressed in the basal layer but in disease may be observed in the more superficial urothelium [269]. Rao reported on the biochemical field changes within the bladder during tumorigenesis [15]. A differential expression of phenotypic biomarkers was observed between the tumor, the area adjacent to the tumor, and the distant, normal-appearing uroepithelium. In this study, G-actin was abnormal in 60% of normal-appearing uroepithelial cells distant from the tumor. These studies emphasize the importance of biochemical field disease and subtle quantitative differences in totally normal-appearing cells. Pathological field changes and associated normal heterogeneity are a crucial component of the molecular basis for bladder cancer. Field biochemical alterations can be used as biomarkers for individual risk assessment and cancer prevention strategies. Protein biochemical normal heterogeneity and field disease are of course, orchestrated through complex signaling pathways driven by genetic and epigenetic factors. I have previously mentioned the work of Czernick, who is currently mapping the phenotypic biomarkers DNA *p53* mutations in the biochemical field, building on the concepts established by Rao [15, 209].

The exogenous exposures and susceptibility factors ultimately determine the premalignant phenotype of the bladder's ecosystem. Important contributing exogenous factors related to bladder cancer include occupational and nonoccupational exposure (e.g. cigarette smoke). The combination of exogenous exposure with DNA may cause adduct formation. Even though a dose response relationship with adducts has been observed, adduct formation does not translate to DNA damage without multiple susceptibility factors. Genetically regulated metabolic products such as benzopyrene potentially may damage DNA [270] but because of the complex interactions, genetic factors alone will not predict individual risks.

The ecosystem of the prostate is anatomically and biochemically more complex than the bladder. The inability of cells in the prostate from one lobe of the gland to seed the opposite lobe facilitates a differential analysis of the organ's microenvironment and distribution of the signaling pathways related to field cancerization and field effects. This is in contrast to the bladder, where the cytokines and clonal seeding in the "closed" compartment confound interpretation. A schematic diagram of the prostate gland and the complexity of its anatomical structure and signaling pathways is given in Figure 6. The prostate consists anatomically of four lobes containing a complex set of glands. The central and transitional zone ducts drain the more central area, while other ducts located in the peripheral zone drain the cancer-prone region. These glands provide the necessary enzymatic and nutritional support for sperm on its journey to fertilization. Understanding the normal anatomy is useful for studying biomarker expression in relation to normal cellular heterogeneity, which potentially exists. For instance, benign growths of the prostate generally develop in the central zone. In contrast, cancer of the prostate arises primarily in the peripheral zone which, fortunately, is located adjacent to the rectum, and is amenable to rectal examination by the educated finger. Normal biomarker levels may vary in different compartments, an area of

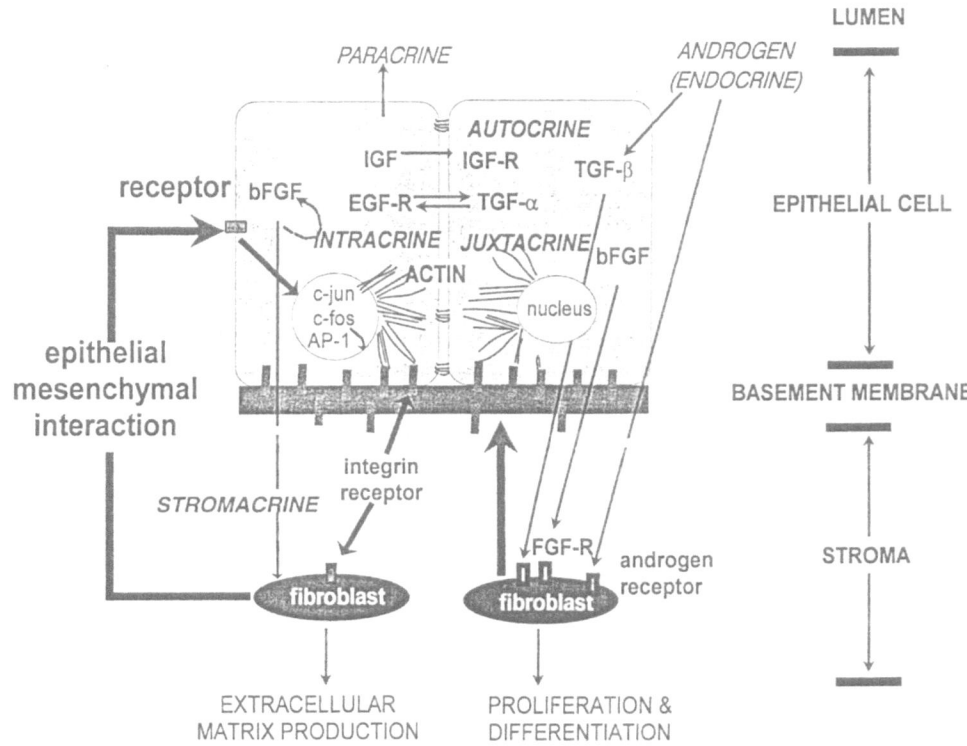

Figure 6. Illustrations of actual and potential modes of growth control reflecting the multiple factors potentially influencing the microecosystem. Adapted from *Biologic Markers in Urinary Toxicology*, 1993.

research for the future, and these variations must be considered in determining biomarker thresholds.

Given the stromal-epithelial architecture of the prostate, it is difficult to visualize how PIN could be multifocal without a change in the microenvironment of the gland prior to the development of PIN. As discussed previously, we have observed a field disease change in the bladder with alterations in biomarkers, and hypothesize that a similar approach may be used to identify individuals at risk for biologically active prostate cancer. Confirmation of the corresponding pathology in the bladder could be achieved with touch preps with cytologic and histopathologic correlation. In the prostate gland, cytological correlations with fine needle aspirations (FNAs) are somewhat more complicated because the cancer within the prostate may be multifocal or without pattern recognition, or definitive cytological morphology definition. However, FNA cytology has been shown to have an accuracy of 85% to 95% in comparison to core biopsies [271, 272]. To facilitate interpretation, biomarkers for specific cell types such as vimentin and cytokerations, may be employed to distinguish stromal from epithelial elements [273]. Interpretation of the biomarker results in this organ system thus requires a careful correlation between histopathological staining and samples obtained by FNA for biomarker analysis. However risk stratification schemas discussed in the section on biomarkers (Tab. 2) may be used to assist in the identification of biomarker results analogous to those used for studying actin in bladder cancer. Understanding an organ and its ecosystem is important in interpreting biomarkers, setting thresholds and optimizing receiver–operator curves (ROC) plots.

A brief review of the biomarker prostate specific antigen (PSA), serves to illustrate the effort and the confounding issues related to the development of a clinically useful biomarker. Normal prostate and malignant prostate epithelial cells contain PSA enzyme which has served as a serum biomarker for prostate cancer. The enzymes escape from the prostate epithelial cells during invasion or cell death, and exist in the serum as free and total bound forms [104]. Detection of biomarker PSA has served as a useful test for detecting prostate cancer in symptomatic patients. Its role as a biomarker for screening is most controversial. The high false-positive and false-negative rates of this biomarker have been acceptable because of the high prevalence of the disease. A report by the National Research Council triggered concerns regarding the contribution of this biomarker as a screening test and its effectiveness for reducing cancer morbidity and mortality [73]. This has become an international issue, and the debate continues regarding the appropriateness of screening for prostate cancer, because of the prolonged natural history of the disease, a high rate of tumor recurrence following radical surgery and the operative mortality and morbidity (incontinence and impotence). Delayed symptomatic therapy has been proposed as an alternative to radical surgical intervention. The high rate of recurrence and the refractory nature of these tumors to therapy is a reflection of the genetic instability. Tribukait has demonstrated increasing genetic instability (aneuploidy) in prostate cancer cases monitored longitudinally with serial biopsies [274]. A trial of delayed treatment *versus* (watchful waiting) screening may predispose the individuals to develop more genetically unstable tumors. Most agree that the PIVOT trial should be completed, while others argue that screening has clearly demonstrated downstaging with earlier detection. Positive lymph node status has decreased from approximately 20% to 3%. Since genetic instability is highly correlated with metastasis, it is intuitive to think that delayed symptomatic management would not be advantageous if the appropriate patients could be selected for operative intervention. Consequently, there is a need to define biomarker changes in the field of the histologically normal prostate gland or in the prostate tumor which signals the development of biologically active disease. Detection of these biomarker alterations should theoretically occur prior to the onset of genetic instability, and thresholds must be established in relation to the organ's ecosystem and the exogenous environment. These are particularly important considerations related to individual risk assessment, targeting chemoprevention and encouraging primary prevention.

A potential approach for defining markers of metastatic risk

The primary result of genetic instability is the malignant, metastatic phenotype. Given that metastasis is a relatively rare event even though circulating tumor cells are relatively common [275, 276], the metastatic phenotype is likely to represent a minority of cells within a tumor. Metastatic cells must also display a number of independent functional traits [277–279], such as weak cell-cell adhesion [280–282], the ability to survive in the circulation and adhere to and subsequently penetrate a capillary bed [283, 284], which implies both mobility on the part of the cancer cell [285] and the ability either to degrade intracellular matrix or stimulate normal cells to degrade matrix [286, 287]. Also required is the capacity for autocrine growth or to use growth signals at the metastatic site [288–291]. Molecular investigations at either the gene or gene product level are identifying the molecular basis of these traits, and it is widely believed that understanding the molecular basis of metastasis will make it possible to predict metastatic potential. This belief may not be warranted because cells lacking any one of these traits are unlikely to be metastatic, though measurement of any single trait is likely to be positively correlated with metastasis. Our research has focused primarily on defining the premalignant phenotype, but it has served to stimulate thought related to defining markers of metastatic risk associated with the genetic phenotype. Understanding mechanisms and selecting markers is further complicated by the likelihood that each trait may be acquired by different molecular pathways. Formally, if there are i traits and j ways to achieve each trait, and if each has an associated correlation, p, with metastasis, then:

(1) $\Sigma p_{ij} = 1.0$

Because the risk is partitioned among all the possible means of achieving the metastatic phenotype, all single markers will be weak predictors of metastatic potential with a power insufficient to formulate major clinical decisions above those delineated by stage and grade. Molecular tools may be too fine if it becomes necessary to identify all j means to identify a particular trait.

One solution to this problem is to focus not on individual molecular traits, but rather upon functional phenotypic markers that identify the traits themselves. In other words, is there a small set of markers that identifies the individual subphenotypes (e.g. a single marker for the capacity for autocrine growth) Finally, consideration must be given as to how such rare cells will be detected. Our hypothesis is that predicting metastatic risk requires several biomarkers in combination using "and-logic." In other words, if two markers together are required, then "and-logic" is being used. One example of such a study was the combination of AMFR (autocrine motility factor receptor) and E-cadherins [292]. This approach is formally equivalent to that seen in cancer epidemiology where relatively weak exposure and susceptibility markers together have very high predictive powers [293].

To define the metastatic phenotype, several traits will have to be investigated to determine the feasibility of developing clinically useful biomarkers for the metastasis phenotype. One model for evaluating the functional metastatic phenotype is to identify a marker associated with a specific function. Motility could be represented by the autocrine motility factor receptor (AMFR), low cellular adhesiveness by E-cadherin, and the ability to degrade extracellular matrix by the ratio of specific metalloproteinases to specific inhibitors. The marker for angiogenesis and matrix degradation could be bFGF. Cytoskeletal changes could be represented by G-actin, which represents a broad phenotypic marker for the malignant phenotype, but has not been specifically investigated as a marker for metastasis. While these may be individually weak, the combination will have high predictive power: if all are present (angiogenic ability, motility, ability to degrade matrix and weak cell-cell interactions), the tumor is likely to have a high metastatic potential.

Tissue transglutaminase is established as a marker for differentiation and apoptosis in a variety of cells and tissues [294]. Retinoids and sodium butyrate (differentiation agents) modify the rate of proliferation and differentiation and induce tissue transglutaminase in a variety of transformed cells and pathological diseases including cancer [294–299]. Metastatic potential has been shown to be inversely proportional to the level of transglutaminase in tumor cells; metastatic cells have lower levels of transglutaminase [300–303]. Transfection of the transglutaminase gene lowers the cellular metastatic potential [304]. In preliminary studies in prostate, we observed reduced levels of tissue transglutaminase in single cells of prostate tissue taken from patients with prostate cancer compared to cells of prostate tissue from patients with BPH [304b]. Thus, combining the biomarkers described here may assist in identifying the metastatic phenotype. Similar preliminary results have been reported for G-actin and DNA [105]. If the combined phenotype is truly a rare event, then finding the phenotype in a heterogeneous primary neoplasm is in itself complex. Studying circulating cells that now can be isolated serves to narrow the complexity of the sampling problem. A study of the metastatic site may be useful for understanding the autocrine and paracrine growth factors. These may be similar, for instance, all tumors which have metastasized to the liver may be very different from those which metastastasize to the bone.

New discoveries about carcinogenesis and cellular differentiation provide a framework for marker selection

The normal bladder, or any other solid organ, represents a complex ecosystem of interacting epithelial and stromal cells whose growth is highly regulated, and the progressive subversion of proliferation, death, and differentiation controls [305–310] leads to the emergence of cells with tumorigenic phenotypes. Some of these altered phenotypes result, singly or together, from genotypic changes, from altered differentiation arising from a changed cytokine and stromal environment [311, 312] or from epigenetic effects [174]. Bladder cancer seems typically to develop by a process of "field disease", frequently involving widespread histopathological or biochemical changes [15] and carrying increased risk for progression and recurrence [313–315].

The genetic molecular events involved in bladder tumorigenesis are being elucidated. As mentioned previously, bladder cancer apparently develops along distinct high- and low-grade pathways [316, 317]. The high-grade pathway results in a distinct series of morphologically evident premalignant changes [16, 313] eventually leading to a flat, invasive lesion. The low-grade pathway does not result in a series of morphological changes, and papillary tumors often emerge from morphologically normal urothelium. The high-grade pathway seems to involve mutations in the p53 suppressor gene and possibly other loci on chromosome 17p as an apparently late step, [187, 205, 318] while loss of a tumor suppressor function on chromosome 9q seems to be an early, obligate step in bladder carcinogenesis of both types [316, 319–321]. Other evidence suggests loss of suppression function may be related to epigenetic effects such as DNA methylation in promoter regions. There is considerable evidence for the possibility of more than a single tumor suppressor gene on chromosome 9 [322].

I have previously discussed the metastatic phenotype related to bladder cancer detections, and when the changes occur during carcinogenesis. Little equivalent information has been collected concerning the metastatic phenotype and when in the course of progression it can be manifested. Metastasis is certainly associated with tumor heterogeneity. Recent studies have shown an interesting effect of heterogeneity; a small minority of cells can affect the entire population. In a model system of mixed cancer cells, the presence of a minority of cells secreting acidic fibroblastic growth factor could increase the tumorigenicity and metastatic potential of the entire population [323]. The synergistic effect observed between elevated AMFR and decreased E-cadherins [292] illustrates that the metastatic phenotype requires multiple factors.

Because many components of, for example, signaling pathways, share common intracellular biochemical components, the possibility of finding markers that reflect alterations in any one of several possible systems would provide higher sensitivity than would using individual signaling pathway components as markers (e.g. growth factor receptors). An example is the use of alterations of the cytoskeleton of the path to carcinogenesis, which has proven to be a powerful marker for assessment of carcinogenic risk [15, 127, 242, 324]. Aberrant DNA ploidy represents an effect of genomic instability and is one of the most powerful markers yet developed, regardless of whether it is used to determine the central tendency of cell populations by flow cytometry [88] or the appearance of rare, aberrant cells as determined by image analysis [15, 87, 325–328]. In comparing the efficacy of genotypic and phenotypic markers, similar considerations hold in that many genotypes, for example, mutations of different codons on the *p53* gene, may share a common phenotype.

In order to be useful clinically, the results of biomarker tests must be definitive enough to select or alter an individual patient's treatment. It is not necessary that definitive answers be provided for all patients; a marker can be clinically useful if a definitive answer is provided for some patients. The requirement that markers have high predictive power pays an important statistical benefit in that their efficacy can be demonstrated in small studies. Indeed, if their efficacy is not demonstrable in a small study, the marker cannot be strong and therefore will not be clinically useful. Moreover, there is also a number of currently used markers, and for a new marker to provide any additional information, it should provide an improvement over what is currently available if the metastatic phenotype is to be defined.

Extrapolation of experimental models to the problem of genetic instability

Studying cancer and normal biomarker expression is highly relevant to individual risk assessment and preventing cancer. There is a scarcity of data pertaining to the point at which tumor heterogeneity and genetic instability develop during tumorigenesis. This is an important theoretical and practical question and is related directly to how early specific classes of chemopreventive agents need to be administered. Cellular heterogeneity is normally present and may be quantitatively differentially expressed during carcinogenesis. Experimental models in whole animals may be useful for investigating how early genetic instability develops, but may not parallel the kinetics or mechanisms of human disease. Although longitudinal studies in high risk cohorts for cancer have unique and numerous advantages, the accessibility of these cohorts is limited. Thus, in addition to animal models, clinical models discussed in the section on the selection on biomarkers may be extremely useful for defining the kinetics of biomarker expression related to tumor heterogeneity.

Animal models have provided useful information for studying tumorigenesis, but few studies have investigated the mechanisms or pre-clinical changes associated with carcinogenesis.

It will be most useful to dissect the mechanisms and onset of tumor heterogeneity and genetic instability in the context of the organ's intact ecosystem. As we previously discussed, there may be considerable cellular heterogeneity in the mediators within normal signaling pathways, and the controlling mechanisms may be different from one species to another. Sexual differences, even in inbred animals, alter the endogenous environment, and are related to the development of cancer. An example is the initiation and promotion of renal cell carcinoma with hydrocarbon exposure in male but not female rats in the gasoline model of carcinogenesis [73]. However, the study of the cells within an organ's ecosystem with intact stromal epithelial interactions, may provide useful information at the cellular *in vivo* level. From both a fiscal and scientific perspective, extrapolation of data from isolated systems to the intact organ and species is paramount. Knowing when to move from one model to the other to confirm initial observations, requires integrated multidisciplinary research groups. In many instances, there is a tendency to overuse a model because of funding pressures even though no new information is being gleaned.

I have previously summarized several *in vitro* models for investigating biomarkers. However, although extremely useful if one is interested in studying quantitative expression, a profound impact of stromal epithelial interactions may be paramount. For example, in the study of a late biomarker of effect, the DD-23 tumor-associated antigen expression was up regulated when cells expressing the marker were grown on a matrix [329]. Biomarkers analyzed for quantitative and qualitative alterations should be very useful in determining which models are most applicable for species, and dose extrapolation. Relevant to biomarker expression is the sequential expression of a biomarker related to tumor heterogeneity and genetic instability.

A study of chemically induced tumors in animals may be informative, but markers in animals may not necessarily be relevant to humans. Similar problems exist with regard to dose selection in animal studies compared to humans. Higher doses of specific carcinogens might result in proliferation secondary to toxicity repair, and explain why non-mutagenic chemicals in the Ames test may be carcinogenic. Another explanation could be the effect of epigenetic factors discussed elsewhere in the text.

Consequently, there are multiple quantitative issues related to extrapolation in general, and specifically, in relation to genetic instability. Dose response modeling is a critical component of cancer risk assessment. The end point for assessment in the past has been disease, but identification of biomarkers expressed at various times (early *versus* late) in carcinogenesis can assist in defining the relevance of an extrapolation model. The problem becomes even more complex if there are multiple different exposures over a protracted interval. Monitoring sequential mutagenic changes is much less complicated than sequential epigenetic effects.

It is useful to expand the concepts of biomarker risk as a model for genetic instability to a conceptual framework outlined in the section on biomarkers. Since many of the mechanisms leading to disease are dependent on multiple variables, it is likely that using biomarkers to evaluate the variable stages of oncogenic process will more effectively result in useful extrapolation. These concepts were discussed in detail in an article on biological markers in urinary toxicology published by the National Research Council [73]. The simplified formula for extrapolation: $P(C) = g (DI) = f_5 (F_4(f_3) f_2(DI,S_2), S_3, S_4), S_5)$ where $P(C)$ is the probability of clinical disease and g(DI) equates to some function of the administered dose. To establish the relationship among the markers (the functions f_2 to f_5), the relationship between the dose and susceptibility factors (S_2 to S_5) for each biomarker is expressed in the above formula. This formula represents a complex series of interactions and the problem of extrapolating from animal data to the human disease. Extrapolation may be made more meaningful by extrapolating from one marker to another rather than between administered dose and disease outcome. At certain points in the continuum, disease analysis between biomarkers of effect may be more informative because the process can be studied in various segments. One could also incorporate into the model genetic and epigenetic effects if markers were defined.

Clinical and epidemiological studies and the mechanism of carcinogenesis (a model study)

Occupationally exposed cohorts at high risk for malignancy provide a unique opportunity to evaluate biomarkers for individual risk assessment, for assessing biomarkers to detect disease, for testing surrogate intermediate endpoints for cancer prevention, and finally, provide a living model for understanding the mechanisms of carcinogenesis. Urine specimens collected longitudinally may be used in nested case-control studies to elucidate the mechanisms of genetic instability and to determine at what point chemopreventive therapy is effective. I have previously discussed how *in vitro* tissue culture and animal studies are helpful for developing methods and testing general concepts. However, there are significant limitations with these systems, as discussed in the section on *Extrapolation of Biomarkers*. Evaluation of biomarkers on cells from patients with previous clinical cancers and at risk for recurrence more closely approximate the carcinogenic process, but may be limited by genetic instability and do not reflect perturbations of the complex network of signaling pathways prior to overt malignancy. The study of occupationally exposed workers monitored over years, allows for monitoring cellular and biochemical alterations not confounded by previously having had the disease.

Historical perspectives in occupational bladder high risk cohorts: The Augusta cohort

In 1981, in conjunction with the National Institute of Occupational Safety and Health (NIOSH) and the Worker's Institute for Occupational Safety and Health (spearheaded by Knut Ringen), a notification and biomarker screening program for workers exposed to aromatic amines was initiated in Augusta, Georgia, USA [330]. This cross-sectional study was a landmark program for the methodological development and notification of workers at risk [176, 330]. Because of the high risk for bladder cancer in this cohort, a community public health based component was incorporated into the study design with the goal of continued surveillance. It was devastating to learn that aniline dye manufacturing, which was known to cause bladder cancer as early as 1895, had been used in the United States, some eighty years later. Presently, these dyes are still consumed in cottage industries in India, China and other countries as well. A major concept that evolved from the Augusta study was that 5C DNA ER correlated with xenobiotic exposure.

5C DNA ER was expressed in the uroepithelial cells in 16 of 74 workers (21.6%) who had been exposed, compared with 15 of 430 workers (3.5%) who had not been exposed. The 5C DNA ER increased in a dose-response manner with duration of exposure from 3.5% to 60%, independent of the age and smoking history. Biomarker expression preceded the occurrence of overt bladder cancer and reflected alterations in genetic instability [145, 328]. Early expression of the bio-marker brought into focus a heightened awareness as to when in the cascade of carcinogeneses a specific phenotypic marker is expressed.

Results also suggest DNA measurements would improve the sensitivity of PAP cytology, but not without sacrificing specificity. In the clinical evaluation, 5C DNA ER subclassified atypias and dysplasias associated with the malignant processes [328]. This has subsequently been confirmed in several other clinical studies [331]

The Drake cohort

Based on our experience with the Augusta cohort, a second study involving the Drake cohort was initiated and has been in progress since 1989. The total study population consists of 374 notified individuals of whom 275 have completed the initial screen and have been followed longitudinally since 1986 [332]. Although based on previous epidemiological studies, the cohort is thought to be at higher risk for bladder cancer; to date one case of bladder cancer (CIS) and one papilloma have been confirmed, and 13 cases of dysplasia have been identified. One important outcome from this study was the inconsistency of biomarker expression in voided uroepithelial samples. However, the cohort has served as a model for longitudinal monitoring, and smoking cessation programs. 5C DNA ER was the primary marker and only two cases have developed bladder cancer over more than eight years of follow-up, but the latency for bladder cancer is only now being reached. Exfoliation of uroepithelial cells with greater than 5C DNA ER, a presumed marker of genetic instability, does not necessarily define genetic instability or preclude effective clinical prevention.

The China cohort: The epidemiological cohort study and preliminary biomarker studies

The original China benzidine cohort consisted of 2,612 workers exposed to benzidine for at least one year in the cities of Tianjing, Shanghai, Jilin, Henan, and Chongqing, between 1945 and 1977. The cohort had previously been identified together with a cohort of nonexposed controls in each city and was studied in China as part of the National Cooperative Group of Occupational Bladder Cancer. Upon completion of the case control study in 1982, 31 bladder cancer cases (30 males and one female) were identified in the exposed group as reported by Bi prior to our pilot study and our longitudinal cohort study [75]. At the conclusion of the epidemiological study, the bladder cancer incidence rates in the exposed and control males were 167.8 and 5.2 per 100,000 workers, respectively. The two incidence rates produced a statistically significant relative risk value of 32.3 [75]. The workers, following the initial epidemiological study, continued to report each year for an annual screening visit that included hematuria testing, physical examination, and

Papanicolaou cytology on voided uroepithelial cells. In 1991, a pilot study was initiated by NIOSH to determine the feasibility of performing a prospective biomarker study on the exposed cohort. This study confirmed that the biomarker studies could be performed on voided exfoliated uroepithelial cells from almost anywhere in the world. Based on clinical studies in patients with bladder cancer, a profile of biomarkers was identified and incorporated into the study design to define individuals at risk for bladder cancer and to improve bladder cancer detection [333].

Selection of biomarkers for the longitudinal cohort study

Biomarkers selected for the China study were based on phase II clinical trials and on the preliminary China pilot study. The biomarker profile was selected as outlined in an earlier paper [15] in which the three markers plus epidermal growth factor receptor (EGFR), p185 (*neu* oncoprotein), and visual cytology were compared in tumor, adjacent field and distant field. Statistical cluster analysis showed that 5C DNA ER, M344 antigen, and G-actin were independent of each other and each seemed to measure a different aspect of carcinogenesis. In this paper we also introduced the concept of "biochemical field disease" in which cells that are on the path to transformation express phenotypic alterations that are not manifested in altered cytology. Subsequently, we have differentiated "field disease," which is the presence of transformed or partially transformed cells in wide areas of the bladder, and "field effect," which is an alteration in the phenotype of genetically normal cells due to the presence of transformed or transforming cells [329]. The combination of M344 antigen and the 5C DNA ER was independently tested as a marker and found to have high sensitivity for bladder cancer [147]. However, these markers also identified a subset of patients with a previous history of cancer and at risk of recurrence due to the presence of field disease.

The cytoskeletal protein G-actin is a quantitative marker representing the shift in the cytoskeleton of transformed cells or cells responding to the altered cytokine milieu caused by the presence of transformed or transforming cells [15, 242, 324, 334]. This latter "field effect" phenomenon means that the abnormal cells themselves may not need to be detected, but may be identified from the fingerprints they leave in the form of phenotypic alterations of normal cells. This effect is so strong that when the set of markers was examined to determine which had the highest sensitivity in predicting recurrence from analysis of a single urine specimen obtained immediately after completion of therapy, G-actin showed an odds ratio of 6.0 (C.I. = 1.26 to 28.56) for recurrence, while the 5C DNA ER nor M344 antigen showed significant odds ratios. Of those patients with positive G-actin following therapy, 67% recurred, while of those who were negative, only 25% recurred (p = 0.032 by Fisher's exact test) [243].

Interim results of the China study

Our initial results with this group have shown that 75% of the workers who developed bladder cancers were initially identified by biomarker analysis as being roughly the 10% at highest risk. Over 92% of the tumors were found within the top two risk strata that comprised 25%–30% of the entire cohort. The goal of these studies was to develop a system of biomarkers to improve the management of bladder cancer in occupationally-exposed groups. The biomarkers would be used in two ways. First would be to identify prevalent cancers in initial screens of high-risk groups with higher sensitivity than is achieved with conventional cytology. The second purpose would be to stratify exposed individuals according to risk so that workers expected to develop cancer in the future could be identified prior to the emergence of a clinically detectable tumor. While specificity is an issue, the main objective is to cast the net widely enough to ensnare future tumors because then the group at low risk can be freed from detailed surveillance. The problem of managing exposed cohorts to prevent bladder cancer death and morbidity is thereby reduced to the size of this smaller cohort. Now, having identified this smaller group of at-risk workers, the next logical step is to administer chemopreventive agents to determine if the biomarkers that identified them as being at high risk are modulated by chemopreventive agents and if the incidence of disease is diminished.

The China cohort using biomarker evaluation

In 1989, a pilot study on three subsets of patients from this initial cohort was undertaken to determine the feasibility of evaluating exogenous risk factors, endogenous risk factors and biological markers to stratify further the exposed workers according to objective biomarker criteria [333]. The results showed that accurate questionnaire data and urine samples can be obtained at remote sites. It also identified two patients in the group with previous exposure history but not previously diagnosed with bladder cancer to have abnormal findings by QFIA cytology and p300 (M344) expression. These two patients were later found to have bladder cancer. Additional observations suggested that premalignant changes related to exposure to benzidine were detectable. The study demonstrated the feasibility of performing molecular marker field studies to define risk in exposed-worker cohorts.

After the feasibility study, urine samples from the entire cohort with matching controls were screened for G-actin, M344 antigen, and for cells with greater than 5C DNA, and stratified on the basis of the findings as described in Table 6. A complex risk algorithm was devised in order to classify subjects into four categories: Very High and High risk (which are treated operationally as one), Moderate and Low risk. Subjects in the Very High and High risk categories were examined by cystoscopy at 6 month intervals. The cohort was then followed with annual visits for three years, and in the fourth year (1995) was entirely re-screened. The High and Very High risk group were monitored annually by cystoscopy and urine specimens. The main finding was that only a single tumor was discovered in the Moderate risk group, and all the others were identified in the Very High and High risk groups. Details of the risk stratification rules were adjusted to optimize the sensitivity and specificity for a single marker or combination of markers after the screen in the first two cities. These data clearly demonstrated that what was an acceptable threshold in one cohort may not be applicable to another for a variety of reasons. It is important to emphasize that the thresholds and risk stratification were established on the basis of previously published clinical studies and preliminary analysis of the distribution of markers in the Chinese population of workers and not after the fact. The only adjustment of threshold that was made was to adjust

Table 6. Rules for risk categorization of biomarker results in China cohort

Risk category	Rules
High	M344 Pos Cells ≥2/10,000 cells
	OR G-actin ≥90 Units AND 5CER ≥0.8
	OR G-actin is extreme (≥140 units)
	OR DNA 5C ER is extreme (≥2.0%)
	OR Papanicolaou cytology is positive
Moderate	NOT already flagged high-risk
	AND G-actin ≥90 Units OR 5C ER ≥0.8
LOW	All values within normal range

upward the 5C DNA ER to increase the specificity, and to add the criterion that a single marker being in the extreme category was sufficient to kick the risk to high values [15, 147, 242].

A total of 12 prevalent cancers were identified and completely evaluated according to the protocol for reviewing slides and quality control and for longitudinal follow-up. An additional 15 incident cancers were identified during the monitoring period together with 19 recurrent cancers.

The most important finding to date is that the biomarker profile is not only much more effective than Papanicolaou cytology for detection of cancers, but the profile is accurate enough to stratify the cohort of exposed workers according to their individual risk. Of the 12 cancers documented in the exposed group, only one was discovered in the initially low-risk group. This individual was completely negative for hematuria, Papanicolaou cytology and the three quantitative markers on 10/91. The worker later became symptomatic and was diagnosed with a grade 4 TCC in April, 1993. Of the other documented cancers in the exposed group, nine occurred in the Very High and High risk groups and two occurred in the Moderate risk group. Interestingly, a single cancer was found in the controls in an individual classified into the High risk group. The improved performance of the QFIA tests over Papanicolaou cytology is evident. Even more interesting was the lack of concordance between QFIA and Papanicolaou cytology. Of the 11 subjects who were positive by QFIA, only two were also positive by Papanicolaou cytology and one was read as atypical. Moreover, by using the stratification scheme to target more aggressive management to individuals at higher risk while offering those at much lower risk a far less expensive and onerous screening program, the total costs and difficulties associated with managing the high-risk cohort may be decreased accordingly.

These results demonstrate that the risk stratification methods do cast the net widely enough to ensnare the potential tumors, in many cases up to five years ahead of time, but often three years prior to detection of the tumor. The risk stratification was confirmed in that the earlier markers for predicting cancer were the moderate risk group >high risk >PAP >hematuria. This gives a high confidence that the group with abnormal markers is the group that is at risk and should be targeted for chemoprevention. The biomarkers represent different aspects of carcinogenesis and are sensitive to different phenomena. It is therefore likely that further information of importance to chemoprevention will be available from these markers. For example, it may well be that samples with a high 5C DNA ER or those with mutations in the *p53* gene may have already developed significant genetic instability and therefore may not be as responsive to chemoprevention as are those tumors that do not display aneuplody (5C DNA ER).

Summary of the China cohort

These studies confirm that biomarkers can be used to identify a group of individuals exposed to benzidine, at least three years in advance of clinically manifested disease. The critical issue is the point at which genetic instability has occurred to a point beyond which conventional cancer therapy is not effective. 5C DNA ER was the single most effective marker for predicting bladder cancer development with a sensitivity of 83.3% and a specificity of 87.5 per cent. One might hypothesize that all individuals with increased 5C DNA ER are at risk for bladder cancer, yet we know based on specificity in asymptomatic controls that approximately 12.5% of these are false positive. Another issue pertaining to the concepts relating to tumor heterogeneity is the interaction of the signaling pathways.

Studying genetic instability in the cancer field may also provide clues as to whether it is an early or late event. Understanding the differences between field disease and field cancerization and the functional pathways is important in the development of strategies for cancer prevention and control. If indeed, genetic instability is driven by primary mutagenic factors, a different approach may be necessary than if epigenetic factors are of primary importance. Once the cascade has been initiated, knowing which one is contributing and when, may alter therapeutic options including the choice of chemopreventive agents. While there is also the tumor suppressor function on chromosome 9 that seems to be an early step in bladder cancer carcinogenesis in both types there is considerable evidence for the possibility that more than a single tumor suppressor gene lies on chromosome 9. Thus, one of the major objectives of future studies is to evaluate further the genotypic and phenotypic alteration in archival cells from the bladder cancer field to understand the genetic and epigenetic alterations involved in the proposed pathways of bladder cancer tumorigenesis. These same approaches may be applied to other organs such as the breast and colon as well.

Combining biomarkers of susceptibility with biomarkers of effect could potentially improve individual risk assessment prior to the onset of genetic instability. Understanding the mechanisms of carcinogenesis is a complex issue involving multiple genetic polymorphism interacting with endogenous and exogenous exposures. Greenwald has summarized the results from twin studies and other observations in animals where exogenous substances can influence gene expression [335]. Macleod has provided several models in which epigenetic events can be perpetuated from one cell generation to another [336]. As mentioned previously, one genetic marker of susceptibility important in the activation or inactivation of bladder carcinogens may be the gene regulating by the slow and fast acetylation pathway [337]. Even though these genetic polymorphisms exist, the kinetics of the reaction may be a rate limiting parameter affecting the clinical and functional importance of these genes, and studying the functional phenotypic susceptibility marker may be primary to defining both biomarkers of susceptibility and effect [338].

A second set of important susceptibility markers may be related to DNA repair. In a case-control study of lung cancer patients and controls, the relative risk for lung cancer was 5.6 times higher in individuals with slow DNA repair [270]. A list of potential biomarkers for measuring genetic instability has been summarized in the previous section. The repository of bladder wash and voided urine samples from the bladder cancer field of patients destined to develop bladder cancer provides a unique opportunity to study the genetic alterations and the associated sequential changes in cancer tumorigenesis, particularly those related to the changes in chromosome 17p and 9p. Furthermore, the response of the bladder cancer field to selected chemopreventive agents might provide insight into when, in the pathway of tumorigenesis, genetic instability occurs, and assist in determining how early chemopreventive agents should be administered to be effective, or when, in the cascade, the induction of apoptosis and cellular differentiation is effective.

Strategies for bladder cancer prevention

This occupationally exposed cohort with the identified surrogate intermediate endpoint bio-markers provides a unique opportunity for evaluating chemopreventive agents. In contrast to clinical cancers that are in remission, the effects of genetic instability may be minimal in this study group. In support of this concept is the increased effectiveness of retinoids in animal model systems with less impressive results in humans when administered 4-HPR [339]. The positive response in animals may be related to the administration of the drug during bladder cancer development in contrast to humans where tumors may display increased genetic instability or a malignant phenotype expressed later in tumorigenesis. Certainly, observations in our laboratory clearly support this hypothesis because a number of malignant tumor lines were resistant to all-trans-retinoic acid (tRA) or 4-HPR [340]. The retinoid 4-HPR has shown strong activity in chemoprevention of bladder cancer in mice and rats prior to the onset of tumor [339, 341], with lower toxicity than tRA [339, 341].

Two important questions remained to be addressed. The first and fundamental question is if the currently administered retinoids such as 4-HPR were administered early enough, would they be effective in the absence of genetic instability? As previously mentioned, we have defined a number of phenotypic markers which are expressed at various stages of bladder cancer tumorigenesis [64, 89, 105, 147, 329, 342, 343]. A number of treatment groups exist. If the currently administered retinoids are effective in normalizing the abnormal phenotypic markers in the cancer field, then this will support the hypothesis that chemopreventive agents must be administered early in the cascade of bladder cancer tumorigenesis. A second alternative is that these differences reflect differences in genetic susceptibility to various chemopreventive agents. A question to be addressed is whether differential drug responsiveness to retinoids reflects a genetic polymorphism or is attributable to heterogeneity associated with carcinogenesis. If cancer prevention drugs need to be administered early, then more emphasis should be placed on studying normal signaling pathways.

Conclusion

Significant advances have been made in understanding the molecular mechanisms of carcinogenesis in the past two decades. In spite of these invaluable advances, the complex networks of
signaling pathways and the development of tumor variability and genetic instability continue to
thwart current therapeutic treatments. Although markers of genetic susceptibility are useful for
defining individuals with inherited genetic disorders, they do not consider endogenous and exogenous risk factors. Because both endogenous and exogenous exposure are difficult to recon-
struct and quantitate and because there is substantial evidence that biomarkers of effect (mutations, mRNA or protein products) are altered years in advance of clinically manifested disease,
efforts should be devoted to defining biomarkers for individual risk assessment. Although
inherited genetic markers are useful for identifying five to 10% of cancers associated with familial cancers, phenotypic biomarkers of effect are a powerful tool for individual risk assessment.
For example, the *BRC-1* gene is present in five to 10% of patients with non-familial breast cancer.
This compares to 75% to 90% of biomarkers of effect which are applicable to all patients who
will develop bladder cancer. Identification of these biomarker alterations in the premalignant field
is possible years in advance of clinically manifested disease. Defining biomarkers of effect incor-
porates epigenetic carcinogens and genetic imprinting into the model. These individuals may be
targeted for chemoprevention. To develop this model further requires defining the relevant biomarker prior to the onset of genetic instability. Less effort should be expended on studying
genetically unstable cancers and our resources should be directed to clarifying the molecular
events of normal signaling pathways, and how the premalignant field differs from normal. Biomarkers of genetic instability may assist in directing this focus, and recent advances in molecular
medicine and biomarkers of susceptibility may increase the specificity of biomarkers of effect in
subsets of patients. These same biomarkers may be used to test and target specific chemopreventive agents.

References

1. Heppner GH (1984) Tumor heterogeneity. *Cancer Res* 44: 2259.
2. Heppner GH and Miller BE (1983) Tumor heterogeneity: biological implications and therapeutic consequences. *Cancer Metastasis Rev* 2: 5.
3. Heppner GH, Loveless SE, Miller FR, Mahoney KH and Fulton AM (1983) Mammary tumor heterogeneity.
   Symposium on Fundamental Cancer Res 36: 209.
4. Heppner GH, Miller BE and Miller FR (1983) Tumor subpopulation interactions in neoplasms. *Biochim
   Biophys Acta* 695: 215.
5. Fearon ER (1997) Human cancer syndromes: clues to the origin and nature of cancer. *Science* 278: 1043.
6. Miller BE, Miller FR, Leith J and Heppner GH (1980) Growth interaction *in vivo* between tumor
   subpopulations derived from a single mouse mammary tumor. *Cancer Res* 40: 3977.
7. Miller BE, Miller FR and Heppner GH (1981) Interactions between tumor subpopulations affecting their
   sensitivity to the antineoplastic agents cyclophosphamide and methotrexate. *Cancer Res* 41: 4378.
8. Miller FR (1983) Tumor subpopulation interactions in metastasis. *Invas Metast* 3: 234.
9. Kerbel RS, Dennis JW, Largarde AE and Frost P (1982) Tumor progression in metastasis: an experimental
   approach using lectin resistant tumor variants. *Cancer Metastasis Rev* 1: 99.
10. Wang N, Yu SH, Liener IE, Hebbel RP, Eaton JW and McKhann CF (1982) Characterization of high- and
    low-metastatic clones derived from a methylcholanthrene-induced murine fibrosarcoma. *Cancer Res* 42: 1046.
11. Woodruff MF (1983) Cellular heterogeneity in tumours. *Brit J Cancer* 47: 589.

12. Yung WK, Shapiro JR and Shapiro WR (1982) Heterogeneous chemosensitivities of subpopulations of human glioma cells in culture. *Cancer Res* 42: 992.
13. Cervantes Saavedra Md (1962) *Adventures of Don Quizote de la Mancha*, New York: Dodd, Mead.
14. Bailar JCI and Gornik HL (1997) Cancer Undefeated. *N Engl J Med* 336: 1569.
15. Rao JY, Hemstreet GP, Hurst RE, Bonner RB, Jones PL, Min KW and Fradet Y (1993) Alterations in phenotypic biochemical markers in bladder epithelium during tumorigenesis. *Proc Natl Acad Sci USA* 90: 8287.
16. Koss LG (1979) Mapping of the urinary bladder: its impact on the concepts of bladder cancer. *Hum Pathol* 10: 533.
17. Slaughter DP, Southwick HW and Smejkal W (1953) "Field cancerization" in oral stratified squamous epithelium: clinical implications of multicentric origin. *Cancer* 6: 963.
18. Kerbel RS (1982) Tumor heterogeneity, invasion and metastasis. June 3–5, 1981, Saskatoon, Sask., Canada. *Invas Metast* 2: 61.
19. Yunis JJ (1983) The chromosomal basis of human neoplasia. *Science* 221: 227.
20. Dexter DL and Calabresi P (1982) Intraneoplastic diversity. *Biochim Biophys Acta* 695: 97.
21. Burnet FM (1970) The concept of immunological surveillance. *Prog Exp Tumor Res* 13: 1.
22. Gross L (1943) Intradermal Immunization of C3H Mice against a Sarcoma That Originated in an Animal of the Same Line. *Cancer Res* 3: 326–333.
23. Gorer PA (1961) The antigenic structure of tumors. *Adv Immunol* 1: 345.
24. Amos DB, Bashir H, Boyle W, MacQueen M and Tiilikainen A (1969) A simple micro cytotoxicity test. *Transplantation* 7: 220.
25. Vanky F, Stjernsward J, Klein G, Steiner L and Lindberg L (1973) Tumor-associated specificity of serum-mediated inhibition of lymphocyte stimulation by autochthonous human tumors. *J Nat Cancer Inst* 51: 25.
26. Hemstreet GP (1978) Renal cell carcinoma: tumor membrane lymphocyte stimulation assay. *Natl Cancer Inst Monogr* 165.
27. Hemstreet GP (1975) Partial biochemical characterization of a lymphocyte-stimulating antigen associated with hypernephroma. ii, (Abstract).
28. Fleuren GJ, Gorter A, Kuppen PJ, Litvinov S and Warnaar SO (1995) Tumor heterogeneity and immunotherapy of cancer. *Immunol Rev* 145: 91.
29. Fialkow PJ (1976) Clonal origin of human tumors. *Biochim Biophys Acta* 458: 283.
30. Fialkow PJ, Jacobson RJ and Papayannopoulou T (1977) Chronic myelocytic leukemia: clonal origin in a stem cell common to the granulocyte, erythrocyte, platelet and monocyte/macrophage. *Amer J Med* 63: 125.
31. Fialkow PJ, Denman AM, Singer J, Jacobson RJ and Lowenthal MN (1978) Human myeloproliferative disorders: clonal origin in pluripotent stem cells. *In*: B Clarkson, PA Marks and JE Till et al. (eds) *Differentiation of normal and neoplastic hematopoietic cell*. Cold Spring Harbor, Cold Spring Harbor Laboratory, New York, pp 131–44.
32. Fialkow PJ, Denman AM, Jacobson RJ and Lowenthal MN (1978) Chronic myelocytic leukemia. Origin of some lymphocytes from leukemic stem cells. *J Clin Invest* 62: 815.
33. Adamson JW, Fialkow PJ, Murphy S, Prchal JF and Steinmann L (1976) Polycythemia vera: stem-cell and probable clonal origin of the disease. *N Engl J Med* 295: 913.
34. Jacobson RJ, Salo A and Fialkow PJ (1978) Agnogenic myeloid metaplasia: a clonal proliferation of hematopoietic stem cells with secondary myelofibrosis. *Blood* 51: 189.
35. Murray RF, Hobbs J and Payne B (1971) Possible clonal origin of common warts (*Verruca vulgaris*). *Nature* 232: 51.
36. Alers JC, Krijtenburg PJ, Vissers CJ, Bosman FT, van der Kwast TH and Van Dekken H (1995) Cytogenetic heterogeneity and histologic tumor growth patterns in prostatic cancer. *Cytometry* 21: 84.
37. Fidler IJ and Hart IR (1982) Biological diversity in metastatic neoplasms: origins and implications. *Science* 217: 998.
38. Owen-Schaub LB, Abraham SR and Hemstreet GP (1986) Phenotypic characterization of murine lymphokine-activated killer cells. *Cell Immunol* 103: 272.
39. Owen-Schaub LB, Hemstreet GP, Hemingway LL, Abraham SR and DeBault LE (1987) Population dynamics of the murine lymphokine activated killer system: precursor frequency and kinetics of maturation and renewal. *Cell Tissue Kinet* 20: 591.
40. Grimm EA, Mazumder A, Zhang HZ and Rosenberg SA (1982) Lymphokine-activated killer cell phenomenon. Lysis of natural killer-resistant fresh solid tumor cells by interleukin 2-activated autologous human peripheral blood lymphocytes. *J Exp Med* 155: 1823.
41. Rosenberg SA, Lotze MT, Muul LM, Chang AE, Avis FP, Leitman S, Linehan WM, Robertson CN, Lee RE, Rubin JT et al (1987) A progress report on the treatment of 157 patients with advanced cancer using lymphokine-activated killer cells and interleukin-2 or high-dose interleukin-2 alone. *N Engl J Med* 316: 889.
42. Rosenberg SA, Lotze MT, Yang JC, Aebersold PM, Linehan WM, Seipp CA and White DE (1989) Experience with the use of high-dose interleukin-2 in the treatment of 652 cancer patients. *Ann Surg* 210: 474.
43. Rosenberg SA (1988) Immunotherapy of patients with advanced cancer using interleukin-2 alone or in combination with lymphokine activated killer cells. *Important Adv Oncol* 217.

44. Whitehead R, Ward D, Hemingway L, Hemstreet GP, Bradley EC and Konrad MW (1990) Subcutaneous recombinant interleukin 2 in a dose-escalating regimen in patients with metastatic renal cell carcinoma. *Cancer Res* 50: 6708–6715.
45. Konrad MW, Hemstreet GP, Hersh EM, Mansell P, Mertelsmann R, Kolitz J and Bradley EC (1990) Pharmacokinetics of recomninant interleukin 2 in humans. *Cancer Res* 50: 2009.
46. Mule JJ, Yang JC, Afreniere RL, Shu SY and Rosenberg SA (1987) Identification of cellular mechanisms operational *in vivo* during the regression of established pulmonary metastases by the systemic administration of high-dose recombinant interleukin 2. *J Immunol* 139: 285.
47. Rosenberg SA (1996) The immunotherapy of solid cancers based on cloning the genes encoding tumor-rejection antigens. *Annu Rev Med* 47: 481.
48. Kuebler JP, Whitehead RP, Ward DL, Hemstreet GP and Bradley EC (1993) Treatment of metastatic renal cell carcinoma with recombinant interleukin-2 in combination with vinblastine or lymphokine-activated killer cells. *J Urol* 150: 814.
49. Lafreniere R and Rosenberg SA (1985) Adoptive immunotherapy of murine hepatic metastases with lymphokine activated killer (LAK) cells and recombinant interleukin 2 (RIL 2) can mediate the regression of both immunogenic and nonimmunogenic sarcomas and an adenocarcinoma. *J Immunol* 135: 4273.
50. Papa MZ, Mule JJ and Rosenberg SA (1986) Antitumor efficacy of lymphokine-activated killer cells and recombinant interleukin 2 *in vivo*: successful immunotherapy of established pulmonary metastases from weakly immunogenic and nonimmunogenic murine tumors of three district histological types. *Cancer Res* 46: 4973.
51. Rosenberg SA (1991) Immunotherapy and gene therapy of cancer. *Cancer Res* 51: 5074 s.
52. Pardoll DM (1995) Paracrine cytokine adjuvants in cancer immunotherapy. *Annu Rev Immunol* 13: 399.
53. Fyfe G, Fisher RI, Rosenberg SA, Sznol M, Parkinson DR and Louie AC (1995) Results of treatment of 255 patients with metastatic renal cell carcinoma who received high-dose recombinant interleukin-2 therapy. *J Clin Oncol* 13: 688.
54. Barinaga M (1997) From Bench Top to Bedside. *Science* 278: 1036.
55. Morales A, Eidinger D and Bruce AW (1976) Intracavitary Bacillus Calmette-Guerin in the treatment of superficial bladder tumors. *J Urol* 116: 180.
56. Lamm DL (1995) BCG immunotherapy for transitional-cell carcinoma *in situ* of the bladder. Oncology 9: 947.
57. Jackson A, Alexandroff A, Fleming D, Prescott S, Chisholm G and James K (1994) Bacillus Calmette-Guerin (BCG) organisms directly alter the growth of bladder tumor cells. *Int J Oncol* 5: 697.
58. Nseyo UO and Lamm DL (1996) Therapy of superficial bladder cancer. *Semin Oncol* 23: 598.
59. Polednak AP (1997) Estimating the prevalence of cancer in the United States. *Cancer* 80: 136.
60. Beck WT, Grogan TM, Willman CL, Cordon-Cardo C, Parham DM, Kuttesch JF, Andreeff M, Bates SE, Berard CW, Boyett JM et al. (1996) Methods to detect P-glycoprotein-associated multidrug resistance in patients' tumors: consensus recommendations. *Cancer Res* 56: 3010.
61. Muller M, Strand S, Hug H, Heinemann EM, Walczak H, Hofmann WJ, Stremmel W, Krammer PH and Galle PR (1997) Drug-induced apoptosis in hepatoma cells is mediated by the CD95 (APO-1/Fas) receptor/ligand system and involves activation of wild-type p53. *J Clin Invest* 99: 403.
62. Friesen C, Herr I, Krammer PH and Debatin KM (1996) Involvement of the CD95 (APO-1/FAS) receptor/ligand system in drug-induced apoptosis in leukemia cells. *Nat Med* 2: 574.
63. Owen-Schaub LB, Zhang W, Cusack JC, Angelo LS, Santee SM, Fujiwara T, Roth JA, Deisseroth AB, Zhang WW, Kruzel E et al (1995) Wild-type human p53 and a temperature-sensitive mutant induce Fas/APO-1 expression. *Mol Cell Biol* 15: 3032.
64. Hemstreet GP, Hurst RE and Bonner RB (1998) Selection and development of biomarkers for bladder cancer. *In*: M Hanausek and Z Walaszek (eds): *Tumor Marker Protocols*. Totowa, NJ: Humana Press, pp 37–60.
65. Kaminski MS, Zasadny KR, Francis IR, Fenner MC, Ross CW, Milik AW, Estes J, Tuck M, Regan D, Fisher S, Glenn SD and Wahl RL (1996) Iodine-131-anti-B1 radioimmunotherapy for B-cell lymphoma. *J Clin Oncol* 14: 1974.
66. DeNardo SJ, O'Grady LF, Richman CM, Goldstein DS, O'Donnell RT, DeNardo DA, Kroger LA, Lamborn KR, Hellstrom KE, Hellstrom I, DeNardo and GL (1997) Radioimmunotherapy for advanced breast cancer using I-131-ChL6 antibody. *Anticancer Res* 17: 1745.
67. DeNardo SJ, Richman CM, Goldstein DS, Shen S, Salako Q, Kukis DL, Meares CF, Yuan A, Welborn JL and DeNardo GL (1997) Yttrium-90/indium-111-DOTA-peptide-chimeric L6: pharmacokinetics, dosimetry and initial results in patients with incurable breast cancer. *Anticancer Res* 17: 1735.
68. Wilder RB, DeNardo GL and DeNardo SJ (1996) Radioimmunotherapy: recent results and future directions. *J Clin Oncol* 14: 1383.
69. Uhlen M and Moks T (1990) Gene fusions for purpose of expression: an introduction. *Methods Enzymol* 185: 129.
70. Nikaido H (1994) Maltose transport system of *Escherichia coli*: an ABC-type transporter. *FEBS Lett* 346: 55.
71. Betton JM and Hofnung M (1994) *In vivo* assembly of active maltose binding protein from independently exported protein fragments. *EMBO J* 13: 1226.

72. DeNardo DA, DeNardo GL, Yuan A, Shen S, DeNardo SJ, Macey DJ, Lamborn KR, Mahe M, Groch MW and Erwin WD (1996) Prediction of radiation doses from therapy using tracer studies with iodine-131-labeled antibodies. *J Nucl Med* 37: 1970.
73. National Research Council (U.S.) Subcommittee on Biologic Markers in Urinary Toxicology Biologic Markers of Effect. *In*: Board on Environmental Studies and Toxicology (ed.): *Biological Markers in Urinary Toxicology*. Washington, DC: National Academy Press, 1995, pp. 81–152.
74. Anonymous (1997) *Application of Biomarkers in Cancer Epidemiology*, Lyon: International Agency for Research on Cancer.
75. Bi WF, Hayes R, Feng P, Qi Y, You X, Zhen J, Zhang M, Qu B, Fu Z, Chen M, Chien HT and Blot WJ (1992) Mortality and incidence of bladder cancer in benzidine-exposed workers in China. Amer. J. Ind. Med. 21: 481.
76. Parry W and Hemstreet GP (1988) Cancer detection by quantitative fluorescence image analysis. *J Urol* 139: 270.
77. Langston AA, Malone KE, Thompson JD, Daling JR and Ostrander EA (1996) BRCA1 mutations in a population-based sample of young women with breast cancer. *N Engl J Med* 334: 137.
78. FitzGerald MG, MacDonald DJ, Krainer M, Hoover I, O'Neil E, Unsal H, Silva-Arrieto S, Finkelstein DM, Beer-Romero P, Englert C, Sgroi DC, Smith BL, Younger JW, Garber JE, Duda RB, Mayzel KA, Isselbacher KJ, Friend SH and Haber DA (1996) Germ-line BRCA1 mutations in Jewish and non-Jewish women with early-onset breast cancer. *N Engl J Med* 334: 143.
79. Rubin H and Xu K (1991) Epigenetic features of spontaneous transformation in the NIH 3T3 line of mouse cells. *Basic Life Sci* 57: 301.
80. Rubin H (1994) Cellular epigenetics: control of the size, shape, and spatial distribution of transformed foci by interactions between the transformed and nontransformed cells. *Proc Natl Acad Sci USA* 91: 1039.
81. Rubin H, Chow M and Yao A (1996) Cellular aging, destabilization, and cancer. *Proc Natl Acad Sci USA* 93: 1825.
82. Rubin H (1985) Cancer as a dynamic developmental disorder. *Cancer Res* 45: 2935.
83. Rubin H (1990) The significance of biological heterogeneity. *Cancer Metastasis Rev* 9: 1.
84. Pilot HC (1963) Metabolic regulatory circuits in carcinogenesis. *Cancer Res* 23: 1694.
85. Bonner RB, Hurst RE, Rao J and Hemstreet GP (1998) Instrumentation, accuracy and quality control in development of quantitative fluorescence image analysis. *In*: M Hanausek and Z Walaszek (eds): *Tumor Marker Protocols*. Totowa, NJ: Humana Press, pp 181–205.
86. Hemstreet GP, West SS, Weems W, Echols CK, McFarland S, Lewin J and Lindseth G (1983) Quantitative fluorescence measurements of AO-stained normal and malignant bladder cells. *Int J Cancer* 31: 577.
87. West SS, Hemstreet GP, Hurst RE, Bass RA, Doggett RS and Schulte PA (1987) Detection of DNA aneuploidy by quantitative fluorescence image analysis: potential in screening for occupational bladder cancer. *In*: K Dillon and M Ho (eds): *Biological monitoring of exposure to chemicals*. Wiley, New York, pp. 327–341.
88. Wheeless LL, Badalament RA, DeVere White RW, Fradet Y and Tribukait B (1993) Consensus review of the clinical utility of DNA Cytometry in bladder cancer. *Cytometry* 14: 478.
89. Hemstreet GP, Bonner RB, Hurst RE and O'Dowd GA (1996) Cytology of Bladder Cancer. *In*: NJ Vogelzang, PT Scardino, WU Shipley, and DS Coffey (eds): *Comprehensive Textbook of Genitourinary Oncology*. Williams and Wilkins, Baltimore, MD, pp. 338–350.
90. Whittemore AS, Wu AH, Kolonel LN, John EM, Gallagher RP, Howe GR, West DW, Teh C-Z and Stamey T (1995) Family history and prostate cancer risk in black, white, and Asian men in the United States and Canada. *Amer J Epidemiol* 141: 732.
91. Anonymous (1997) *Food, Nutrition, and the Prevention of Cancer: a global perspective*, BANTA Book Group, Menasha, WI.
92. Jones PA and Taylor SM (1980) Cellular differentiation, cytidine analogs and DNA methylation. *Cell* 20: 85.
93. Marshall A and Hudson J (1998) Microchip arrays. *Nat Biotechnol* 16: 27.
94. Clifton KH (1996) Comments on the evidence in support of the epigenetic nature of radiogenic initiation. *Mutat Res* 350: 77.
94b. Feinberg AP (1998) Genomic imprinting and cancer. *In*: B Vogelstein and KW Kinzler (eds): *The genetic basis of human cancer*. McGraw-Hill, New York, Health Professions Divisions, pp 95–107.
95. Caspersson T, Lomakka G and Caspersson O (1960) Quantitative cytochemical methods for the study of tumor cell populations. *Biochem Pharmacol* 4: 113.
96. Hemstreet GP, Hurst RE, Bass R and Rao JY (1990) Quantitative fluorescence image analysis in bladder cancer screening. *J Occup Med* 32(9): 822.
97. Zhang L, Zhou W, Velculescu VE, Kern SE, Hruban RH, Hamilton SR, Vogelstein B and Kinzler KW (1997) Gene expression profiles in normal and cancer cells. *Science* 276: 1268.
98. Duluc I, Jost B and Freund JN (1993) Multiple levels of control of the stage- and region-specific expression of rat intestinal lactase. *J Cell Biol* 123: 1577.

99. Sood R, Bear C, Auerbach W, Reyes E, Jensen T, Kartner N, Riordan JR and Buchwald M (1992) Regulation of CFTR expression and function during differentiation of intestinal epithelial cells. *EMBO J* 11: 2487.

100. Mettlin C, Littrup PJ, Kane RA, Murphy GP, Lee F, Chesley A, Badalament R and Mostofi FK (1994) Relative sensitivity and specificity of serum prostate specific antigen (PSA) level compared with age-referenced PSA, PSA density, and PSA change: Data from the American Cancer Society National Prostate Cancer Detection Project. *Cancer* 74: 1615.

101. Morgan TO, Jacobsen SJ, McCarthy WF, Jacobson DJ, McLeod DG and Moul JW (1996) Age-specific reference ranges for prostate-specific antigen in black men. *N Engl J Med* 335: 304.

102. Whittemore AS, Lele C, Friedman GD, Stamey T, Vogelman JH and Orentreich N (1995) Prostate-specific antigen as predictor of prostate cancer in black men and white men. *J Nat Cancer Inst* 87: 354.

103. Crawford ED, DeAntoni EP and Ross CA (1996) The role of prostate-specific antigen in the chemoprevention of prostate cancer. *J Cell Biochem* 63: 149.

104. Lilja H, Cockett AT and Abrahamsson PA (1992) Prostate specific antigen predominantly forms a complex with alpha 1-antichymotrypsin in blood. Implications for procedures to measure prostate specific antigen in serum. *Cancer* 70: 230.

105. Hemstreet GP, Rao JY, Hurst RE, Bonner RB, Waliszewski P, Grossman HB, Liebert M and Bane BL (1996) G-actin as a Risk Factor and Modulatable Endpoint for Cancer Chemoprevention Trials. *J Cell Biochem* 255: 197.

106. Hemstreet GP, Hurst RE and Asal NR (1993) Biologic markers in the genitourinary system. *In*: PA Schulte and FP Perera (eds): *Molecular Epidemiology: Principles and Practices*. Academic Press, San Diego, pp. 469–495.

107. Folkman J and Shing Y (1992) Angiogenesis. *J Biol Chem* 267: 10931.

108. Bashkin P, Doctrow S, Klagsbrun M, Svahn CM, Folkman J and Vlodavsky I (1989) Basic fibroblast growth factor binds to subendothelial extracellular matrix and is released by heparitinase and heparin-like molecules. *Biochemistry* 28: 1737.

109. Folkman J (1997) Addressing Tumor Blood Vessels. *Nat Biotechnol* 15: 510.

110. Folkman J (1971) Tumor angiogenesis: therapeutic implications. *N Engl J Med* 285: 1182.

111. Pasqualini R, Koivunen E and Ruoslahti E (1997) αv Intergrins as Receptors for Tumor Targeting by Circulating Ligands. *Nat Biotechnol* 15: 542.

112. Vogelstein B, Fearon E, Hamilton S, Kern S, Preisinger AC, Leppert M et al (1988) Genetic alterations during colorectal tumor development. *N Engl J Med* 319: 525.

113. Cohen SM and Ellwein LB (1993) Use of cell proliferation data in modeling urinary bladder carcinogenesis. *Environ Health Perspect* 101 Suppl. 5: 111.

114. Waliszewski P (1994) Mathematical Methods in Molecular Biology. *Biotechnolgia* 26: 7.

115. Bohr VA (1995) DNA repair fine structure and its relations to genomic instability. *Carcinogenesis* 16: 2885.

116. Luce MC, Marra G, Chauhan DP, Laghi L, Carethers JM, Cherian SP, Hawn M, Binnie CG, Kam-Morgan LN, Cayouette MC et al (1995) *In vitro* transcription/translation assay for the screening of hMLH1 and hMSH2 mutations in familial colon cancer. *Gastroenterology* 109: 1368.

117. Luce MC, Binnie CG, Cayouette MC and Kam-Morgan LN (1996) Identification of DNA mismatch repair gene mutations in hereditary nonpolyposis colon cancer patients. *Int J Cancer* 69: 50.

118. Anonymous (1996) Statement of the American Society of Clinical Oncology: genetic testing for cancer susceptibility, Adopted on February 20, 1996. *J Clin Oncol* 14: 1730.

119. Leach FS, Nicolaides NC, Papadopoulos N, Liu B, Jen J, Parsons R, Peltomäki P, Sistonen P, Aaltonen LA, Nyström-Lahti M et al. (1993) Mutations of a mutS homolog in hereditary nonpolyposis colorectal cancer. *Cell* 75: 1215.

120. Papadopoulos N, Nicolaides NC, Wei YF, Ruben SM, Carter KC, Rosen CA, Haseltine WA, Fleischmann RD, Fraser CM, Adams MD et al (1994) Mutation of a mutL homolog in hereditary colon cancer. *Science* 263: 1625.

121. Nicolaides NC, Papadopoulos N, Liu B, Wei YF, Carter KC, Ruben SM, Rosen CA, Haseltine WA, Fleischmann RD, Fraser CM et al (1994) Mutations of two PMS homologues in hereditary nonpolyposis colon cancer. *Nature* 371: 75.

122. Fishel R, Lescoe MK, Rao MR, Copeland NG, Jenkins NA, Garber J, Kane M and Kolodner R (1993) The human mutator gene homolog MSH2 and its association with hereditary nonpolyposis colon cancer [published erratum appears in *Cell* 1994 Apr 8; 77(1): 167]. *Cell* 75: 1027.

123. Bronner CE, Baker SM, Morrison PT, Warren G, Smith LG, Lescoe MK, Kane M, Earabino C, Lipford J, Lindblom A et al (1994) Mutation in the DNA mismatch repair gene homologue hMLH1 is associated with hereditary non-polyposis colon cancer. *Nature* 368: 258.

124. Fang WH, Li GM, Longley M, Holmes J, Thilly W and Modrich P (1993) Mismatch repair and genetic stability in human cells. Cold Spring Harb. *Symp Quant Biol* 58: 597.

125. Scheffner M, Werness BA, Huibregtse JM, Levine AJ and Howley PM (1990) The E6 oncoprotein encoded by human papillomavirus types 16 and 18 promotes the degradation of p53. *Cell* 63: 1129.

126. Dyson N, Howley PM, Munger K and Harlow E (1989) The human papilloma virus-16 E7 oncoprotein is able to bind to the retinoblastoma gene product. *Science* 243: 934.
127. Hemstreet GP, Rao JY, Hurst RE, Bonner RB, Jones PL, Vaidya AM, Fradet Y, Moon RC and Kelloff GJ (1992) Intermediate endpoint biomarkers for chemoprevention. *J Cell Biochem* Suppl. 16I: 93.
128. Larson AA, Kern S, Sommers RL, Yokota J, Cavenee WK and Hampton GM (1996) Analysis of replication error (RER+) phenotypes in cervical carcinoma. *Cancer Res* 56: 1426.
129. Blackburn EH (1991) Structure and function of telomeres. *Nature* 350: 569.
130. Rhyu MS (1995) Telomeres, telomerase, and immortality. *J Nat Cancer Inst* 87: 884.
131. Holt SE, Wright WE and Shay JW (1996) Regulation of telomerase activity in immortal cell lines. *Mol Cell Biol* 16: 2932.
132. Piatyszer MA, Kim NW, Weinrich SL, Hiyama K, Hiyama E, Wright WE and Shay JW (1995) Detection of Telomerase Activity in Human Cells and Tumors by a Telomeric Repeat Amplification Protocol(TRAP). *Meth Cell Science* 17: 1.
133. Sommerfeld HJ, Meeker AK, Piatyszek MA, Bova GS, Shay JW and Coffey DS (1996) Telomerase activity: a prevalent marker of malignant human prostate tissue. *Cancer Res* 56: 218.
134. Zhu X, Kumar R, Mandal M, Sharma N, Sharma HW, Dhingra U, Sokoloski JA, Hsiao R and Narayanan R (1996) Cell cycle-dependent modulation of telomerase activity in tumor cells. *Proc Natl Acad Sci USA* 93: 6091.
135. Sharma HW, Maltese JY, Zhu X, Kaiser HE and Narayanan R (1996) Telomeres, telomerase and cancer: is the magic bullet real? *Anticancer Res* 16: 511.
136. Saluz H and Jost JP (1993) Major techniques to study DNA methylation. In: JP Jost and HP Saluz (eds): *DNA Methylation: Molecular Biology and biological Significance.* Birkhäuser Verlag, Basel, pp. 11–26.
137. Sardi I, Dal Canto M, Bartoletti R and Montali E (1997) Abnormal c-myc oncogene DNA methylation in human bladder cancer: Possible role in tumor progression. Eur. Urol. 31: 224.
138. Bird A (1992) The Essentials of DNA Methylation. *Cell* 70: 5.
139. Ogawa O (1996) Disruption of genomic imprinting in human carcinogenesis. *Hum Cell* 9: 37.
140. Malkin A (1987) Biochemical and immunologic diagnosis of cancer. Prostatic cancer. Tumour Biol. 8(2–3): 113.
141. Zingg JM, Pedraza-Alva G and Jost JP (1994) MyoD1 promoter autoregulation is mediated by two proximal E-boxes. *Nucl Acid Res* 22: 2234.
142. Bruhat A and Jost JP (1996) Phosphorylation/dephosphorylation of the repressor MDBP-2-H1 selectively affects the level of transcription from a methylated promoter *in vitro. Nucl Acid Res* 24: 1816.
143. Mass MJ and Wang L (1997) Arsenic alters cytosine methylation patterns of the promoter of the tumor suppressor gene p53 in human lung cells: a model for a mechanism of carcinogenesis. *Mutat Res* 386: 263.
144. Makos M, Nelkin BD, Reiter RE, Gnarra JR, Brooks J, Isaacs W, Linehan M and Baylin SB (1993) Regional DNA hypermethylation at D17S5 precedes 17p structural changes in the progression of renal tumors. *Cancer Res* 53: 2719.
145. Schulte PA, Ringen K, Altekruse EB, Gullen W, Hemstreet GP and Stringer W (1984) Interaction of aromatic amines and cigarette smoking in bladder cancer, preliminary findings. *Amer J Epidemiol* 120: 482.
146. Driscoll HK, Adkins CD, Chertow TE, Cordle MB, Matthews KA and Chertow BS (1997) Vitamin A stimulation of insulin secretion: Effects on transglutaminase mRNA and activity using rat islets and insulin-secreting cells. *Pancreas* 15: 69.
147. Bonner RB, Hemstreet GP, Fradet Y, Rao JY, Min KW and Hurst RE (1993) Bladder cancer risk assessment with quantitative fluorescence image analysis of tumor markers in exfoliated bladder cells. *Cancer* 72: 2461.
148. Hopman A, Moesker O, Smeets A, Pauwels R, Vooijs G and Ramaekers FCS (1991) Numerical chromosome 1, 7, 9, and 11 aberrations in bladder cancer detected by *in situ* hybridization. *Cancer Res* 51(2): 644.
149. Wheeless LL, Reeder JE, Han R, O'Connell MJ, Frank IN, Cockett AT and Hopman AH (1994) Bladder irrigation specimens assayed by fluorescence *in situ* hybridization to interphase nuclei. *Cytometry* 17: 319.
150. Zitzelsberger H, Szücs S, Weier H-U, Lehmann L, Braselmann H, Enders S, Schilling A, Breul J, Höfler H and Bauchinger M (1994) Numerical abnormalities of chromosome 7 in human prostate cancer detected by fluorescence *in situ* hybridization (FISH) on paraffin-embedded tissue sections with centromere-specific DNA probes. *J Pathol* 172: 325.
151. Bryant P, Davies P and Wilson D (1991) Detection of human papillomavirus DNA in cancer of the urinary bladder by *in situ* hybridisation. *Brit J Urol* 68(1): 49.
152. Nederlof PM, van der Flier S, Wiegant J, Raap AK, Tanke HJ, Ploem JS and van der Ploeg M (1990) Multiple fluorescence *in situ* hybridization. *Cytometry* 11: 126.
153. Oka K, Ishikawa J, Bruner JM, Takahashi R and Saya H (1991) Detection of loss of heterozygosity in the p53 gene in renal cell carcinoma and bladder cancer using the polymerase chain reaction. *Mol Carcinogen* 4: 10.
154. Saran KK, Gould D, Godec CJ and Verma RS (1996) Genetics of bladder cancer. *J Molec Med* 74: 441.
155. Ittmann MM (1996) Loss of heterozygosity on chromosomes 10 and 17 in clinically localized prostate carcinoma. *Prostate* 28: 275.
156. Decker HJ, Gemmill RM, Neumann HP, Walter TA and Sandberg AA (1989) Loss of heterozygosity on 3p in a renal cell carcinoma in von Hippel-Lindau syndrome. *Cancer Genet Cytogenet* 39: 289.

157. Kovacs G, Wilkens L, Papp T and de Riese W (1989) Differentiation between papillary and nonpapillary renal cell carcinomas by DNA analysis. *J Nat Cancer Inst* 81: 527.
158. Horikawa I and Oshimura M (1991) Tumor-suppressor genes. *Gan to Kagaku Ryoho* 18: 153.
159. Field JK (1996) Genomic instability in squamous cell carcinoma of the head and neck. *Anticancer Res* 16: 2421.
160. Knudson AG, Jr (1989) Hereditary cancers disclose a class of cancer genes. *Cancer* 63: 1888.
161. Knudson AG, Jr and Strong LC (1972) Mutation and Cancer. *J Nat Cancer Inst* 48: 313.
162. Knudson AG, Jr (1989) Nakahara memorial lecture. Hereditary cancer, oncogenes, and anti-oncogenes. *Int. Symp. Princess Takamatsu Cancer Res. Fund.* 20: 15.
163. Li FP, Fraumeni JF, Jr Mulvihill JJ, Blattner WA, Dreyfus MG, Tucker MA and Miller RW (1988) A cancer family syndrome in twenty-four kindreds. *Cancer Res* 48: 5358.
164. Greenblatt MS, Bennett WP, Hollstein M and Harris CC (1994) Mutations in the p53 tumor suppressor gene: clues to cancer etiology and molecular pathogenesis. *Cancer Res* 54: 4855.
165. Malkin D, Li FP, Strong LC, Fraumeni JF, Jr Nelson CE, Kim DH, Kassel J, Gryka MA, Bischoff FZ, Tainsky MA et al (1990) Germ line p53 mutations in a familial syndrome of breast cancer, sarcomas, and other neoplasms. *Science* 250: 1233.
166. Nigro JM, Baker SJ, Preisinger AC, Jessup JM, Hostetter R, Cleary K, Bigner SH, Davidson N, Baylin S, Devilee P et al (1989) Mutations in the p53 gene occur in diverse human tumour types. *Nature* 342: 705.
167. Levine AJ (1993) The tumor suppressor genes. *Annu Rev Biochem* 62: 623.
168. Popescu NC, Zimonjic DB, Leventon-Kriss S, Bryant JL, Lunardi-Iskandar Y and Gallo RC (1996) Deletion and translocation involving chromosome 3 (p14) in two tumorigenic Kaposi's sarcoma cell lines. *J Nat Cancer Inst* 88: 450.
169. Sugawa N and Ueda S (1996) The reliability of the differential polymerase chain reaction compared to restriction fragment length polymorphism for the detection of gene loss in primary tumors. *Cancer Lett* 99: 139.
170. Kushner BH and Cheung NK (1996) Allelic loss of chromosome 1p in neuroblastoma. *N Engl J Med* 334: 1608.
171. Olsson H and Borg A (1996) Genetic predisposition to breast cancer. *Acta Oncol* 35: 1.
172. Marcus JN, Watson P, Page DL, Narod SA, Lenoir GM, Tonin P, Linder-Stephenson L, Salerno G, Conway TA and Lynch HT (1996) Hereditary breast cancer: pathobiology, prognosis, and BRCA1 and BRCA2 gene linkage. *Cancer* 77: 697.
173. Radford DM and Zehnbauer BA (1996) Inherited breast cancer. Surgical Clinics of North America 76: 205.
174. Prehn RT (1994) Cancers beget mutations *versus* mutations beget cancers. *Cancer Res* 54: 5296.
175. Rubin H (1992) Adaptive evolution of degrees and kinds of neoplastic transformation in cell culture. *Proc Natl Acad Sci USA* 89: 977.
176. Schulte PA, Ringen K, Hemstreet GP and Ward E (1987) Occupational cancer of the urinary tract. *Occupational Medicine: State of the Art Reviews* 2: 85.
177. Landrigan PJ (1996) The prevention of occupational cancer. *CA Cancer J Clin* 46: 67.
178. Perera F, Santella R, Brandt-Rauf PW, Kahn S, Jiang W, Tang D and Mayer JL (1990) The role of molecular epidemiology in cancer prevention. *Int. Symp. Princess Takamatsu Cancer Res. Fund.* 21: 339.
179. Barrios L, Miro R, Caballin MR, Fuster C, Guedea F, Subias A and Egozcue J (1990) Chromosome instability in bladder carcinoma patients. *Cancer Genet Cytogenet* 49: 107.
180. Hsu TC (1983) Genetic instability in the human population: a working hypothesis. *Hereditas* 98: 1.
181. Uchida T, Wang CX, Wada CK, Iwamura M, Egawa S and Koshiba K (1996) Microsatellite instability in transitional cell carcinoma of the urinary tract and its relationship to clinicopathological variables and smoking. *Int J Cancer* 69: 142.
182. Levine AJ (1997) p53, the cellular gatekeeper for growth and division. *Cell* 88: 323.
183. Oliner JD, Kinzler KW, Meltzer PS, George DL and Vogelstein B (1992) Amplification of a gene encoding a p53-associated protein in human sarcomas. *Nature* 358: 80.
184. Weinberg WC, Azzoli CG, Chapman K, Levine AJ and Yuspa SH (1995) p53-mediated transcriptional activity increases in differentiating epidermal keratinocytes in association with decreased p53 protein. *Oncogene* 10: 2271.
185. el-Deiry WS, Tokino T, Velculescu VE, Levy DB, Parsons R, Trent JM, Lin D, Mercer WE, Kinzler KW and Vogelstein B (1993) WAF1, a potential mediator of p53 tumor suppression. *Cell* 75: 817.
186. Moll UM, LaQuaglia M, Benard J and Riou G (1995) Wild-type p53 protein undergoes cytoplasmic sequestration in undifferentiated neuroblastomas but not in differentiated tumors. *Proc Natl Acad Sci USA* 92: 4407.
187. Sidransky D, Von Eschenbach A, Tsai YC, Jones P, Summerhayes I, Marshall F, Paul M, Green P, Hamilton SR, Frost P et al (1991) Identification of p53 gene mutations in bladder cancers and urine samples. *Science* 252: 706.
188. Blount PL, Ramel S, Raskind WH, Haggitt RC, Sanchez CA, Dean PJ, Rabinovitch PS and Reid BJ (1991) 17p allelic deletions and p53 protein overexpression in Barrett's adenocarcinoma. *Cancer Res* 51: 5482.

189. Dolcetti R, Doglioni C, Maestro R, Gasparotto D, Barzan L, Pastore A, Romanelli M and Boiocchi M (1992) p53 over-expression is an early event in the development of human squamous-cell carcinoma of the larynx: genetic and prognostic implications. *Int J Cancer* 52: 178.
190. Lin J, Teresky AK and Levine AJ (1995) Two critical hydrophobic amino acids in the N-terminal domain of the p53 protein are required for the gain of function phenotypes of human p53 mutants. *Oncogene* 10: 2387.
191. el-Deiry WS, Harper JW, O'Connor PM, Velculescu VE, Canman CE, Jackman J, Pietenpol JA, Burrell M, Hill DE, Wang Y et al (1994) WAF1/CIP1 is induced in p53-mediated G1 arrest and apoptosis. *Cancer Res* 54: 1169.
192. Harper JW, Adami GR, Wei N, Keyomarsi K and Elledge SJ (1993) The p21 Cdk-interacting protein Cip1 is a potent inhibitor of G1 cyclin-dependent kinases. *Cell* 75: 805.
193. Deng C, Zhang P, Harper JW, Elledge SJ and Leder P (1995) Mice lacking p21CIP1/WAF1 undergo normal development, but are defective in G1 checkpoint control. *Cell* 82: 675.
194. Waldman T, Kinzler KW and Vogelstein B (1995) p21 is necessary for the p53-mediated G1 arrest in human cancer cells. *Cancer Res* 55: 5187.
195. Zhan Q, Lord KA, Alamo I, Jr Hollander MC, Carrier F, Ron D, Kohn KW, Hoffman B, Liebermann DA and Fornace AJ, Jr (1994) The gadd and MyD genes define a novel set of mammalian genes encoding acidic proteins that synergistically suppress cell growth. *Mol Cell Biol* 14: 2361.
196. Kastan MB, Zhan Q, el-Deiry WS, Carrier F, Jacks T, Walsh WV, Plunkett BS, Vogelstein B and Fornace AJ, Jr (1992) A mammalian cell cycle checkpoint pathway utilizing p53 and GADD45 is defective in ataxia-telangiectasia. *Cell* 71: 587.
197. Haupt Y, Rowan S, Shaulian E, Vousden KH and Oren M (1995) Induction of apoptosis in HeLa cells by trans-activation-deficient p53. *Gene Develop* 9: 2170.
198. Oltvai ZN and Korsmeyer SJ (1994) Checkpoints of dueling dimers foil death wishes. *Cell* 79: 189.
199. Miyashita T and Reed JC (1995) Tumor suppressor p53 is a direct transcriptional activator of the human bax gene. *Cell* 80: 293.
200. Cairns P, Tokino K, Eby Y and Sidransky D (1994) Homozygous deletions of 9p21 in primary human bladder tumors detected by comparative multiplex polymerase chain reaction. *Cancer Res* 54: 1422.
201. Keen AJ and Knowles MA (1994) Definition of two regions of deletion on chromosome 9 in carcinoma of the bladder. *Oncogene* 9: 2083.
202. Williamson MP, Elder PA, Shaw ME, Devlin J and Knowles MA (1995) p16 (CDKN2) is a major deletion target at 9p21 in bladder cancer. *Hum Mol Genet* 4: 1569.
203. Cairns P, Polascik TJ, Eby Y, Tokino K, Califano J, Merlo A, Mao L, Herath J, Jenkins R, Westra W et al (1995) Frequency of homozygous deletion at p16/CDKN2 in primary human tumours. *Nat Genet* 11: 210.
204. Olopade OI, Pomykala HM, Hagos F, Sveen LW, Espinosa R, 3rd Dreyling MH, Gursky S, Stadler WM, Le Beau MM and Bohlander SK (1995) Construction of a 2.8-megabase yeast artificial chromosome contig and cloning of the human methylthioadenosine phosphorylase gene from the tumor suppressor region on 9p21. *Proc Natl Acad Sci USA* 92: 6489.
205. Olumi AF, Tsai YC, Nichols PW, Skinner DG, Cain DR, Bender LI and Jones PA (1990) Allelic loss of chromosome 17p distinguishes high grade from low grade transitional cell carcinomas of the bladder. *Cancer Res* 50: 7081.
206. Sauter G, Deng G, Moch H, Kerschmann R, Matsumura K, De Vries S, George T, Fuentes J, Carroll P, Mihatsch MJ et al (1994) Physical deletion of the p53 gene in bladder cancer. Detection by fluorescence *in situ* hybridization. *Amer J Pathol* 144: 756.
207. Reznikoff CA, Belair CD, Yeager TR, Savelieva E, Blelloch RH, Puthenveettil JA and Cuthill S (1996) A molecular genetic model of human bladder cancer pathogenesis. *Semin Oncol* 23: 571.
208. Hruban RH, van der Riet P, Erozan YS and Sidransky D (1994) Brief report: molecular biology and the early detection of carcinoma of the bladder – the case of Hubert H. Humphrey. *N Engl J Med* 330: 1276.
209. Chaturvedi V, Li L, Hodges S, Johnston D, Ro JY, Logothetis C, von Eschenbach AC, Batsakis JG and Czerniak B (1997) Superimposed histologic and genetic mapping of chromosome 17 alterations in human urinary bladder neoplasia. *Oncogene* 14: 2059.
210. Harney JV, Liebert M, Ethier SP, Stein JA, Wedemeyer GA, Washington R et al (1991) Down regulation of epidermal growth factor receptor in cultured human normal urothelial cells and in low and high grade human bladder cancer cell lines. *J Urol* 145: 311A.
211. Chi SG, White RWD, Meyers FJ, Siders DB, Lee F and Gumerlock PH (1994) p53 in prostate cancer: Frequent expressed transition mutations. *J Nat Cancer Inst* 86: 926.
212. Heidenberg HB, Sesterhenn IA, Gaddipati JP, Weghorst CM, Buzard GS, Moul JW and Srivastava S (1995) Alteration of the tumor suppressor gene p53 in a high fraction of hormone refractory prostate cancer. *J Urol* 154: 414.
213. Levine AJ, Wu MC, Chang A, Silver A, Attiyeh EF, Lin J and Epstein CB (1995) The spectrum of mutations at the p53 locus. Evidence for tissue-specific mutagenesis, selection of mutant alleles, and a "gain of function" phenotype. *Ann N Y Acad Sci* 768: 111.
214. Moch H, Sauter G, Mihatsch MJ, Gudat F, Epper R and Waldman FM (1994) p53 but not erbB-2 expression is associated with rapid tumor proliferation in urinary bladder cancer. *Hum Pathol* 25: 1346.

215. Runnebaum IB, Kieback DG, Tong XW and Kreienberg R (1993) p53 gain-of-function mutation in codon 175 is a rare event in human breast cancer. *Hum Mol Genet* 2: 1501.
216. Hsiao M, Low J, Dorn E, Ku D, Pattengale P, Yeargin J and Haas M (1994) Gain-of-function mutations of the p53 gene induce lymphohematopoietic metastatic potential and tissue invasiveness. *Amer J Pathol* 145: 702.
217. Lowe SW, Ruley HE, Jacks T and Housman DE (1993) p53-dependent apoptosis modulates the cytotoxicity of anticancer agents. *Cell* 74: 957.
218. Lowe SW, Schmitt EM, Smith SW, Osborne BA and Jacks T (1993) p53 is required for radiation-induced apoptosis in mouse thymocytes. *Nature* 362: 847.
219. Smith ML, Chen IT, Zhan Q, Bae I, Chen CY, Gilmer TM, Kastan MB, O'Connor PM and Fornace AJ, Jr (1994) Interaction of the p53-regulated protein Gadd45 with proliferating cell nuclear antigen. *Science* 266: 1376.
220. Sasaki M, Honda T, Yamada H, Wake N, Barrett JC and Oshimura M (1994) Evidence for multiple pathways to cellular senescence. *Cancer Res* 54: 6090.
221. Lindqvist B and Wahlin A (1975) Differential count of urinary leucocytes and renal epithelial cells by phase contrast in microscopy. *Acta Med Scand* 198(6): 505.
222. Langkilde NC, Wolf H and Orntoft TF (1991) Lewis antigen expression in benign and malignant tissues from RBC Le(a-b-) cancer patients. *Brit J Haematol* 79: 493.
223. Limas C (1991) Quantitative interrelations of Lewis antigens in normal mucosa and transitional cell bladder carcinomas. *J Clin Pathol* 44: 983.
224. Strohman RC (1997) The coming Kuhnian revolution in biology. *Nat Biotechnol* 15: 194.
225. McBride TJ, Preston BD and Loeb LA (1991) Mutagenic spectrum resulting from DNA damage by oxygen radicals. *Biochemistry* 30: 207.
226. Floyd RA and Carney JM (1996) Nitrone radical traps (NRTs) protect in experimental neurodegenerative diseases. *In*: Chapman, CW Olanow, P Jenner and M Youssim (eds): *Neuroprotective approaches to the treatment of Parkinson's disease and other neurodegenerative disorders*. Academic Press Limited, pp. 69–90.
227. el-Naggar AK, van Dekken HD, Ensign LG and Pathak S (1994) Interphase cytogenetics in paraffin-embedded sections from renal cortical neoplasms. Correlation with cytogenetic and flow cytometric DNA ploidy analyses. *Cancer Genet Cytogenet* 73: 134.
228. Jacobson MD (1996) Reactive oxygen species and programmed cell death. *Trends Biochem Sci* 21: 83.
229. Schreck R, Rieber P and Baeuerle PA (1991) Reactive oxygen intermediates as apparently widely used messengers in the activation of the NF-kappa B transcription factor and HIV-1. *EMBO J* 10: 2247.
230. Crawford D, Zbinden I, Amstad P and Cerutti P (1988) Oxidant stress induces the proto-oncogenes c-fos and c-myc in mouse epidermal cells. *Oncogene* 3: 27.
231. Nose K, Shibanuma M, Kikuchi K, Kageyama H, Sakiyama S and Kuroki T (1991) Transcriptional activation of early-response genes by hydrogen peroxide in a mouse osteoblastic cell line. *Eur J Biochem* 201: 99.
232. Jaruga P, Zastawny TH, Skokowski J, Dizdaroglu M and Olinski R (1994) Oxidative DNA base damage and antioxidant enzyme activities in human lung cancer. *FEBS Lett* 341: 59.
233. Swaim MW and Pizzo SV (1988) Methionine sulfoxide and the oxidative regulation of plasma proteinase inhibitors. *J Leukocyte Biol* 43: 365.
234. Johnson D and Travis J (1979) The oxidative inactivation of human alpha-1-proteinase inhibitor. Further evidence for methionine at the reactive center. *J Biol Chem* 254: 4022.
235. Wolff SP, Garner A and Dean RT (1986) Free radicals, lipids and protein degradation. *Trends Biochem Sci* 11: 27.
236. Floyd RA (1990) Role of oxygen free radicals in carcinogenesis and brain ischemia. *FASEB J* 4: 2587.
237. Feig DI, Sowers LC and Loeb LA (1994) Reverse chemical mutagenesis: Identification of the mutagenic lesions resulting from reactive oxygen species-mediated damage to DNA. *Proc Natl Acad Sci* 91: 6609.
238. National Institute of Health and Division of Research Grants (1988) Oxy radicals in carcinogenesis – a chemical pathology study section workshop. *Cancer Res* 48: 3882.
239. Toyokuni S, Okamoto K, Yodoi J and Hiai H (1995) Persistent oxidative stress in cancer. *FEBS Lett* 358: 1.
240. Ramaekers FC, Moesker O, Huysmans A, Schaart G, Westerhof G, Wagenaar SS, Herman CJ and Vooijs GP (1985) Intermediate filament proteins in the study of tumor heterogeneity: an in-depth study of tumors of the urinary and respiratory tracts. *Ann N Y Acad Sci* 455: 614.
241. Roberts ES, Vaz AD and Coon MJ (1992) Role of isozymes of rabbit microsomal cytochrome P-450 in the metabolism of retinoic acid, retinol, and retinal. *Mol Pharmacol* 41: 427.
242. Rao JY, Hemstreet GP, Hurst RE, Bonner RB, Min KW and Jones PL (1991) Cellular F-actin levels as a marker for cellular transformation: correlation with bladder cancer risk. *Cancer Res* 51: 2762.
243. Hemstreet GP, Rao JY, Hurst RE, Bonner RB, Mellott J and Rooker GM (1998) Biomarkers in monitoring for efficacy of immunotherapy and chemoprevention of bladder cancer with dimethylsulfoxide. *Cancer Detection Prev*; in press.

244. Barboro P, Alberti I, Sanna P, Parodi S, Balbi C, Allera C and Patrone E (1996) Changes in the cytoskeletal and nuclear matrix proteins in rat hepatocyte neoplastic nodules in their relation to the process of transformation. *Exp Cell Res* 225: 315.
245. Cohen SM and Ellwein LB (1991) Genetic errors, cell proliferation, and carcinogenesis. *Cancer Res* 51: 6493.
246. Martin SJ and Green DR (1995) Protease activation during apoptosis: death by a thousand cuts? *Cell* 82: 349.
247. Huot J, Houle F, Spitz D and Landry J (1996) HSP27 Phosphorylation-mediated Resistance against Actin Fragmentation and Cell Death Induced by Oxidative Stress. *Cancer Res* 56: 273.
248. Hinshaw DB, Sklar LA, Bohl B, Schraufstatter IU, Hyslop PA, Rossi MW, Spragg RG and Cochrane CG (1986) Cytoskeletal and morphologic impact of cellular oxidant injury. *Amer J Pathol* 123: 454.
249. Bellomo G and Mirabelli F (1992) Oxidative stress and cytoskeletal alterations. *Ann N Y Acad Sci* 663: 97.
250. Bellomo, G, Mirabelli F, Vairetti M, Iosi F and Malorni W (1990) Cytoskeleton as a target in menadione-induced oxidative stress in cultured mammalian cells. I. Biochemical and immunocytochemical features. *J Cell Physiol* 143: 118.
251. Palladini G, Finardi G and Bellomo G (1996) Modifications of Vimentin Filament Architecture and Vimentin-Nuclear Interactions by Cholesterol Oxides in 73\73 Endothelial Cells. *Exp Cell Res* 223: 83.
252. Palladini G, Finardi G and Bellomo G (1996) Disruption of Actin Microfilament Organization by Choelsterol Oxides in 73\73 Endothelial Cells. *Exp Cell Res* 223: 72.
253. Hinshaw DB, Armstrong BC, Burger JM, Beals TF and Hyslop PA (1988) ATP and microfilaments in cellular oxidant injury. *Amer J Pathol* 132: 479.
254. Mirabelli F, Salis A, Marinoni V, Finardi G, Bellomo G, Thor H and Orrenius S (1988) Menadione-induced bleb formation in hepatocytes is associated with the oxidation of thiol groups in actin. *Arch Biochem Biophys* 264: 261.
255. Liu ZR, Wilkie AM, Clemens MJ and Smith CW (1996) Detection of double-stranded RNA-protein interactions by methylene blue-mediated photo-crosslinking. *RNA* 2: 611.
256. Hagen TM, Huang S, Curnutte J, Fowler P, Martinez V, Wehr CM, Ames BN and Chisari FV (1994) Extensive oxidative DNA damage in hepatocytes of transgenic mice with chronic active hepatitis destined to develop hepatocellular carcinoma. *Proc Natl Acad Sci USA* 91: 12808.
257. Floyd RA (1990) The role of 8-hydroxyguanine in carcinogenesis. *Carcinogenesis* 11: 1447.
258. Okamoto K, Toyokuni S, Kim WJ, Ogawa O, Kakehi Y, Arao S, Hiai H and Yoshida O (1996) Overexpression of human mutT homologue gene messenger RNA in renal-cell carcinoma: evidence of persistent oxidative stress in cancer. *Int J Cancer* 65: 437.
259. Legrand-Poels S, Bours V, Piret B, Pflaum M, Epe B, Rentier B and Piette J (1995) Transcription factor NF-κB is activated by photosensitization generation oxidative DNA damages. *J Biol Chem* 270: 6925.
260. Wang C, Mayo MW and Baldwin AS (1996) TNF- and cancer therapy-induced apoptosis: potentiation by inhibition of NF-κB. *Science* 274: 784.
261. Okamoto M, Kawai K, Reznikoff CA and Oyasu R (1996) Transformation *in vitro* of a nontumorigenic rat urothelial cell line by hydrogen peroxide. *Cancer Res* 56: 4649.
262. Sun Y (1990) Free radicals, antioxidant enzymes, and carcinogenesis. *Free Radical Biol Med* 8: 583.
263. Parsons CL, Boychuk D, Jones S, Hurst RE and Callahan H (1990) Bladder surface glycosaminoglycans: an epithelial permeability barrier. *J Urol* 143: 139.
264. Kadlubar FF and Badawi AF (1995) Genetic susceptibility and carcinogen-DNA adduct formation in human urinary bladder carcinogenesis. *Toxicol Lett* 82–83: 627.
265. Badawi AF, Hirvonen A, Bell DA, Lang NP and Kadlubar FF (1995) Role of aromatic amine acetyltransferases, NAT1 and NAT2, in carcinogen-DNA adduct formation in the human urinary bladder. *Cancer Res* 55: 5230.
266. Romkes-Sparks M, Mnuskin A, Chern HD, Persad R, Fleming C, Sibley GN, Smith P, Wilkinson GR and Branch RA (1994) Correlation of polymorphic expression of CYP2D6 mRNA in bladder mucosa and tumor tissue to *in vivo* debrisoquine hydroxylase activity. *Carcinogenesis* 15: 1955.
267. Gonzalez FJ and Gelboin HV (1993) Role of human cytochrome P-450s in risk assessment and susceptibility to environmentally based disease. *J Toxicol Environ Health* 40: 289.
268. Kawajiri K and Fujii-Kuriyama Y (1991) P450 and human cancer. *Jpn J Cancer Res* 82: 1325.
269. Messing EM, Hanson P, Ulrich P and Erturk E (1987) Epidermal growth factor – interactions with normal and malignant urothelium: *in vivo* and *in situ* studies. *J Urol* 138: 1329.
270. Wei Q, Cheng L, Hong WK and Spitz MR (1996) Reduced DNA repair capacity in lung cancer patients. *Cancer Res* 56: 4103.
271. Raica M and Bajan F (1991) Fine needle aspiration of the prostate: a histo-cytological correlation. *Rom J Morphol Embryol* 37(3–4): 137.
272. Mondal A, Ghosh E and Ghose A (1990) The role of transrectal fine needle aspiration cytology in the diagnosis of prostatic nodules suspicious of malignancy a study of 126 cases. *Indian J Pathol Microbiol* 33(1): 23.
273. Nagle RB (1996) Intermediate filament expression in prostate cancer. *Cancer Metastasis Rev* 15: 473.

274. Adolfsson J and Tribukait B (1990) Evaluation of tumor progression by repeated fine needle biopsies in prostate adenocarcinoma: modal deoxyribonucleic acid value and cytological differentiation. *J Urol* 144: 1408.

275. Gomella L, White J, McCue P, Byrne D and Mulholland S (1993) Screening for occult nodal metastasis in localized carcinoma of the prostate. *J Urol* 149(4): 776.

276. Wood DP, Jr Banks ER, Humphreys S, McRoberts JW and Rangnekar VM (1994) Identification of bone marrow micrometastases in patients with prostate cancer. *Cancer* 74: 2533.

277. Kerbel R (1989) Towards an understanding of the molecular basis of the metastatic phenotype. *Invas Metast* 9: 329.

278. Fidler IJ (1991) The biology of human cancer metastasis. *Acta Oncol* 30: 669.

279. Aznavoorian S, Murphy AN, Steller-Stevenson WG and Liotta LA (1993) Molecular aspects of tumor cell invasion and metastasis. *Cancer* 71: 1368.

280. Albelda SM and Buck CA (1990) Integrins and other cell adhesion molecules. *FASEB J* 4: 2868.

281. Johnson JP (1991) Cell adhesion molecules of the immunoglobulin supergene family and their role in malignant transformation and progression to metastatic disease. *Cancer Metastasis Rev* 10: 11.

282. Schipper JH, Frixen UH, Behrens J, Unger A, Jahnke K and Birchmeier W (1991) E-cadherin expression in squamous cell carcinomas of head and neck: inverse correlation with tumor dedifferentiation and lymph node metastasis. *Cancer Res* 51: 6328.

283. Poggi A, Stella M and Donati MB (1993) The importance of blood cell-vessel wall interactions in tumour metastasis. *Bailliere Clin Haematol* 6: 731.

284. Klienman HK and Kibbey MC (1991) Basement Membrane Regulation of Tumor Growth and Metastasis. *J NIH Res* 3: 63.

285. Stracke ML, Aznavoorian SA, Beckner ME, Liotta LA and Schiffmann E (1991) Cell motility, a principal requirement for metastasis. *EXS* 59: 147.

286. Stetler-Stevenson WG, Liotta LA and Kleiner DE, Jr (1993) Extracellular matrix 6: role of matrix metalloproteinases in tumor invasion and metastasis. *FASEB J* 7: 1434.

287. van den Hooff A (1991) The role of stromal cells in tumor metastasis: a new link. *Cancer Cells* 3: 186.

288. Gleave ME, Hsieh JT, Wu HC, Hong SJ, Zhau HE, Guthrie PD and Chung LW (1993) Epidermal growth factor receptor-mediated autocrine and paracrine stimulation of human transitional cell carcinoma. *Cancer Res* 53: 5300.

289. Ware JL (1993) Growth factors and their receptors as determinants in the proliferation and metastasis of human prostate cancer. *Cancer Metastasis Rev* 12: 287.

290. Wright JA, Turley EA and Greenberg AH (1993) Transforming growth factor beta and fibroblast growth factor as promoters of tumor progression to malignancy. *Crit Rev Oncogen* 4: 473.

291. Lu C and Kerbel RS (1994) Cytokines, growth factors and the loss of negative growth controls in the progression of human cutaneous malignant melanoma. *Curr Opin Oncol* 6: 212.

292. Otto T, Birchmeier W, Schmidt U, Hinke A, Schipper J, Rübben H and Raz A (1994) Inverse relation of E-cadherin and autocrine motility factor receptor expression as a prognostic factor in patients with bladder carcinomas. *Cancer Res* 54: 3120.

293. Shields P and Harris C (1991) Molecular epidemiology and the genetics of environmental cancer. *JAMA* 266(5): 681.

294. Greenberg CS, Birckbichler PJ and Rice RH (1991) Transglutaminases: Multifunctional cross-linking enzymes that stabilize tissues. *FASEB J* 5: 3071.

295. Lee KN, Birckbichler PJ, Patterson MK, Jr Conway E and Maxwell M (1987) Induction of cellular transglutaminase biosynthesis by sodium butyrate. *Biochim Biophys Acta* 928: 22.

296. Lichti U, Ben T and Yuspa SH (1985) Retinoic acid-induced transglutaminase in mouse epidermal cells is distinct from epidermal transglutaminase. *J Biol Chem* 260: 1422.

297. Hague A, Manning AM, Hanlon KA, Huschtscha LI, Hart D and Paraskeva C (1993) Sodium butyrate induces apoptosis in human colonic tumour cell lines in a p53-independent pathway: implications for the possible role of dietary fibre in the prevention of large-bowel cancer. *Int J Cancer* 55: 498.

298. D'Argenio G, Cosenza V, Sorrentini I, De Ritis F, Gatto A, Delle Cave M, D'Armiento FP and Mazzacca G (1994) Butyrate, mesalamine, and factor XIII in experimental colitis in the rat: effects on transglutaminase activity. *Gastroenterology* 106: 399.

299. Fukuda K, Kojiro M and Chiu JF (1994) Differential regulation of tissue transglutaminase in rat hepatoma cell lines McA-RH7777 and McA-RH8994: relation to growth rate and cell death. *J Cell Biochem* 54: 67.

300. Barnes RN, Bungay PJ, Elliott BM, Walton PL and Griffin M (1985) Alterations in the distribution and activity of transglutaminase during tumour growth and metastasis. *Carcinogenesis* 6: 459.

301. Delcros JG, Bard S, Roch AM, Quash G, Poupon MF and Korach S (1986) Transglutaminase activity and putrescine-binding capacity in cloned cell lines with different metastatic potential. *FEBS Lett* 196: 325.

302. Hand D, Elliott BM and Griffin M (1987) Correlation of changes in transglutaminase activity and polyamine content of neoplastic tissue during the metastatic process [published erratum appears in *Biochim Biophys Acta* 1987 Dec 10;931(3): 385]. *Biochim Biophys Acta* 930: 432.

303. Knight CR, Rees RC, Elliott BM and Griffin M (1990) The existence of an inactive form of transglutaminase within metastasising tumours. *Biochim Biophys Acta* 1053: 13.

304. Johnson TS, Knight CR, el-Alaoui S, Mian S, Rees RC, Gentile V, Davies PJ and Griffin M (1994) Transfection of tissue transglutaminase into a highly malignant hamster fibrosarcoma leads to a reduced incidence of primary tumour growth. *Oncogene* 9: 2935.

304b. Birckbichler PJ, Bonner RB, Kong J, Rowland TC, Hurst RE, Bane BL, Pitha JV and Hemstreet GP (1998) Identification of field effect changes in tissue transglutaminase expression in prostate cancer: potential for risk assessment and early detection. *submitted.*

305. Weinberg R (1989) Oncogenes, antioncogenes, and the molecular bases of multistep carcinogenesis. *Cancer Res* 49: 3713.

306. Pienta K, Partin A and Coffey DS (1989) Cancer as a disease of DNA organization and dynamic cell structure. *Cancer Res* 49: 2525.

307. Tzen C, Estervig DN, Minoo P, Filipak M, Maercklein P, Hoerl B and Scott R (1988) Differentiation, cancer, and anticancer activity. *Biochem Cell Biol* 66: 478.

308. Heldin C, Betscholz C, Claesson-Welsh, l and Westermark B (1987) Subversion of growth regulatory pathways in malignant transformation. *Biochim Biophys Acta* 907: 219.

309. Couture J and Hansen M (1991) Recessive genes in tumorigenesis. *Cancer Bull* 43: 41.

310. Kastan MB, Onyekwere O, Sidransky D, Vogelstein B and Craig RW (1991) Participation of p53 protein in the cellular response to DNA damage. *Cancer Res* 51: 6304.

311. Ruoslahti E and Yamaguchi Y (1991) Proteoglycans as modulators of growth factors. *Cell* 64: 867.

312. Nathan C and Sporn M (1991) Cytokines in context. *J Cell Biol* 113: 981.

313. Koss LG (1979) Tumors of the urinary tract and prostate. *In* LG Koss (ed.): *Diagnostic cytology and its histologic basis.* J.B. Lippincott, Philadelphia, pp. 749–811.

314. Heney NM, Ahmed S, Flanagan MJ, Frable W, Corder MP, Hafermann MD and Hawkins IR (1983) Superficial bladder cancer: progression and recurrence. *J Urol* 130: 1083.

315. Norming U, Nyman C and Tribukait B (1989) Comparative flow and cytometric deoxyribonucleic acid studies on exophytic tumor and random mucosal biopsies in untreated carcinoma of the bladder. *J Urol* 142: 1442.

316. Presti JC, Jr Reuter VE, Galan T, Fair WR and Cordon-Cardo C (1991) Molecular genetic alterations in superficial and locally advanced human bladder cancer. *Cancer Res* 51: 5405.

317. Karnauchow PN (1994) Screening for prostate cancer. *Lancet* 343: 1437.

318. Fujimoto K, Yamada Y, Okajima E, Kakizoe T, Sasaki H, Sugimura T and Terada M (1992) Frequent association of p53 gene mutation in invasive bladder cancer. *Cancer Res* 52: 1393.

319. Tsai YC, Nichols PW, Skinner DG and Jones PA (1990) Allelic losses of chromosomes 9, 11, and 17 in human bladder cancer. *Cancer Res* 50: 44.

320. Hursting S, Thornquist M and Henderson M (1990) Types of dietary fat and the incidence of cancer at five sites. *Prev Med* 19(3): 242.

321. Spruck CH, III, Ohneseit PF, Gonzalez-Zulueta M, Esrig D, Miyao N, Tsai YC, Lerner SP, Schmütte C, Yang AS, Cote R et al. (1994) Two molecular pathways to transitional cell carcinoma of the bladder. *Cancer Res* 54: 784.

322. Ruppert JM, Tokino K and Sidransky D (1993) Evidence for two bladder cancer suppressor loci on human chromosome 9. *Cancer Res* 53: 5093.

323. Jouanneau J, Moens G, Bourgeois Y, Poupon MF and Thiery JP (1994) A minority of carcinoma cells producing acidic fibroblast growth factor induces a community effect for tumor progression. *Proc Natl Acad Sci USA* 91: 286.

324. Rao JY, Hurst RE, Bales WD, Jones PL, Bass RA, Archer LT and Hemstreet GP (1990) Cellular f-actin levels as a marker for cellular transformation: relationship to cell division and differentiation. *Cancer Res* 50: 2215.

325. Bass RA, Hemstreet GP, Honker NA, Hurst RE and Doggett RS (1987) DNA Cytometry and cytology by quantitative fluorescence image analysis in symptomatic bladder cancer patients. *Int J Cancer* 40(5): 698.

326. Rhodes S, Hurst RE, Rollins SA, Jones PL, Hemstreet GP, Detrisac CJ, Thomas CF, Moon RC and Kelloff GJ (1991) DNA ploidy and p21 protein levels in tissue sections as end-point markers in animal carcinogenesis trials. *Biol Monitor* 1: 61.

327. Hurst RE, Petrone R, Bass RA, Hemstreet GP, Detrisac CL, Thomas CF et al (1991) Quantitative biochemical markers of DNA hyperploidy as end-point indicators in chemical risk assessment and chemoprevention studies. *Biol Monitor* 1: 5.

328. Hemstreet GP, Schulte PA, Ringen K, Stringer W and Altekruse EB (1988) DNA hyperploidy as a marker for biological response to bladder to carcinogen exposure. *Int J Cancer* 42: 817.

329. Bonner RB, Liebert M, Hurst RE, Grossman HB, Bane BL, Hemstreet GP and (1996) Marker Network for Bladder Cancer Characterization of the DD23 Tumor-Associated Antigen for Bladder Cancer Detection and Recurrence Monitoring. *Cancer Epidem Biomarker Prev* 5: 971.

330. Schulte PA, Ringen K, Hemstreet GP, Aktekruse E, Gullen W, Patton M, Allsbrook W, Crosby J, West SS, Witherington R et al. (1985) Risk assessment of a cohort exposed to aromatic amines, initial results. *J Occup Med* 27: 115.

331. Slaton JW, Dinney CPN, Veltri RW, Miller MC, Liebert M, O'Dowd GJ and Grossman HB (1997) Deoxyribonucleic acid ploidy enhances the cytological, prediction of recurrent transitional, cell carcinoma of the bladder. *J Urol* 158: 806.
332. Lose G, Frandsen B, Hojensgard J, Jespersen J and Astrup T (1983) Chronic interstitial cystitis: increased levels of eosinophil cationic protein in serum and urine and an ameliorating effect of subcutaneous heparin. *Scand J Urol Nephrol* 17(2): 159.
333. Bi W, Rao J, Hemstreet GP, Fang P, Asal NR, Zang M, Min KW, Ma Z, Lee E, Li G, Hurst RE, Bonner RB, Weng Y, Fradet Y and Yin S (1993) Field molecular epidemiology. Feasibility of monitoring for the malignant bladder cell phenotype in a benzidine-exposed occupational cohort. *J Occup Med* 35(1): 20.
334. Rao JY, Bonner RB, Hurst RE, Qiu WR, Reznikoff CA and Hemstreet GP (1997) Quantitative changes in cytoskeletal and nuclear actin levels during cellular transformation. *Int J Cancer* 70: 423.
335. Greenwald P (1996) Cancer risk factors for selecting cohorts for large-scale chemoprevention trials. *J Cell Biochem* Suppl. 25: 29.
336. MacLeod MC A (1996) Possible Role in Chemical Carcinogenisis for Epigenetic, Heritable Changes in Gene Expression. *Mol Carcinogen* 15: 241.
337. Niedel J, Kuhn L and Vanderbard G (1983) Phobol Diester Receptor Copurified with Protein Kinase C. *Proc Natl Acad Sci USA* 80: 36.
338. Rothman N, Bhatnagar VK, Hayes RB, Zenser TV, Kashyap SK, Butler MAX, Bell DA, Lakshmi V, Jaeger M, Kashyap R et al (1996) The impact of interindividual variation in NAT2 activity on benzidine urinary metabolites and urothelial DNA adducts in exposed workers. *Proc Natl Acad Sci USA* 93: 5084.
339. Moon RC, Detrisac CJ, Thomas CF and Kelloff GJ (1992) Chemoprevention of experimental bladder cancer. *J Cell Biochem Suppl* 16I: 134.
340. Waliszewski P, Waliszewska M, Niekrasz M, Gordon AN, Hemstreet GP and Hurst RE (1996) Alterations in expression of steroid-retinoid superfamily genes in human bladder cancer cell lines. *Proc Amer Assn Cancer Res* 37: 233.
341. Moon RC, McCormick DL and Mehta RG (1983) Inhibition of carcinogenesis by retinoids. *Cancer Res* 43(Suppl): 2469 s.
342. Bane BL, Rao J and Hemstreet GP (1996) Pathology and Staging of Bladder Cancer. *Semin Oncol* 23: 546.
343. Rao JY, Hemstreet GP, Hurst RE, Bonner RB and Fradet Y (1993) Mapping of bladder cancer tumorigenesis with biochemical markers. *Cytometry Suppl.* 6: 33.
344. Kennedy AR (1985) Evidence that the first step leading to carcinogen-induced malignant transformation is a high frequency, common event. *Carcinogenesis; a Comprehensive Survey* 9: 355.
345. Kennedy AR (1991) Is there a critical target gene for the first step in carcinogenesis? *Environ Health Perspect* 93: 199.
346. Boothman DA, Meyers M, Fukunaga N and Lee SW (1993) Isolation of x-ray-inducible transcripts from radioresistant human melanoma cells. *Proc Natl Acad Sci USA* 90: 7200.
347. Feinberg AP, Gehrke CW, Kuo KC and Ehrlich M (1988) Reduced genomic 5-methylcytosine content in human colonic neoplasia. *Cancer Res* 48: 1159.
348. Holliday R (1991) Mutations and epimutations in mammalian cells. *Mutat Res* 250: 351.
349. Yao A and Rubin H (1994) A critical test of the role of population density in producing transformation. *Proc Natl Acad Sci USA* 91: 7712.
350. Chisari FV, Klopchin K, Moriyama T, Pasquinelli C, Dunsford HA, Sell S, Pinkert CA, Brinster RL and Palmiter RD (1989) Molecular pathogenesis of hepatocellular carcinoma in hepatitis B virus transgenic mice. *Cell* 59: 1145.
351. Rosette C and Karin M (1995) Cytoskeletal control of gene expression: depolymerization of microtubules activates NF-kappa B. *J Cell Biol* 128: 1111.

Subject index